CW00816016

Applie
for Pu
and Research

Handbooks in Health Economic Evaluation Series

Series editors: Alastair Gray and Andrew Briggs

Applied Health Economics for Public Health Practice and Research

Edited by

Rhiannon T. Edwards and Emma McIntosh

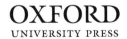

OXFORD
UNIVERSITY PRESS

OXFORD
UNIVERSITY PRESS

Great Clarendon Street, Oxford, OX2 6DP,
United Kingdom

Oxford University Press is a department of the University of Oxford.
It furthers the University's objective of excellence in research, scholarship,
and education by publishing worldwide. Oxford is a registered trade mark of
Oxford University Press in the UK and in certain other countries

Published in the United States of America by Oxford University Press
198 Madison Avenue, New York, NY 10016, United States of America

British Library Cataloguing in Publication Data

Data available

Library of Congress Control Number: 2018966912

ISBN 978–0–19–873748–3

Printed and bound by
CPI Group (UK) Ltd, Croydon, CR0 4YY

Series preface

Economic evaluation in health care is a thriving international activity that is increasingly used to allocate scarce health careresources. Economic evaluation is a subject within which applied and methodological research, teaching, and publications are flourishing. Several widely respected texts are already well established in the market, so what is the rationale for not just one more book but for a series? We believe that the books in the series Handbooks in Health Economic Evaluation share a strong distinguishing feature, which is to cover as much as possible of this broad field with a much stronger practical flavour than existing texts, using plenty of illustrative material and worked examples. We hope that readers will use this series not only for authoritative views on the current practice of economic evaluation and likely future developments but also for practical and detailed guidance on how to undertake an analysis. The books in the series are textbooks, but first and foremost they are handbooks.

Our conviction that there is a place for the series has been nurtured by the continuing success of two short courses we helped develop—Advanced Methods of Cost-Effectiveness Analysis, and Advanced Modelling Methods for Economic Evaluation. Advanced Methods was developed in Oxford in 1999 and has run several times a year ever since, in Oxford, Canberra, and Hong Kong. Advanced Modelling was developed in York and Oxford in 2002 and has also run several times a year ever since, in Oxford, York, Glasgow, and Toronto. Both courses were explicitly designed to provide computer-based teaching that would take participants through the theory but also the methods and practical steps required to undertake a robust economic evaluation or construct a decision-analytic model to current standards. The proof of concept was the strong international demand for the courses—from academic researchers, government agencies, and the pharmaceutical industry—and the very positive feedback on their practical orientation.

Thus, the original concept of the Handbooks series, as well as many of the specific ideas and illustrative material, can be traced to these courses. The Advanced Modelling course is in the phenotype of the first book in the series, Decision Modelling for Health Economic Evaluation, which focuses on the role and methods of decision analysis in economic evaluation. The Advanced Methods course has been an equally important influence on Applied Methods of Cost-Effectiveness, the third book in the series which sets out the key elements of analysing costs and outcomes, calculating cost-effectiveness, and reporting results. The concept was then extended to cover several other important topic areas. First, the design, conduct, and analysis of economic evaluations alongside clinical trials have become a specialized area of activity with distinctive methodological and practical issues, and its own debates and controversies. It seemed worthy of a dedicated volume, hence the second book in the series, *Economic Evaluation in Clinical Trials*. Next, while the use of cost–benefit analysis in health care has spawned a substantial literature, this is mostly theoretical, polemical, or focused on specific issues such as willingness to pay. The fourth book in the series, *Applied Methods of Cost–Benefit Analysis in Health care*, fills an important gap in the literature by providing a comprehensive guide to the theory but also the practical conduct of cost–benefit analysis, again with copious illustrative material and worked out examples. This fifth book on the economics of public health is is an increased relflection of the need for society to focus on prevention of ill-health and disability in the face of rising demands upon health and social care systems. Economic evaluation of population focused public health interventions raisies additional challenges on the design, conduct and reporting of such interventions, over and above the evaluation of clinical interventions. Many public health interventions are delivered outside of the health sector in schools, work places and the natural environment. Spillover effects mean that the benefits and costs of such interventions are felt across many sectors spanning health care, housing, transport and the judicial system. This book accompanied by a short course, *Applied Health Economics for Public Health Practice and Research*, run annually since 2013 at Bangor University attracting delegates, health economists, public health professionals and a wide range of related occupations from around the United Kingdom, Europe, and the world.

Each book in the series is an integrated text prepared by several contributing authors, widely drawn from academic centres in the United Kingdom, the United States, Australia, and elsewhere. Part of our role as editors has been to foster a consistent style, but not to try to impose any particular line: that would have been unwelcome and also unwise amidst the diversity of an evolving field. News and information about the series, as well as supplementary material for each book, can be found at the series website: <http://www.herc.ox.ac.uk/books>.

Alastair Gray
Oxford
Andrew Briggs
Glasgow

Web resources

In addition to worked examples in the text, readers of this book can download datasets and programs for Stata® for Windows (Stata Corporation, College Station, Texas, United States) that provide examples of the analysis of cost and quality-adjusted life years, estimation of sampling uncertainty for the comparison of cost and effect, and calculation of sample size and power for cost-effectiveness analysis in clinical trials.

Materials for the book are maintained at the following web addresses: <http://www.uphs.upenn.edu/dgimhsr/eeinct.htm and <http://www.herc.ox.ac.uk/ books/trials.shtml>.

More information is available on the websites. We anticipate that the web-based material will be expanded and updated over time.

Acknowledgements

I undertook my training in health economics at the University of Calgary with Professor Malcolm Brown and the University of York with Professor Alan Williams. The opportunities to take part in the exchange of ideas through the Health Economics Study Group (HESG) in the UK in my early career were extremely formative. My first job was as lecturer in Health Economics in the department of public health at the University of Liverpool where Professor John Ashton and Dr Ruth Hussey introduced me to the principles of the Healthy Cities movement. I moved to North Wales in 1997 to set up the Centre for Health Economics and Medicines Evaluation (CHEME) at Bangor University, which I now co-direct with Professor Dyfrig Hughes. I am indebted to Dyfrig, Professor Ceri Philips, and Professor David Cohen, and more recently Professor Deb Fitzsimmons and Dr Pippa Anderson for their encouragement and our shared goal of helping to develop health economics in Wales. Over the years, I gained a great deal of practical experience by working with colleagues in Public Health Wales and the Welsh government on topics ranging from the economic evaluation of exercise on prescription, parenting programmes for children at risk of developing conduct disorder, and the ventilation of homes of children with asthma. I learned a great deal about pragmatic trial design and statistical analysis in health economics from Professor Ian Russell and Dr Daphne Russell. With an opportunity to spread my wings, in 2004/05 my interest in the economics of public health inspired me to study the 'business case for prevention' in the US health care system through a Commonwealth Fund Harkness Fellowship in health policy, which took our family to Seattle. I want to thank Professor Robert Reid and Dr Dean Roehl for many discussions about public health relating to the United States, Canada, and the United Kingdom through this Fellowship and our continued friendship.

Reflecting on the methodological challenges when conducting public health evaluation set out by Smith and Petticrew in 2010, Rutter and colleagues (2017), and Squires and colleagues (2016), namely to see the whole wood rather than individual trees, to link public health to economic growth, health, and well-being and recognize its impact on inequality, this book outlines current practice and future directions. There is a clear need to widen the evaluative space in which the economics of public health is explored. As editors, and against a background of research funding realities and constraints, we believe that use of contemporary micro-economic evaluation methods to evaluate public health interventions complements this wider societal perspective which acknowledges the need for a breadth in outcome measurement, understanding of the complex causal pathways of public health interventions, their many spillover effects, and a need for a truly multi-sectoral perspective of analysis.

My co-editor, Emma McIntosh, and I want to thank the contributing authors of this book who have helped to demonstrate the ways in which a range of methods in economic evaluation are being applied in novel ways to the evaluation of public health interventions to support decision making.

I want to acknowledge the support of my mother Eleri, husband Paul, and children Will and Non, and reflect on my father Richard's role as a doctor and scientist in guiding me towards a career in health economics. I want to thank Ann Lawton for administrative help and for speaking Welsh with me every day—diolch yn fawr. I want to acknowledge the invaluable help of the people who have read for me over the years: Alison Shaw, Allison Gash, Jackie Williams-Bulkeley, and Bethany Fern Anthony. Finally, my guide dog Jazz should receive a mention as she has enabled me to travel widely and independently during the course of writing and editing this book.

Rhiannon T. Edwards

Contents

Abbreviations

ABM	agent-based modelling		DALY	disability-adjusted life year
ACE	adverse childhood experience		DCE	discrete choice experiment
AMR	antimicrobial resistance		DES	discrete event simulation
ATE	average treatment effect		EED	Economic Evaluation Database
BMI	body mass index		ESR	electronic staff records
BFI	Baby-Friendly initiative		EV	equivalent variation
BFWS	Breastfeeding Welcome Scheme		FTE	full-time equivalent
BPSP	Breastfeeding Peer Support Programme		GAF	global assessment of functioning
BRE	Building Research Establishment		GDP	gross domestic product
CABE	Commission for Architecture and the Built Environment		GDPR	General Data Protection Regulations
			GNI	gross national income
CBA	cost–benefit analysis		HACT	Housing Associations' Charitable Trust
CCA	cost–consequence analysis			
CCG	clinical commissioning group		HALE	healthy adjusted life expectancy
CE	cost effectiveness		HALY	health-adjusted life year
CEA	cost-effectiveness analysis		HDI	human development index
CEAC	cost-effectiveness acceptability curve		HES	Hospital Episode Statistics
			HESG	Health Economics Study Group
CHARISMA	Children's Health in Asthma: Research to Improve Status through Modifying Accommodation		HIA	Health Impact Assessment
			HPCF	Healthy Pupils Capital Fund
			HPV	human papilloma virus
CHEERS	Consolidated Health Economic Evaluation Reporting Standards		HRG	Health Resource Group
			HTA	Health technology assessment
CHEME	Centre for Health Economics and Medicines Evaluation		HRQoL	health-related quality of life
			HSCIC	Health & Social Care Information Centre
CI	confidence interval			
CMA	cost-minimization analysis		HIU	health utilities index
CPHE	Centre for Public Health Excellence		ICECAP_A	ICEpop CAPability measure for Adults
CRD	Centre for Reviews and Dissemination		ICECAP_O	ICEpop CAPability measure for Older people
CS	consumer surplus		ICER	incremental cost-effectiveness ratio
CUA	cost–utility analysis			
CV	contingent valuation		ICUR	incremental cost–utility ratio
CVD	cardiovascular disease		IHDI	inequality-adjusted human development index

HIS	Integrated Household Survey		PSSRU	Personal Social Services Research Unit
ISPOR	International Society for Pharmacoeconomics and Outcomes Research		QALYs	quality-adjusted life years
			QoL	quality of life
IY	Incredible Years		RCT	randomized controlled trial
MAU	multi-attribute utility		ROI	return on investment
MCA	multi-criteria analysis		RP	revealed preference
MCDA	multi-criteria decision making		RPL	random parameter logit
MRC	Medical Research Council		SACS	Sociology and Complexity Science
MRS	marginal rate of substitution			
MSC	musculoskeletal condition		SAIL	Secure Anonymized Information Linkage
MXL	mixed logit			
NHB	net health benefit		SAP	Standard Assessment Procedure
NICE	National Institute for Health and Care Excellence		SDQ	Strengths and Difficulties Questionnaire
NMB	net monetary benefit		SG	standard gamble
NOAA	National Oceanic Administrative Association		SHIP	Scottish Informatics System
			SIB	social impact bonds
NRT	nicotine replacement therapy		SP	stated preference
OCAP	Operationalising the Capabilities		SPDCE	stated preference discrete choice experiment
OECD	Organisation for Economic Co-operation and Development		SROI	social return on investment
			SSLP	Sure Start Local Programme
OR	odds ratio		SSB	sugar-sweetened beverage
OT	occupational health		SSW	Stop Smoking Wales
OXAP	Oxford Capabilities Questionnaire		STI	sexually transmitted infection
			SWF	social welfare function
PA	physical activity		TTO	time trade-off
PBMA	programme budgeting and marginal analysis		VA	visual analogues
			VOI	value of information
PDG	Programme Development Group		WCVSN	West and Central Voluntary Sector Network
PHE	Public Health England			
PHI	public health initiative		WI	workplace intervention
PPIC	Pareto-improvement criterion		WTA	willingness to accept
PSA	probabilistic sensitivity analysis		WTP	willingness to pay
PSS	personal social services		YLD	years lost due to disability
			YLL	years of life lost

Title and editors

Health Economics for Public Health Practice and Research

Rhiannon T. Edwards is Professor of Health Economics and the founding Director of health economics research at Bangor University. She is Co-Director of the Centre for Health Economics and Medicines evaluation (CHEME), Bangor University. She was a Commonwealth Fund Harkness Fellow in Health Policy to the United States in 2004/ 05. She is Fellow of the Learned Society of Wales and an Honorary Member of the UK Faculty of Public Health.

Emma McIntosh is Professor of Health Economics, Deputy Director of the Health Economics and Health Technology Assessment (HEHTA) team at the Institute of Health & Wellbeing at the University of Glasgow and Director of the NIHR Global Health Research Group on Arthritis. Emma has an MSc in Health Economics and a PhD in Economics. Prior to joining HEHTA Emma worked at the University of Oxford's Health Economics Research Centre (HERC) where she completed the 4th book in this series entitled 'Applied Methods of Cost-Benefit Analysis in Health'. Emma has also previously held posts at the University of Aberdeen and the Personal Social Services Research Unit (PSSRU) at the University of Kent.

Contributors

Robert Atenstaedt Consultant in Public Health Medicine at Public Health Wales, Visiting Professor at Glyndwr University and Honorary Senior Lecturer, Bangor University

Camilla Baba Research Assistant, Health Economics and Health Technology Assessment (HEHTA), University of Glasgow

Willings Botha Research Fellow in Health Economics at the National Perinatal Epidemiology and Statistics Unit (NPESU), University of New South Wales

Kathleen Boyd Senior Lecturer in Health Economics, Health Economics and Health Technology Assessment (HEHTA), University of Glasgow

Nathan Bray Lecturer in Health care Improvement, Bangor University and Health and Care Research Wales Fellow

Joanna M. Charles Research Fellow in Health Economics Centre for Health Economics and Medicines Evaluation (CHEME), Bangor University

Ned Hartfiel Research Officer at Centre for Health Economics and Medicines Evaluation (CHEME), Bangor University

Alice Jones Independent social impact consultant; Alice has a Doctorate in Business Administration from Nottingham Business School

Carys Jones Research Fellow in Health Economics Centre for Health Economics and Medicines Evaluation (CHEME), Bangor University

Huw Lloyd-Williams PhD student, Centre for Health Economics and Medicines Evaluation (CHEME), Bangor University

Hazel Squires Senior Research Fellow, School of Health and Related Research, University of Sheffield

Eira Winrow PhD student and Research Project Support Officer, Centre for Health Economics and Medicines Evaluation (CHEME), Bangor University

Olivia Wu Professor of Health Technology Assessment and and Director of Health Economics and Health Technology Assessment (HEHTA), University of Glasgow

Seow Tien Yeo Research Fellow in Health Economics, Centre for Health Economics and Medicines Evaluation (CHEME), Bangor University

Chapter 1

Introduction to public health and public health economics

Rhiannon T. Edwards and
Robert Atenstaedt

1.1 Public health economics: An historical perspective

Health economics is the study of how society uses scarce resources to meet our health care needs. Economic evaluation asks whether a particular health care intervention is worth producing, weighting up its cost and benefits relative to the benefits that could be produced by using scarce resources to produce other health care interventions (Drummond et al., 2015). What happens, however, when we start to talk about using wider societal resources to prevent ill health and disability? An emerging applied subdiscipline of health economics is increasingly referred to as 'public health economics', which may be defined as how society uses scarce resources to meet our preventive health care needs, improve health, and reduce inequalities in health (Edwards et al., 2016).

This fifth book in the series Handbooks in Health Economic Evaluation aims to provide a practical and contemporary guide to economic evaluation of public health interventions (PHIs). The book is specifically written for health economists who may have been traditionally working in health technology assessment (HTA), turning their hand to the health economic component of PHI evaluation, and equally, for public health practitioners interested in health economics. Economic evaluation, as a component of the wider subdiscipline of health economics, began in the early 1960s assisted by the theoretical developments of Selma Mushkin (1958) 'Toward a Definition of Health Economics' and later, her work on the notion of health as an 'investment' (Mushkin, 1962), where she proposed health and education as joint investments in an individual, making that individual more effective as a producer and consumer in society. Mushkin defined health economics as a broader science concerned with the optimum use of scarce economic resources for the care of the sick and the promotion of health, taking into account competing uses of these resources. It was during this period that more formal economic evaluations in health care were being developed, initially as basic economic analyses where the value of improved health was measured in terms of increased labour production (Blumenschein and Johannesson, 1996). Nowadays, the science of economic evaluation employs more refined methods to measure health changes in terms of, for example, quality and length of life as measured by quality-adjusted life years (QALYs) gained or the broader valuation of attributes of health care goods and services using stated preference methods. Adjacent to this development of the economics of health grew the paradigm of 'evidence-based medicine' (Cochrane, 1972). Archie Cochrane advocated the use of randomized controlled trials (RCTs) in medical research to underpin evidence-based practice. HTA grew alongside this movement. HTA can be defined as a multidisciplinary activity that systematically examines the safety, clinical efficacy and effectiveness, cost, cost-effectiveness, organizational implications, social consequences, and legal and ethical considerations of the application of a given health technology. The term 'health technology' covers a range of methods used to promote health, prevent and treat disease, and improve rehabilitation and long-term care. Given this definition, a health technology includes drugs, medical devices, or clinical/surgical procedures (Draborg et al., 2005; Raftery and Powell, 2013; Goodman, 2014; Drummond et al., 2015), (Velasco-Garrido and Busse, 2005; Nielsen et al., 2011) but also preventive PHIs. Health economists interested in reconstructing the 'missing' market in health care developed methods of economic evaluation of medical technologies, often conducted alongside RCTs (Ramsey et al., 2005; Drummond et al., 2015).

Twenty years ago, Williams (1993), Phelps (1995), Fuchs (2000), and Maynard and Kanavos (2000) set out their visions for health economics for the next two decades, entirely focused on health care as a means of producing better health. These commentators envisaged the subdiscipline focusing, over the coming decades, on: healthcare as a production function; improving the structure and finance of health care systems; increased use of routinely collected data in economic evaluation; the increased institutionalization of economic evidence in policy (as borne out with the establishment of the National Institute for Health and Care Excellence (NICE)) in the United Kingdom; and growing interest in behavioural economics as a basis for incentive structures for health care professionals.

In the 1980s and 1990s, it was argued that these visions of the future of mainstream health economics were very much about 'healthcare economics' rather than 'health economics'. Growing interest in the wider determinants of health, and causes of inequalities in health, would need a 'paradigm shift' from 'healthcare economics' to 'health economics' (Weinstein and Stason, 1976; Warner and Murt, 1984; Mooney and McGuire, 1988; Mooney, 1992; Kenkel, 2000; Edwards, 2001). In thinking about public health we must begin by thinking about inter-generational, environmental, and economic sustainability. Today, as economists or HTA practitioners, we need to be aware that we are implicitly accepting the status quo in terms of the distribution of wealth in society and the relative distribution of resources across government departments. Developing interest in the application of methods of economic evaluation to the appraisal of PHIs has been evidenced by the burgeoning publications in this area. Public health is about preventing ill health and reducing inequalities in health across the population life course by delivering interventions, often outside traditional health care settings (in this book we mainly refer to the UK NHS as such a health care setting). PHI initiatives are just as likely to take place in settings such as homes, schools, workplaces, and the community. Indeed, it is often this public health 'context' which creates complexity in economic evaluation alongside the potential complexity of the interventions themselves. In this sense, throughout the book we will often refer to the methodology of economic evaluation of PHIs as akin to the economic evaluation of 'complex interventions' (see Chapter 3).

In the United Kingdom in the 1960s, economic evaluation of health care programmes grew out of general public sector policy economics, responding, in a UK context, to a demand from the NHS to address resource allocation issues within a culture of evidence-based medicine (Williams, 1972; Sackett et al., 1996). In the 1990s and 2000s, economic evaluation of health care programmes remained within a 'medical model' of health care (Phelps, 1995; Fuchs, 2000) with a focus on the increasing efforts to standardize methods of evaluation (Ramsey et al., 2005; Drummond et al., 2008; Drummond et al., 2015). However, paradigms began to change with a focus on 'health economic evaluation' rather than 'health services economics' (Edwards, 2001), which we argue underpins the current interest in applying techniques of economic evaluation to the evaluation of PHIs. Indeed, this 'health economic' evaluation is arguably still a narrow approach to the multi-sector impacts likely to arise through PHIs, and as such, the need for systems evaluations is advocated as a useful approach (Smith and Petticrew, 2010).

1.2 **Rationale for the book**

Coincidentally, the very first cost–benefit analysis (CBA) in health care was of the 1875 Public Health Act aimed at preventing cholera (Calkins, 1891). However, more contemporary economic evaluation of PHIs developed from the Wanless report (Wanless, 2004) as well as a growing awareness of increasing pressure on the NHS being attributable to lifestyle choices causing ill health in the population.

The rule of rescue means that patients ill or dying today will take precedence over potential patients in the future and the public health case for prevention, as evidenced by the balance of spending between treatment and prevention in the NHS (Edwards et al., 2013). This book is a response to growing interest in the need for economic evaluation of PHIs in the face of escalating costs to the NHS and the wider economy, resulting, in part, from an upstream socio-economic gradient of ill-health and disability, compounded by our health-harming choices in lifestyles. In part, then, this paradigm shift from 'health services economics' to 'health economics' has already happened, requiring a far more multi-sectoral approach to thinking about health than has been the case and now the application of methods of economic evaluation, including economic evaluation within systems approaches, to the evaluation of PHIs.

The purpose of economic evaluation is to support informed, evidence-based decision-making in public policy relating to health. One of the key advantages of economic evidence is that it can support transparent prioritization of services intended to improve public health. Many PHIs are 'complex' in nature and the implications of this complexity will be discussed in Chapter 3 of this book.

Recent commentators including Kelly et al (2005), Weatherly et al (2009), Payne et al (2013), and Edwards and colleagues (2013) have argued that economists evaluating PHIs should measure a full range of costs and outcomes, going beyond (but sometimes including) QALYs (an index of life years gained weighted to reflect health-related quality of life) to take account of inter-sectoral stakeholders. These authors have also highlighted the need to address inequalities in health in these evaluations. Others go further, arguing for a systems approach to economic evaluation of PHIs (Midgley, 2006).

This book argues that health economic evaluation may have come full circle from its roots in broad public sector policy economics and that we may find it useful to think in this broader paradigm with respect to public health or population health economics. A review of published sources of technical guidance on the application of economic evaluation methods to the appraisal of PHIs found most evaluations to be focused on, and to measure, health outcomes such as QALYs (Edwards et al., 2013). Recent guidance from NICE, together with the views and insights of health economists working in the evaluation of PHIs, means that there is now a greater appetite for exploring wider methods of economic evaluation rooted, theoretically, in welfare economics. Specifically, we are talking about greater use of broader frameworks of economic evaluation, namely CBA, consideration of less theoretical but practical spin-off methods such as social return on investment (SROI), and adopting systems thinking and methods to our design and evaluation.

This book acknowledges the contribution of *Promoting Health, Preventing Disease: The Economic Case* (McDaid et al., 2015), which consolidates economic evidence on a range of public health topics spanning smoking, alcohol, physical activity, nutrition, child health, road-related injuries, and improving mental health (in particular, preventing depression). This book, the fifth publication in the series 'Handbooks in Health Economic Evaluation', offers a methodological guide and case studies to provide health economists and public health practitioners with the tools to design and conduct economic evaluations of PHIs.

Chapter 2 of this book introduces the concept of the supply and demand of prevention goods, services, and environments; market failure for these goods, services, and environments; and the need for economic evaluation. In this context, market failure is defined as a situation in which the allocation of goods and services by a free market is not efficient, this can lead to a net social welfare loss. The chapter introduces those new to methods of economic evaluation to the traditional approach to measuring cost-effectiveness with some explanation of the theoretical and mathematical basis for the calculation of incremental cost-effectiveness ratios (ICERs). The subsequent chapters take readers through various methods of economic evaluation with practical case studies, covering a wide range of PHIs.

1.3 Population health and public health

Population health is concerned with the study of socio-economic and environmental influences on physical and mental health and well-being, with reference to a range of upstream influences such as early life experiences including adverse childhood experiences (Bellis et al., 2013). A key aim of population health research is to understand how and why ill health varies within and between populations and across the life course, and how to improve the health of the public through clinical or PHIs, including those that may be delivered outside conventional health services (MRC, 2008).

Public health was originally defined as the science and art of preventing disease, prolonging life, and promoting health through the organized efforts and informed choices of society, organizations, public and private, communities, and individuals (Winslow, 1920). This definition has been simplified and adopted by the UK Faculty of Public Health of the Royal College of Physicians, which regulates the public health profession and its standards in the United Kingdom (Faculty of Public Health, 2014). The definition encapsulates the multi-disciplinary nature of public health and necessitates a collective effort, taking a population perspective to improving health.

For the purposes of this book we could equally use the terms 'population health' or 'public health' but have chosen to use the latter as we are primarily concerned with how governments, and other agencies, use scarce resources in order to promote better health (Kindig, 2007).

1.4 **The history of public health**

A number of overlapping phases, or 'waves', of public health improvement initiatives in the United Kingdom have been described in papers by Hanlon and colleagues (2011) and Davies and team (2014). These waves are summarized in Table 1.1. The first wave, from 1830 to 1900, was largely a response to the social disruptions which followed the Industrial Revolution, and was concerned with improving environmental conditions. This effort included the provision of clean drinking water, improved sanitation, and better food safety, coupled with legislation which aimed to improve working conditions and protect children. The second wave, from 1890 to 1950, saw the emergence of scientific medicine, including the embedding of 'germ theory' and implementation

Table 1.1 The five waves of public health in the United Kingdom

Wave	Date	Public Health Developments
First Wave	1830–1900	◆ Improved environmental conditions—e.g. water/sanitation, child protection. ◆ Post Industrial Revolution—concentrated on civil and social order.
Second Wave	1890–1950	◆ Emergence of scientific medicine—antibiotics and vaccinations.
Third Wave	1940–1980	◆ Emergence of the UK welfare state: NHS, social security, social housing, universal education.
Fourth Wave	1960–present	◆ Effective health care interventions prolong life. ◆ Focus on risk factors and lifestyle. ◆ Social inequalities in health examined.
Fifth Wave	The future	◆ Focus on health assets. ◆ Boosting value of health for individuals. ◆ Incentives needed for health behaviours—promoting healthy food and lifestyle choices as the default.

Sources: data from Hanlon et al., 2011 and Davies et al., 2014.

of measures to combat infectious disease such as vaccination and antibiotics. The third wave, from 1940 to 1980, saw the expansion of the welfare state, including the establishment of the NHS, the provision of social security, and universal education. Preventive efforts began to focus on the individual. The fourth wave, from 1960 to the present, has been characterized by a shift in focus from human biology to the importance of social and psychological aspects as determinants of health and well-being. For example, the first International Conference on Health Promotion in November 1986 led to the development of the Ottawa Charter for Health Promotion, which signalled recognition of the many wider influences on health and illness and outlined five key planks of successful health promotion/improvement (WHO, 1986). More recently, due to the challenges arising from increasing rates of obesity, health inequalities, and a decline in well-being, combined with an exponential growth in population, energy use, and expenditure, it has been argued by Hanlon and colleagues (2011) that a 'fifth wave' of public health development is needed, one that is radically different from its predecessors. This approach could involve a focus on health assets, boosting the value of health for individuals and implementing incentives for healthy behaviour, making the most of social media and e-health technology, promoting healthy food and lifestyle choices as a default, and reducing factors which create an environment and culture which encourages unhealthy behaviour (Davies et al., 2014). Aligned with this we also believe there is a significant role for Government policies aimed at industry (e.g. food and drink manufacturers), such a the recent 'sugar tax'.

A potential sixth wave is becoming known as 'precision public health', which can be thought of as the use of data to guide interventions that benefit populations more efficiently. It requires robust primary surveillance data, the tracking of geographical distribution of risk factors, disability, and disease, and the capacity to act on this information (Desmond-Hellmann, 2016). We will return to this topic in the final chapter of this book as it has implications for the future economic evaluation of PHIs tailored for specific population groups.

1.5 Domains of public health practice

Broadly, there are three generally accepted domains within which public health practitioners currently work. They are:

- **Health improvement**—this is concerned with improving the health and well-being of the population and reducing health inequalities utilizing health promotion and community development approaches. Those working in this discipline seek to influence the lifestyle and socio-economic, physical, and cultural environment of populations, communities, and individuals.

- **Health protection**—this focuses on preventing the transmission of communicable diseases, and protecting the population against environmental health hazards. Those working in health protection may be involved in disease monitoring, managing disease outbreaks, and dealing with other incidents that threaten the population's health and well-being. An example of this would be vaccination programmes for flu, rotavirus, human papilloma virus (HPV), and herpes zoster.

- **Improving services**—in the United Kingdom, this domain of public health is concerned with the commissioning, planning, and evaluation of services. Areas within which practitioners work include: quality improvement and clinical governance, patient safety, equity of service provision, and prioritization of health services.

Practice within these three domains is supported by public health intelligence. This discipline includes surveillance, monitoring, and assessment of health and the determinants of health, and the development of the public health evidence base and knowledge.

Since April 2013, much of the public health function in England has moved to local government although a specialist workforce, including a group of health economists, has been retained within Public Health England, an executive agency sponsored by the Department of Health. In Wales, Scotland, and Northern Ireland the public health function remains mainly within the NHS.

1.6 The social determinants of health

It is now widely accepted that health is not just an outcome of genetic or biological processes but is strongly influenced by social and economic conditions and lifestyle choices. These influences are known as the 'social determinants of health' or the 'wider determinants of health'. In the classic Dahlgren and Whitehead (1991) model of health (Figure 1.1), a series of enveloping circles are seen radiating outwards from the individual who is placed at the core. The person, possessed of certain intrinsic characteristics (age, gender, ethnicity, and genetics) is immediately surrounded by

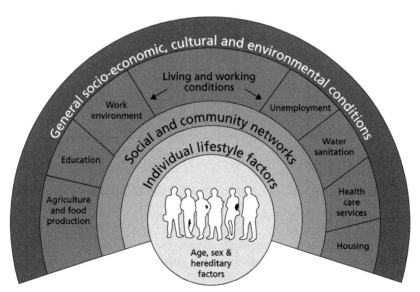

Figure 1.1 Determinants of health.
Reproduced with permission from Dahlgren G, Whitehead M. (1991). Policies and Strategies to Promote Social Equity in Health. Stockholm, Sweden: Institute for Futures Studies. Available at: <https://www.iffs.se/policies-and-strategies/>.

layers of influences on health that could theoretically be modified, radiating out from lifestyle and behavioural factors (e.g. smoking and alcohol consumption). At a wider level, the person is placed in a wider social world comprising social networks and social support that can also affect an individual's health. A further layer of influence outside this relates to living and working environments and education. Finally, general socio-economic, cultural, and environmental factors are placed on the outside. Public health aims to work 'upstream', focusing on these wider circumstances that produce unhealthy behaviours such as social and economic conditions. This is in contrast to 'downstream' interventions that are designed to optimize access to care services in order to mitigate the negative impacts of these socio-economic conditions on individuals.

1.7 **Inequalities in health**

A key objective of public health programmes is to work towards reducing inequalities in health across groups in the population. There is a clear social gradient in life expectancy and health-related quality of life across socio-economic groups in the United Kingdom. The review 'Fair Society, Healthy Lives' (Marmot et al., 2010) highlights that education levels, supportive family and community networks, social capital, and parenting skills are unequally distributed across groups in society, and that this results in differing health outcomes for individuals within and across these groups. The more disadvantaged the neighbourhood, the more likely it is to have social and environmental characteristics presenting risks to health. These characteristics include poor housing, higher rates of crime, poorer air quality, a lack of green spaces and places for children to play, and more risks to safety from traffic. Professor Sir Michael Marmot, famous for stating that 'medicine is failed prevention' (Marmot et al., 2010), advocated an upstream approach across the whole of the life course. Marmot identified six specific priorities to reduce health inequalities. These priorities advocate giving each child the best start in life; enabling all children, young people, and adults to maximize capabilities and have control over their lives; creating fair employment and good work for all; ensuring a healthy standard of living for all; creating healthy sustainable places and communities, and strengthening ill health prevention (Marmot et al., 2010).

1.8 **The assets-based approach to public health**

For many years, improving population health has focused on what makes people ill and trying to prevent or reduce these factors. This is known as the deficits approach. More recently, public health has started to consider the asset-based approach to health and well-being. Asset-based approaches concentrate on the assets that people and communities employ such as time, people, and infrastructure to remain well and to bounce back from adversity. Furthermore, health assets can act at the individual, community, and organizational levels (Morgan and Ziglio, 2007).

There is increasing policy and academic interest in asset-based approaches as a means to develop and deliver interventions for improving health and reducing health inequalities. Asset-based approaches are characterized where end-users are directly engaged in the development and delivery of services. The rationale is to foster a 'do with' culture and that by utilizing the knowledge, skills, and experiences of recipients, services will then be more appropriate, effective, and sustainable. The traditional 'deficit approach' is characterized by a 'do to' culture, where health professionals identify perceived need and provide standardized services. This deficit approach is perceived to have failed by those advocating asset-based approaches. It is contended that asset-based approaches are required to address the enduring problem of health inequalities (McLean and McNeice, 2012). Asset-based working is not novel. Related concepts that have been in use for some time include community empowerment, co-production, and community ownership. Examples of interventions that may be characterized as taking an asset-based approach include leadership programmes, employability schemes, and time banking to encourage volunteering. The concept of 'empowerment' is at the heart of asset-based working: working with individuals and communities to enable them to take more control over their lives and communities. The role of empowerment is addressed further in Chapter 6 of this book.

Asset-based working may involve project-specific approaches which can be highly responsive to local conditions. However, the approach still utilizes assets (e.g. people, time, physical assets) and develops interventions (e.g. employability schemes) with the ultimate aim to increase health and well-being over a period of time. In this sense, asset-based working should be amenable to economic evaluation. However, to date there is little evidence in relation to the cost-effectiveness of such assets-based approaches for the improvement of population health (Lawson and McIntosh, 2013).

The assets-based approach has been the premise of the World Health Organization (WHO) Healthy Cities Movement internationally (Taylor, 2010). In 1988, the first WHO International Healthy Cities Conference was held in Liverpool in the United Kingdom (Ashton, 2009).

1.9 Social norms and the concept of nudge and choice architecture

The British public is now used to the absence of smoking in public places. Legislation in 2007 to prohibit smoking in all public places has been one of the most important interventions to reduce smoking rates in the United Kingdom in recent years (Goodman et al., 2009; Heim et al., 2009; Hyland et al., 2009; Akhtar et al., 2010). Being able to eat out with young children in a pub or restaurant without the fear of the effect of passive smoking is now an accepted social norm. Alongside legislation to improve public health, there has been growing interest in the concept of 'nudge' (Sunstein and Thaler, 2012) and 'choice architecture' (Hollands et al., 2013) in terms of influencing social norms without legislation and via the use of social media. Examples of these could include the influence that the popular TV chef Jamie Oliver has had on improving the quality of school meals or Hugh Fearnley-Whittingstall's campaign to make productive use of fruit and vegetables currently wasted by British supermarkets. Choice architecture is about intervening to design the choices that people face in their everyday lives. An example of this can be seen in the placement of fruit in a more prominent position than chocolate in a self-service cafeteria.

1.10 **Strategies for prevention of ill-health**

The ultimate goal of public health is the prevention of disease; this can be considered on a number of levels (Donaldson and Donaldson, 2003):

Primary prevention—this approach aims to prevent the onset of disease through the control of exposure to risk factors. For example, careful weight control prevents obesity which in itself is a risk factor for many conditions including heart disease and diabetes.

Secondary prevention—this approach looks to halt the progression of a disease once it is established through early detection of disease followed by effective treatment. Screening is a major component of secondary prevention; for example, breast screening for women to detect early changes which may advance to breast cancer.

Tertiary prevention—this approach is concerned with the rehabilitation of individuals with an established disease to reduce or eliminate long-term impairments and disabilities. For example, a person identified as having type 2 diabetes will have regular blood glucose checks to monitor control of their disease and prevent complications.

There is also **primordial prevention**; this aims to prevent future disease by influencing its social determinants (Farquhar, 1999).

There are two main approaches to prevention: targeting a whole population whether they are exposed to risk factors or not, or tackling only those identified as being at high risk. The strengths and weaknesses of the high risk and population approaches are shown in Table 1.2.

The influential epidemiologist Geoffrey Rose clearly showed that a preventive measure that brings large benefits to the community may offer little to each participating person (Rose, 1985, 1992). For example, to prevent one death due to a motor vehicle accident many hundreds of people must wear seat belts. Conversely, although individuals who are at high risk may benefit from interventions specifically targeted at them, the effect on the overall incidence of the disease will be limited in the absence of a population-oriented intervention. This has been termed the 'prevention paradox' (Rose, 1981). For this reason, a combination of population and approaches to high-risk individuals is usually most effective. This approach was taken, for example, in the successful project undertaken in North Karelia in Finland in the 1970s to reduce mortality from cardiovascular disease (Puska, 2002). A paper published by the Foundation in Genomics & Population Health argues that Rose's 'high-risk strategy', a clinically oriented approach to preventive medicine, may be modified by segmenting the population by risk (e.g. genetic risk) into a number of individual strata, to each of which differential interventions may be applied (Burton et al., 2012). This is called 'stratified prevention' and they argue that this approach would lead to advantages in efficiency, effectiveness, and harm minimization.

Table 1.2 Strengths and weaknesses of strategies for prevention

	High risk approach	Population approach
Strengths	◆ Intervention may be matched to the specific requirements of the individual ◆ Selectivity may increase the cost-effective use of resources ◆ May prevent interference with those who are not at special risk ◆ May be adopted within the economic, ethical, and cultural values as well as the organizational structures of the health care system	◆ The effects on society of a distributional shift may be significant ◆ It may be more appropriate and sustainable to obtain a general change in societal behavioural norms than to try to change socially conditioned behaviours in individuals
Weaknesses	◆ Prevention may become medicalized ◆ The input to overall control of a disease may be small ◆ The preventive intervention may be unsustainable or behaviourally/culturally inappropriate ◆ May have a weak capability to foresee who will benefit from intervention	◆ May give only a small benefit to each participant ◆ Needs significant changes in economics and societal functioning, which often makes changes unlikely ◆ People generally favour 'paying' as late as feasible, and to have the benefit as soon as possible

Reproduced with permission from Porta, M. Ed. (2008) A dictionary of epidemiology, 5th Ed. New York, USA: Oxford University Press. Copyright © 2008 OUP.

1.11 Public health economics in the developing world

As Western societies grapple with the economics of public health it is interesting to note that there may be much to be learned from the evidence of the economics of investing in public health preventative interventions in the developing world.

At a micro-economics level there has been a body of literature modelling the cost-effectiveness of, for example, primary care midwifery services and training local village midwives (Walker et al., 2002). Numerous research studies on preventing communicable diseases such as malaria and studies on willingness to pay for preventive measures such as insecticide-treated nets (Trapero-Bertran et al., 2013) provide excellent examples. Likewise, there have been important reviews of the evidence base of economic evaluations of non-communicable diseases (Mulligan et al., 2006). In addition to identifying clear gaps in the literature, Mulligan et al found that the quality of studies was often poor and resource allocation decisions made by local and global policy-makers on the basis of this evidence could be misleading.

Given the costs of undertaking economic evaluation studies in developing country settings, there has been interest in both pooling data and exploring the transferability of findings from one developing country to another (Walker and Fox-Rushby, 2000).

At a macro-economic level, health economists and economists more generally have explored data in order to develop theories about the relationship between investing in improving health, particularly child health, and the impact on economic growth in gross domestic product (GDP), identifying the drivers of change such as child educational attainment, household income, global statistics on savings and expenditure (Bloom et al., 2004).

Most notably, there has been a shift in emphasis in the focus of provision of aid to developing countries on investment in 'the first 1000 days of life' (from conception to two years). Economists have identified large potential returns on investment of US$138 per US$1 invested (Hoddinott, Rosegrant, and Torero, 2012).

1.12 Concepts of efficiency in health economics and three important economic questions relevant to public health

Students of health economics learn about three economic questions which face all economies from simple barter economies to the most sophisticated free-market economies. With respect to a government or public sector role in public health these questions are:

1. What public health goods, services, and environments should society produce?
2. What technical means of production should be used to produce these public health goods, services, and environments?
3. How should these public health goods, services, and environments be distributed between members of society?

Question 1 is based on the concept of 'allocative efficiency', a concept that aims to maximize social welfare in relation to defined societal goals, through choices about how scarce resources may best be used. Question 2 is based on the concept of 'technical efficiency', which explains the relationship between inputs and outputs in a production process. Question 3 is based on our choice of principles of equity or fairness.

The answers to these three questions will depend on the prevailing political leanings of government, social norms, and, we hope, evidence of effectiveness and cost-effectiveness (Phillips, 2008; LGA and DoH, 2012; Edwards et al., 2013).

1.13 Studies of the costs of various risk factors

In the United Kingdom, we are used to hearing in the media about the enormous cost to the NHS and to the wider economy of health-harming behaviours and associated illnesses such as alcohol harm (Department of Health, 2008). Such staggering figures outine the sheer scale of a specific problem and convey a message that the consequences of risk factors resulting from health harming behaviours are not just to the NHS but are far more wide reaching across the whole economy, to families, communities, employers, the judicial system, and across government. Table 1.3 illustrates this with estimates of the annual cost of alcohol misuse in England.

Table 1.3 Cost of alcohol misuse in England to the NHS and the wider economy

Cost to individuals and families/household (e.g. loss of income, informal care costs)	£26.4 billion
Cost to public health services/care services	£ 3.5 billion
Cost to other public services (e.g. criminal justice system costs, education and social services costs)	£2.7 billion
Cost to employers (e.g. absenteeism)	£9.2 billion
Human costs (disability-adjusted life years (DALYs))	£27.5 billion
Total	£69.2 billion

Based on CPI from ONS up to September 2018.
Retrieved from: <https://www.ons.gov.uk/economy/inflationandpriceindices/datasets/consumerpriceinflation>
Source: data from Department Of Health, 2008 – inflated to 2015 costs. Copyright © 2015 Department of Health, HMS Government.

What these estimates of the total cost of such health-harming behaviours, to the NHS and the wider economy, fail to show, however, is the relationship between the marginal costs and marginal benefits of investing in prevention and treatment programmes. We will return to the concept of the margin in Chapter 2. For now, suffice it to say that the concept of the margin in economics is the idea that we are interested in the marginal or incremental benefit that can be achieved, and at what marginal or incremental cost. Conversely, if we are talking about disinvestment, it is the incremental loss of this disinvestment (Guest et al., 2013).

1.14 The purpose and methods of economic evaluation applied to public health

There is a strong recognition within health care of the need to consider scarcity of resources and opportunity cost. Every choice, action, or decision about the use of resources has an associated foregone opportunity, namely the value of those resources in their next-best use. Economic evaluation provides a framework for identifying the costs and benefits of different options for delivering goods and services. What is different about the health economics of PHIs is that many of the influences on the health of the population lie outside the reach of the NHS and traditional models of the delivery of public health services. This has led government, in light of the high costs to both the NHS and the wider economy of many health-harming behaviours, to call, over the last decade, for evidence on the cost-effectiveness of specific interventions to prevent and treat health-harming behaviours. Also for evidence on the wider financial return on investment of investing in PHIs wherever these are delivered, within the NHS or across wider society.

1.15 The UK's NICE public health reference case

The UK's NICE provides national guidance and advice to improve health and social care. NICE was originally set up in 1999 as the National Institute for Clinical Excellence, a special health authority, to reduce variation in the availability and quality of NHS treatments and care. In 2005, after merging with the Health Development

Agency, NICE began developing public health guidance to help prevent ill health and promote healthier lifestyles.

NICE has published a reference case for the evaluation for new drugs and clinical health programmes (NICE, 2013). The reference case takes an NHS perspective and proposes the measure of outcomes in QALYs. NICE supports the use of health-state valuation for QALY calculations based on EQ-5D. The EQ-5D is a generic preference-based health-related quality of life instrument (EuroQoL Group, 2015), discussed further in Chapters 2 and 8 in this book. The Institute proposes the extrapolation of costs and benefits, if possible, over a lifetime. It also proposes that all costs and benefits are discounted at 3.5 per cent and that uncertainties are fully explored through an economic model and sensitivity analysis (NICE, 2013).

The Centre for Public Health Excellence (CPHE) at NICE produced a supplemented reference case for the economic evaluation of PHIs (NICE, 2009, and subsequently updated online in 2012 and 2014). Instead of an NHS perspective, in recognition that costs and benefits of PHIs may span over many sectors of the economy, the NICE public health reference case proposes the use of a public sector perspective (Public sector, including the NHS and PSS, or local government Societal perspective (where appropriate)).

The reference case acknowledges that QALYs, as an outcome measure, may fail to capture the full range of benefits across these sectors from a PHI and so it has instead proposed the use of alternative outcome measures. Increased attention is placed on the potential usefulness of broader CBAs and cost–consequence analysis (CCA) frameworks discussed in Chapters 9 and 10 of this book. NICE also undertook a cost impact study exploring the potential of SROI and return on investment (ROI) methods which measures pound for pound the financial return on investment of a PHI (NICE, 2011).

In summary, NICE has recommended the use of CCA, and where possible cost–utility analysis (CUA), in order to make it possible to compare the relative cost-effectiveness of PHIs compared with medical interventions such as new drugs. This also makes it theoretically possible to compare the cost-effectiveness of PHIs with the NICE threshold of £20,000–£30,000 per QALY, as was undertaken by Owen and colleagues in 2011 (this paper is reproduced in full in Chapter 8 of this book). NICE and Public Health England, in particular, are developing a series of ROI tools to support local government with decisions about where to spend resources to improve public health. Examples of these tools are presented in Chapter 11 of this book. NICE has recommended the use of a variety of time horizons and discount rates in order to take into account the fact that PHIs that yield benefits far into the future are affected by discounting future benefits when costs are incurred today. NICE has also proposed sensitivity analyses which use a lower discount rate of 1.5 per cent for both costs and outcomes in the evaluation of some PHIs (NICE 2014). The cost impact report proposed the use of other techniques not usually used in economic evaluation of medical technologies such as multi-criteria decision-making (MCDA) discussed in Chapter 13 of this book and also the potential of capability measures (discussed in Chapter 6) as an alternative to QALYs in capturing wider health outcomes from PHIs. Finally, this report proposed the wider application of programme budgeting and marginal analysis (PBMA) in the prioritization of PHIs. We present a case study of how PBMA has been applied to public health in Chapter 14 of this book.

What may be clear to readers from this description of the NICE public health reference case is that, in terms of evaluating the cost-effectiveness of PHIs, health economists need the skills to undertake a range of techniques of evaluation. We have tried, in the subsequent chapters of this book, to describe these various approaches with case studies drawn from our work in public health economics over the last ten years.

1.16 Should we expect PHIs to save money?

The increasing use of return on investment (ROI) approaches (including the development of an ROI toolkit by Public Health England) represents a growing expectation that PHIs 'need' to demonstrate that these initiatives will save money for society in the long run. This is interesting as decisions to fund surgical interventions or a new drug are not routinely subjected to this expectation of 'invest to save' (Edwards et al., 2013). Woolf and colleagues (2009), in a US context, argue that there is a need to distinguish between measuring the intermediate outcome of a PHI (e.g. the number of people who stop smoking in response to a particular intervention, as opposed to the wider long-term social benefits of reduced prevalence of smoking in society) and associated long-term economic benefits (reduced deaths from lung cancer and increased economic productivity). They (Woolf et al., 2009) argue that there is a need to look at the cost-effectiveness of a public health prevention intervention in the same way as a clinical intervention—mindful that it may well have much wider benefits, not just expect it to be cost saving, hence levelling the playing field between public health and clinical interventions in terms of making a claim on finite public resources.

There is, however, evidence that PHIs can save money at the same time as reducing inequalities, as shown by Anopa and colleagues (2015) in their cost analysis of a national nursery tooth-brushing intervention. Figure 1.2 shows the annual costs of implementing the intervention and the resulting cost savings arising (due to avoided treatments) from the national toothbrushing intervention in pre-school children in Scotland. This research also revealed that the highest expected savings, hence health gains (as per avoided treatments for tooth decay), were observed in the most disadvantaged children. Figure 1.3 shows the results of the population-standardized analysis by deprivation category, with the most disadvantaged children (Depcat7) gaining the greatest cost savings (avoided treatments) post intervention.

1.17 Public spending across the life course

Figure 1.4 shows representative profiles for tax, public services, and welfare spending for the United Kingdom. It shows that in early life, people consume a relatively large amount of health care and state-funded education. Parents can claim child benefits and child tax credits during this period. In early years, children contribute little to tax revenues through their income and spending. During working age, people consume fewer public services whilst paying more tax, and, in some cases, receiving welfare benefits. In later life, people are more likely to consume more health care and social care and claim pensioner benefits, for example the state pension, but pay less tax as their incomes and spending fall (OBR, 2015).

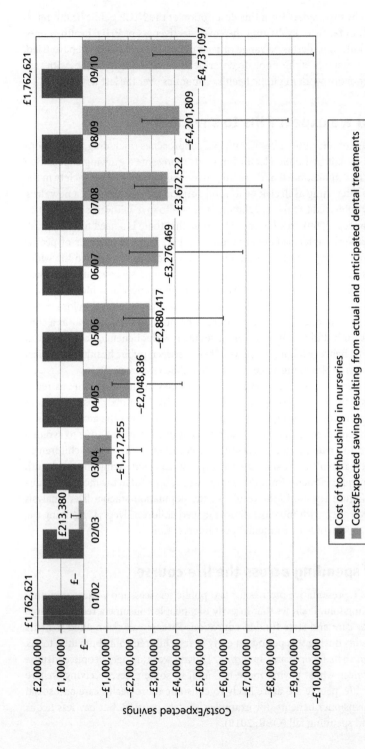

Figure 1.2 Annual cost of nursery toothbrushing programme and costs/expected savings resulting from actual and anticipated dental treatments—in comparison with 2001/02 dental treatment costs.

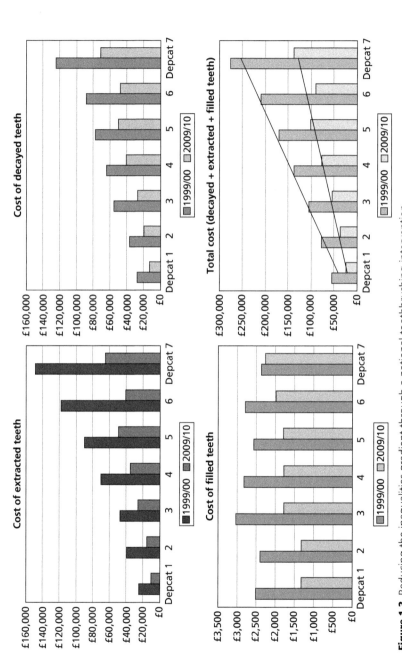

Figure 1.3 Reducing the inequalities gradient through a national toothbrushing intervention.

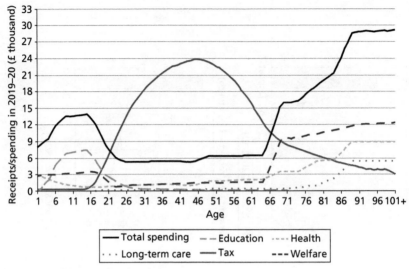

Figure 1.4 Public spending in relation to age.
Reproduced from Office for Budget Responsibility. (2016), Fiscal sustainability report. London, UK: Office for Budget Responsibility. Copyright © 2016 Office for Budget Responsibility. Published under the Open Government Licence.

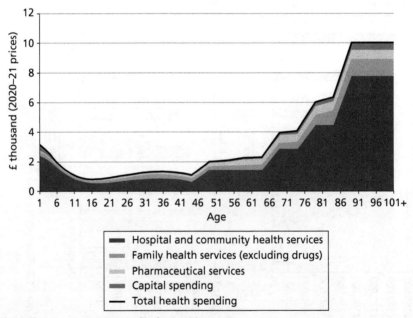

Figure 1.5 Representative profile for health spending.
Reproduced from Office for Budget Responsibility. (2016). Fiscal sustainability analytical paper: Fiscal sustainability and public spending on health. Copyright © 2016 Office for Budget Responsibility. Published under the Open Government Licence.

Focusing on health care spending, Figure 1.5 shows UK health spending across the life course for hospital and community services, family health services (excluding drugs), pharmaceutical services, and capital spending (Licchetta and Stelmach, 2016).

These figures clearly show that the bulk of total public spending, and health and welfare spending in particular, increase dramatically with age, with relatively little spent in the early years of life.

1.18 **The economic case for investment in early years**

Neuroscience research shows that environment and experiences have an impact on brain development in early years (Perry, 2002) There is an increasing amount of evidence that investing public resources in evidence-based programmes and practice to intervene and create the best conditions for early childhood development can be less costly and more effective than tackling the resulting consequences of poor conditions in later life (McDaid et al., 2015; Edwards et al., 2016).

Some of the most convincing evidence has come from the United States. James Heckman, a Nobel prize-winning Chicago economist, provides evidence that investment in pre-school produces a return on investment of between US$7 and US$10 for every US$1 invested (Heckman, 2012). This is attributed to better outcomes in health, education, sociability, economic productivity, and reduced crime.

Figure 1.6 shows returns to a unit dollar invested, assuming that one dollar is invested at each age from birth (Heckman, 2008).

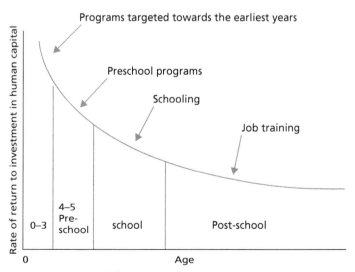

Figure 1.6 Returns to a unit dollar invested in pre-school in the United States.
Reproduced with permission from Heckman, J.J., 2008. The case for investing in disadvantaged young children. *ifo DICE Report*.6(2), 3–8. Copyright © 2008 © ifo Institute.

1.19 The role of the health economist in applying methods of economic evaluation to PHIs

As economists, or HTA practitioners, we need to be aware that we are implicitly accepting the status quo in terms of the distribution of wealth in society and the relative distribution of resources across government departments. The discipline of health economics highlights the fact that decisions about resource use involve choices that essentially represent trade-offs in the use of public sector resources, trade-offs between different groups in society, and trade-offs between different stages in the life course (Edwards et al., 2016). Professor Tony Culyer, in a distillation of his most influential writings, refers to the health economist as the 'dispassionate analyst' (Culyer, 2012). This is the health economist in a 'positive' role, presenting evidence of the marginal benefit for each marginal pound devoted to any particular intervention to promote better health. This role is rather different from what Culyer referred to in 1989 as 'normative health economics', which is a role where setting out options for the allocation of resources in itself can shape government policy (Culyer, 1989). In his discussion of extra-welfarism, in which characteristics such as health or happiness might be added in explicitly to a social welfare function (discussed further in Chapter 2 of this book) alongside individual utility, Culyer puts forward the idea that certain goods are merit goods. Consumption of these goods is so important, for example health education about health-harming products or behaviours, that they should be provided by government above and beyond what the market might bear. As the health economist rolls up her/his sleeves, and helps with any decision-making process about resource use in public health, they essentially move between generating empirical estimates of the relative cost-effectiveness of using resources in different ways to a more normative role about what would be an improvement or more desirable allocation of resources to achieve public health goals. In the United Kingdom, public health has traditionally only received 4 per cent of the NHS budget, and in times of financial recession, the temptation for commissioning groups and health boards is to disinvest in public health in order to meet the needs of acutely ill patients of today (Donaldson, 2010). Ambulances outside accident and emergency departments make the front page of newspapers, interventions to promote tooth brushing amongst socially deprived children do not.

1.20 Study design, modelling, and the basis for economic evaluation of PHIs

Figure 1.7 shows the range of study designs that can be used in clinical and health services research and which are relevant to the design of effectiveness studies that underpin economic evaluations of PHIs. Later chapters outline how economic evaluations can be conducted alongside the various research designs, typically analytic methods including experimental randomized controlled trials (RCTs) and observational such as natural experiments to evaluate the impact of policy interventions.

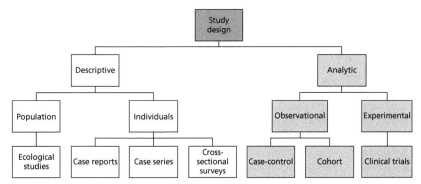

Figure 1.7 Types of research and evaluation studies.

Summary of Chapter 1

◆ In thinking about public health we must begin by thinking about intergenerational, environmental, and economic sustainability.

◆ As economists or HTA practitioners, we need to be aware that we are implicitly accepting the status quo in terms of the distribution of wealth in society and the relative distribution of resources across government departments.

◆ As public health practitioners we need to acknowledge that we are starting from a position of moving from the fourth to fifth wave of public health.

◆ There is much to be learned from public health economics in developing countries including research in global health economics.

◆ In terms of research methodology we need to recognize that many public health economics interventions are complex in nature, often requiring behavioural change by the individual, and effected by the context in which they are delivered.

◆ We would be wise to consider the role of the health economist—as the dispassionate analyst, or as the benevolent paternalist, helping to shape choice architecture of public policy that has the potential to impact the health of the population.

◆ There is a need to compare the cost-effectiveness of nudge and choice architecture as part of behavioural economics versus government legislation (or as a complement to) in achieving public health goals.

◆ We need to place great emphasis on equity, starting with identifying who benefits and who loses.

References

Akhtar, P.C., Haw, S.J., Levin, K.A., Currie, D.B., Zachary, R., and Currie, C.E., 2010. Socioeconomic differences in second-hand smoke exposure among children in Scotland after introduction of the smoke-free legislation. *Journal of Epidemiology & Community Health*, 64(4): 341–6.

Anopa, Y., McMahon, A., Conway, D., Ball, G., McIntosh, E., and MacPherson, L., 2015 Improving child oral health: Cost analysis of a national nursery toothbrushing programme. *PLoS ONE*, **10**(8): e0136211.

Ashton, J.R., 2009. From healthy towns 1843 to Healthy Cities 2008. *Public Health*, *123*(1): e11–e13.

Bellis, M.A., Lowey, H., Leckenby, N., Hughes, K., and Harrison, D., 2013. Adverse childhood experiences: Retrospective study to determine their impact on adult health behaviours and health outcomes in a UK population. *Journal of Public Health*, *36*(1): 81–91.

Bloom, D. E., Canning, D., and Jamison, D.T., 2004. Health, wealth, and welfare in health and development: Why investing in health is critical for achieving economic development goals. A compilation of articles from Finance and Development. Washington D.C.: International Monetary Fund.

Blumenschein, K. and Johannesson, M., 1996. Economic evaluation in health care: A brief history and future directions. *Pharmacoeconomics*, *10*(2): 114–22.

Burton, H., Sagoo, G.S., Pharoah, P., and Zimmern, R.L., 2012. Time to revisit Geoffrey Rose: Strategies for prevention in the genomic era? *Italian Journal of Public Health*, *9*(4): e8665-1-9.

Calkins, G, 1891. Results of sanitary legislation in England since 1875. *Publications of the American Statistical Association*, *2*(14): 297–303.

Cochrane, A., 1972. *Effectiveness and Efficiency: Random Reflections on Health Services*. London: The Nuffield Provincial Hospital Trust.

Culyer, A.J., 1989. The normative economics of health care finance and provision. *Oxford Review of Economic Policy*, *5*(1): 34–58.

Culyer, A.J., 2012. *The Humble Economist*. York: University of York and Office of Health Economics.

Dahlgren, G. and Whitehead, M., 1991. *Policies and Strategies to Promote Social Equity in Health*. Stockholm: Institute for Future Studies.

Davies, S.C., Winpenny, E., Ball, S., Fowler, T., Rubin, J., and Nolte, E., 2014. For debate: A new wave in public health improvement. *Lancet*, *384*(9957): 1889–95.

Department of Health, 2008. *The Cost of Alcohol Harm to the NHS in England: An Update to the Cabinet Office (2003) Study*. London: Department of Health.

Desmond-Hellmann, S., 2016. Progress lies in precision. *Science*, *353*(6301): 731.

Donaldson, L.J. and Donaldson, R.J., 2003. *Essential Public Health*. Berkshire: Radcliffe Publishing.

Donaldson, C., Bate, A., Mitton, C., Dionne, F., and Ruta, D., 2010. Rational disinvestment. *Quarterly Journal of Medicine*, *103*(10): 801–7.

Draborg, E., Gyrd-Hansen, D., Poulsen, P.B., and Horder, M., 2005. International comparison of the definition and the practical application of health technology assessment. *International Journal of Technology Assessment in Health Care*, *21*(1): 89–95.

Drummond, M.F., Sculpher, M.J., Claxton, K., Stoddart, G.L., and Torrance, G.W., 2015. *Methods for the Economic Evaluation of Health Care Programmes*. Oxford: Oxford University Press.

Drummond, M.F., Schwartz, J.S., Jönsson, B., Luce, B.R., Neumann, P.J., Siebert, U., and Sullivan, S.D., 2008. Key principles for the improved conduct of health technology assessments for resource allocation decisions. *International Journal of Technology Assessment in Health Care*, *24*(3): 244–58.

Edwards, R.T., 2001. Paradigms and research programmes: Is it time to move from health care economics to health economics? *Health Economics*, *10*(7): 635–49.

Edwards, R.T., Charles, J.M., and Lloyd-Williams, H., 2013. Public health economics: A systematic review of guidance for the economic evaluation of PHIs and discussion of key methodological issues. *BMC Public Health*, *13*(1): 1001.

Edwards, R.T., Bryning, L., and Lloyd-Williams, H., 2016. *Transforming Young Lives across Wales: The Economic Argument for Investing in Early Years*. Bangor: Bangor University, Centre for Health Economics and Medicines Evaluation.

EuroQoL, 2015. *EQ-5D. User Guide version 5.1.* <https://euroqol.org/wp-content/uploads/2016/09/EQ-5D-3L_UserGuide_2015.pdf> (Accessed 22 October 2018).

Faculty of Public Health. What Is Public Health? Retrieved from <http://fph.org.uk/what_is_public_health> (Accessed 10 October 2014).

Farquhar, J.W., 1999. Primordial prevention: The path from Victoria to Catalonia. *Preventive Medicine*, *29*(6): S3–S8.

Fuchs, V.R., 2000. The future of health economics. *Journal of Health Economics*, *19*(2): 141–57.

Goodman, P.G., Haw, S., Kabir, Z., and Clancy, L., 2009. Are there health benefits associated with comprehensive smoke-free laws. *International Journal of Public Health*, *54*(6): 367–78.

Goodman, C.S., 2014. *HTA 101: Introduction to Health Technology Assessment*. Bethesda, MD: National Library of Medicine.

Guest, C., Ricciardi, W., Kawachi, I., and Lang, I. (eds), 2013. *Oxford Handbook of Public Health Practice*. Oxford: Oxford University Press.

Hanlon, P., Carlisle, S., Hannah, M., Reilly, D., and Lyon, A., 2011. Making the case for a 'fifth wave' in public health. *Public Health*, *125*(1): 30–6.

Heckman, J.J., 2008. Schools, skills, and synapses. *Economic inquiry*, *46*(3): 289–324.

Heckman, J.J., 2012. Invest in early childhood development: Reduce deficits, strengthen the economy. *The Heckman Equation*. <https://heckmanequation.org/resource/invest-in-early-childhood-development-reduce-deficits-strengthen-the-economy> (Accessed 10 October 2018).

Heim, D., Ross, A., Eadie, D., MacAskill, S., Davies, J.B., Hastings, G., and Haw, S., 2009. Public health or social impacts? A qualitative analysis of attitudes toward the smoke-free legislation in Scotland. *Nicotine & Tobacco Research*, *11*(12): 1424–30.

Hoddinott, J., Rosegrant, M., and Torero, M., 2012. Hunger and malnutrition. <http://www.copenhagenconsensus.com/sites/default/files/Hunger+and+Malnutrition.pdf> (Accessed 10 October 2018).

Hollands, G.J., Shemilt, I., Marteau, T.M., Jebb, S.A., Kelly, M.P., Nakamura, R., Suhrcke, M., and Ogilvie, D., 2013. Altering micro-environments to change population health behaviour: Towards an evidence base for choice architecture interventions. *BMC Public Health*, *13*(1): 1218.

Hyland, A., Hassan, L.M., Higbee, C., Boudreau, C., Fong, G.T., Borland, R., Cummings, K.M., et al., 2009. The impact of smokefree legislation in Scotland: Results from the Scottish ITC Scotland/UK longitudinal surveys. *European Journal of Public Health*, *19*(2): 198–205.

Kelly, M.P., McDaid, D., Ludbrook, A., and Powell, J., 2005. *Economic Appraisal of PHIs*. London: Health Development Agency.

Kenkel, D.S., 2000. Prevention. In: A.J. Culyer and J.P. Newhouse (eds), *Handbook of Health Economics*. Amsterdam: Elsevier, pp. 1675–720.

Kindig, D.A., 2007. Understanding population health terminology. *The Milbank Quarterly*, *85*(1): 139–61.

Lawson, K. and McIntosh, E., 2013. *A Review of the Economic Evidence for Asset-Based Approaches for Health Improvement: Findings and Recommendations*. Report commissioned by the Glasgow Centre for Population Health.

Local Government Association (LGA) and UK Department of Health (DoH), 2012. From transition to transformation in public health: Resource Sheet 2: Understanding Public Health. London: Local Government Association.

Licchetta, M. and Stelmach, M. (2016). *Fiscal Sustainability Analytical Paper: Fiscal Sustainability and Public Spending on Health*. London: Office for Budget Responsibility. <http://budgetresponsibility.org.uk/docs/dlm_uploads/Health-FSAP.pdf> (Accessed 10 October 2018).

Marmot, M.G., Allen, J., Goldblatt, P., Boyce, T., McNeish, D., Grady, M., and Geddes, I., 2010. Fair society, healthy lives: Strategic review of health inequalities in England post-2010. The Marmot Review: London.

Maynard, A. and Kanavos, P., 2000. Health economics: An evolving paradigm. *Health Economics*, *9*(3): 183–90.

McDaid, D., Sassi, F., and Merkur, S., 2015. *Promoting Health, Preventing Disease: The Economic Case*. European Observatory on Health Systems and Policies Series. Maidenhead: Open University Press.

McLean, J. and McNeice, V., 2012. *Assets in Action: Illustrating Asset Based Approaches for Health Improvement*. Glasgow: Glasgow Centre for Population Health.

Medical Research Council (MRC), 2008. Economic Impact Reporting Framework. <http://www.mrc.ac.uk/publications/browse/economic-impact-report-2008-09/> (Accessed 10 October 2018).

Midgley, G. (2006). Systemic intervention for public health. *American Journal of Public Health*, *96*: 466–72.

Mooney, G.H. and McGuire, A., 1988. *Medical Ethics and Economics in Health Care*. Oxford: Oxford University Press.

Mooney, G., 1992. *Economics, Medicine and Health Care* (2nd edn). London: Harvester Wheatsheaf.

Morgan, A. and Ziglio, E., 2007. Revitalising the evidence base for public health: an assets model. *Promotion & Education*, *14*(2_suppl): 17–22.

Mulligan, J.A., Walker, D., and Fox-Rushby, J., 2006. Economic evaluations of non-communicable disease interventions in developing countries: A critical review of the evidence base. *Cost Effectiveness and Resource Allocation*, *4*(1): 7.

Mushkin, S. J., 1958. Toward a definition of health economics. *Public Health Reports*, *73*(9): 785–93.

Mushkin S. J., 1962. Health as an Investment. *Journal of Political Economy*, *70*(2), suppl. 1: 129–57.

National Institute for Health and Care Excellence, 2009. Methods for the Development of NICE Public Health Guidance (2nd edition). London: NICE.

National Institute for Health and Care Excellence, 2011. Supporting Investment in Public Health: Review of Methods for Assessing Cost Effectiveness, Cost Impact and Return on Investment. London: NICE.

National Institute for Health and Care Excellence, 2014. Developing NICE Guidelines: The Manual. London: NICE.

National Institute for Health and Care Excellence, 2013. Guide to the Methods of Technology Appraisal. London: NICE.

Nielsen, C.P., Funch, T.M., and Kristensen, F.B., 2011. Health technology assessment: research trends and future priorities in Europe. *Journal of Health Services Research & Policy*, *16*(2): 6–15.

Office for Budget Responsibility, 2015. *Fiscal Sustainability Report*. <http://budgetresponsibility.org.uk/docs/dlm_uploads/49753_OBR-Fiscal-Report-Web-Accessible.pdf (Accessed 10 October 2018).

Owen, L., Morgan, A., Fischer, A., Ellis, S., Hoy, A., and Kelly, M.P., 2011. The cost-effectiveness of PHIs. *Journal of Public Health*, *34*(1): 37–45.

Payne, K., McAllister, M., and Davies, L.M., 2013. Valuing the economic benefits of complex interventions: When maximising health is not sufficient. *Health Economics*, *22*(3): 258–71.

Perry, B. D., 2002. Childhood experience and the expression of genetic potential: What childhood neglect tells us about nature and nurture. *Brain and Mind*, *3*: 79–100.

Phelps, C.E., 1995. Perspectives in Health Economics. *Health Economics*, *4*(5): 335–53.

Phillips, C.J., 2008. *Health Economics: An Introduction for Health Professionals*. London: John Wiley & Sons.

Porta, M. (ed.), 2008. *A Dictionary of Epidemiology*. Oxford: Oxford University Press.

Puska, P., 2002. Successful prevention of non-communicable diseases: 25 year experiences with North Karelia Project in Finland. *Public Health Medicine*, *4*(1): 5–7.

Raftery, J. and Powell, J., 2013. Health technology assessment in the UK. *Lancet*, *382*(9900): 1278–85.

Ramsey, S., Willke, R., Briggs, A., Brown, R., Buxton, M., Chawla, A., Cook, J., et al., 2005. Good research practices for cost-effectiveness analysis alongside clinical trials: the ISPOR RCT-CEA Task Force report. *Value in Health*, *8*(5): 521–33.

Rose, G., 1981. Strategy of prevention: lessons from cardiovascular disease. *British Medical Journal*, *282*: 1847–51.

Rose, G., 1985. Sick individuals and sick populations. *International Journal of Epidemiology*, *14*: 32–8.

Rose, G., 1992. The Strategy of Preventive Medicine. Oxford: Oxford University Press.

Sackett, D.L., Rosenberg, W.M., Gray, J.M., Haynes, R.B., and Richardson, W.S., 1996. Evidence based medicine: what it is and what it isn't. *BMJ (Clinical Research edition)*, *312*(7023): 71–2.

Smith, R.D. and Petticrew, M., 2010. Public health evaluation in the twenty-first century: Time to see the wood as well as the trees. *Journal of Public Health*, **32**(1): 2–7.

Sunstein, C.R. and Thaler, R.H., 2012. *Nudge: Improving Decisions About Health, Wealth and Happiness*. London: Penguin.

Taylor, M. 2010. The Healthy Cities Movement: Working Paper on the Lancet Commission for Healthy Cities. <https://www.ucl.ac.uk/healthy-cities/outputs/Working_Paper> (Accessed 10 October 2018).

Trapero-Bertran, M., Mistry, H., Shen, J., and Fox-Rushby, J., 2013. A systematic review and meta-analysis of willingness-to-pay values: The case of malaria control interventions. *Health Economics (United Kingdom)*, *22*(4): 428–50. http://bura.brunel.ac.uk/handle/2438/10019

Velasco-Garrido, M. and Busse, R., 2005. *Health Technology Assessment: An Introduction to Objectives, Role of Evidence, and Structure in Europe.* Geneva: WHO Regional Office for Europe.

Walker, D., McDermott, J.M., Fox-Rushby, J., Tanjung, M., Nadjib, M., Widiatmoko, D., and Achadi, E., 2002. An economic analysis of midwifery training programmes in South Kalimantan, Indonesia. *Bulletin of the World Health Organization, 80*(1): 47–55.

Walker, D. and Fox-Rushby, J.A., 2000. Economic evaluation of communicable disease interventions in developing countries: A critical review of the published literature. *Health Economics, 9*(8): 681–98.

Wanless, D., 2004. *Securing Good Health for the Whole Population.* London: HM Stationery Office

Warner, K.E. and Murt, H.A. 1984. Economic incentives for health. *Annual Review of Public Health 5*: 107–33.

Weatherly, H., Drummond, M., Claxton, K., Cookson, R., Ferguson, B., Godfrey, C., Rice, N., et al., 2009. Methods for assessing the cost-effectiveness of PHIs: key challenges and recommendations. *Health Policy, 93*(2): 85–92.

Weinstein, M.C. and Stason, W.B. 1976. *Hypertension: A Policy Perspective.* Cambridge, MA: Harvard University Press.

Williams, A., 1972. Cost-benefit analysis: Bastard science? And/or insidious poison in the body politick? *Journal of Public Economics, 1*(2): 199–225.

Williams, A., 1993. Priorities and research strategy in health economics for the 1990s. *Health Economics, 2*(4): 295–302.

Winslow, C.E., 1920. The untilled fields of public health. *Science, 51*(1306): 23–33.

Woolf, S.H., Husten, C.G., Lewin, L.S., Marks, J.S., Fielding, J.E., and Sanchez, E.J., 2009. *The Economic Argument for Disease Prevention: Distinguishing Between Value and Savings.* Washington, DC: Partnership for Prevention.

World Health Organization, 1986. *Ottawa Charter for Health Promotion.* Geneva: World Health Organization.

Chapter 2

The supply and demand of preventive goods and services and the need for economic analysis

Seow Tien Yeo, Huw Lloyd-Williams, and Rhiannon T. Edwards

2.1 Medicine is failed prevention

Professor Sir Michael Marmot has said that 'medicine is failed prevention'. This chapter looks at the nature of preventive goods and services and the extent to which they can produce cost efficiencies and health gains for health care organizations. For this purpose, preventive goods and services are defined as measures taken for disease prevention, as opposed to disease treatment (Leavell and Clark, 1979). The main tenet, as explained here, is the fact that in economic theory, prevention goods and services are different from normal goods and services (Wagstaff, 1986). As a consequence, they first need to be provided in a different way and, second need to be evaluated differently. In this chapter we first introduce some concepts of basic micro-economics, outlining ideas of rational choice and preferences, giving context to the concept of demand. We then go on to describe how the provision of prevention goods and services requires government intervention in order for optimal provision to take place. The second part of the chapter focuses on the methods of economic evaluation of prevention goods and services.

2.2 Micro-economic theory of utility, rational choice, and demand and supply

Micro-economics is the study of how individuals and organisations made decisions. Individuals are assumed to be rational economic actors satisfying some axiomatic assumptions about economic rationality. The most important of these are *completeness* and *transitivity* (Mankiw, 2011). Completeness assumes that all pairs of alternative choices can be compared with each other, that is, if the choice set is A and B, an individual can prefer A to B, or B to A, or is indifferent between A and B. Transitivity implies that if A is preferred to B, and B preferred to C, then A is preferred to C. Individual preference can be presented in terms of an indifference curve, which is based on the

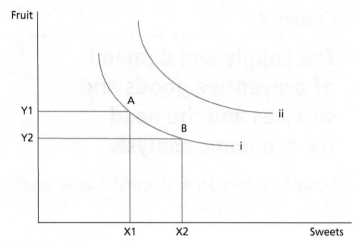

Figure 2.1 Indifference curves
Reproduced courtesy of Huw Lloyd-Williams.

concept of utility. Utility, in economics, is a measure of the satisfaction gained by the consumer of a good. The utility function is a curve on a plane that assigns a number to choice combinations of two goods. An indifference curve joins the points at which the consumer has equal utility for each possible choice, that is, the point at which the consumer is 'indifferent' between different choice combinations of both goods. Figure 2.1 shows an indifference curve 'i' that shows the relationship between two goods, fruit and sweets. Along the indifference curve we have points whereby the consumer is indifferent between combinations of fruit and sweets.

Choice set Y1X1, or point A on the indifference curve, where the consumer chooses Y1 amount of fruit and X1 amount of sweets, has the same level of utility, or satisfaction, as choice set Y2X2, or point B. The further we move away from the origin (i.e. co-ordinates (0,0)), the higher utility level that indifference curve represents. Thus, each point on indifference curve 'ii' yields a greater level of utility than indifference curve 'i'.

Economics is about making the most of limited resources. The way economists factor this in is through what is called a budget constraint. A budget constraint can be represented by a straight line which connects different price combinations that satisfy a given budget. In other words, it is what the consumer can afford at different prices of fruit and sweets. In Figure 2.2 it is the line MN. The consumer wants to get the most she can out of her given budget. In economic terms, she wants to 'maximize her utility subject to her budget constraint'. In other words, to get the most she can with her money.

The aim of a consumer, therefore, in economic terms, is to maximize utility subject to a budget constraint. The consumer is trying to extract as much utility as she can from her available budget. In economics, the calculation performed uses calculus to optimize the indifference function subject to the budget constraint. In other words, the optimal position is the choice set between fruit and sweets where the indifference curve is tangential to the budget constraint—point A in Figure 2.2. Note that

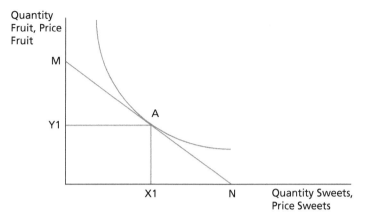

Figure 2.2 Maximizing utility subject to budget constraint.
Reproduced courtesy of Huw Lloyd-Williams.

for this example, it is the budget assigned for the purchase of fruit and sweets. This budget could be increased (with an opportunity cost for other things in life) to achieve a higher level of utility.

The concept of demand in economics relates to how much of a 'good' or 'service' consumers want to buy at each possible price. Consumers or 'demanders of goods and services' could be members of the public or, for the purposes of this book, members of the population, public health service users, or patients. The nature of demand for normal goods is that the relationship between a products' quantity demanded and price is represented by a downward sloping curve. The higher the price, the less quantity of the product is demanded. Conversely, the lower the price, the higher quantity is demanded. Demand has a close relationship with consumer choice as described earlier. Figure 2.3 shows the relationship between demand curves and indifference curves, or how we can derive a demand curve from an indifference curve. There is a relationship between preferences and actual demand for a good or service, and this is shown in Figure 2.3 where we can go from a situation where there is a reduction in relative prices between fruit and sweets and this fall in price causes quantity demanded to increase.

We see that as the price of sweets decreases in relation to fruit, the budget line shifts from Y0X3 to Y0X4. This means that for any given quantity of fruit, more sweets can be bought and consumed because the price is lower. This translates into the demand curve where a lower price increases the demand for sweets. This is because the demand curve is downward sloping—higher price, lower demand, and lower price, higher demand.

Care must be taken to distinguish between the level of demand itself and quantity demanded. A shift along the demand curve, that is, from points A to B, is a change in quantity demanded—as price decreases from PX1 to PX2 so quantity demanded rises from X1 to X2. However, an external influence such as a successful advertising campaign can cause demand itself to shift and this can be shown as a shift in the demand curve itself as shown in Figure 2.4. This shows that for any given price demand is now higher.

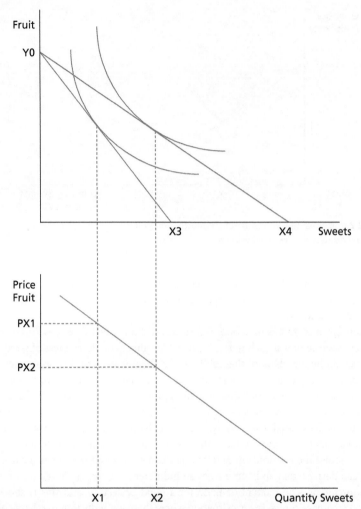

Figure 2.3 Deriving a demand curve from an indifference curve.
Reproduced courtesy of Huw Lloyd-Williams.

While the theory of demand is based on consumer preference and choice, the theory of supply is rooted in decisions made in producing goods and services (Mankiw, 2011). The supply of a good or service is also related to the price of the product, but rather than a downwards sloping curve, as is seen with demand, the supply curve is upward sloping, meaning that as the price of a product increases, suppliers are willing to supply more of the product. If we plot the demand and supply curve for a particular product on the same graph we can then introduce the concept of market equilibrium. This is a situation where demand is equal to supply in a market so what is demanded is what is supplied and there is no waste or inefficiencies in the system.

The interaction, where the demand function crosses the supply function, signifies at which price and quantity this market is in equilibrium. In Figure 2.5 this is at point

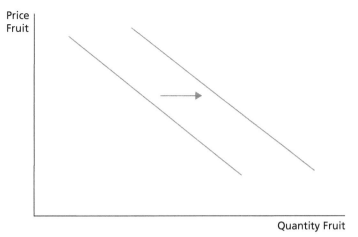

Figure 2.4 The demand curve shifts to the right.
Reproduced courtesy of Huw Lloyd-Williams.

P1Q1. At this point the quantity demanded is equal to the quantity supplied. At any price above P1, the quantity supplied is greater than quantity demanded and so there is said to be an excess of supply. When this is the case suppliers will react to their excess stock by reducing its price in order to be able to offload it and hence the price will tend towards the equilibrium again. If the price is lower than P1 then there will be excess demand—demand will be greater than supply. When this is the case the price will tend upwards towards the equilibrium as sellers run down their stocks in a response to excessive demand, triggering a rise in price. This price mechanism is sometimes re-ferred to as the 'invisible hand' of the free market. This term was first coined by Adam

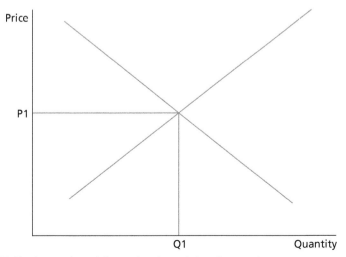

Figure 2.5 The interaction of demand and supply in a free market.
Reproduced courtesy of Huw Lloyd-Williams.

Smith in his book *An Inquiry into the Nature and Causes of the Wealth of Nations* in 1776. This is where market forces combine to provide efficient allocations of goods and services—situations where there is the optimal level of provision of goods and services and no under- or over-provision.

Another concept that should be introduced to the non-economist reader is the idea of 'elasticity of demand'. This is a measure of how responsive demand is to changes in price or income. The demand curve, as we have established, is downward sloping, signifying that more quantity is demanded at lower prices. What happens, however, when the price of a good changes? How will consumers behave? A measure of what happens to quantity demanded following a price change is known as the elasticity of that demand. It is calculated as the change in quantity demanded divided by the change in price. In other words, it is measured as the value of the slope of the demand curve. For example, if price increases by 10 per cent and then quantity demanded falls by 20 per cent, the price elasticity of demand is calculated as follows in Figure 2.6.

There is a negative sign in front of the formula to take account of the inverse relationship between quantity demanded and price. An elasticity greater than 1 means the product is *elastic*, meaning that a change in price will bring about an even greater change in demand. An elasticity of less than 1 refers to a good that is price *inelastic*, so that a change in price will be associated with a lesser change in quantity demanded. An elasticity of 1 refers to a good that has *unit elasticity*; that is, the change in quantity demanded is equal to the change in price. Elastic goods and services tend to be those with close substitutes so that a small increase in price, for example, would lead to a larger reduction in quantity demanded since people would substitute this good for another, similar product at a lower price. Inelastic demand occurs when goods and services are necessities or addictive. People will still buy cigarettes, for example, when the price goes up. Demand for cigarettes might fall as the price rises but not by as much as the concomitant rise in price (Perucic, 2012).

2.3 Market failure and the economic case for prevention

Preventive goods and services include such things as government policies, education, and information, and environments designed specifically to prevent ill-health and promote healthy behaviours. This section will explore why it is the case that left to

$$\text{Price Elasticity of Demand} = -\frac{\text{\% Change in quantity of good demanded}}{\text{\% Change in price of good}}$$

$$= -\frac{-20\%}{10\%}$$

$$= 2$$

Figure 2.6 Calculating the elasticity of demand.

market mechanisms alone, these goods and services would be under-provided and their optimal allocation will not be fulfilled. When thinking about preventive goods and services there are three key economic questions to address:

1. What preventive goods and services should be produced?
2. What technical methods should be used to produce these goods and services?
3. How should access to preventive goods and services be distributed between individuals in society?

Market failure refers to a situation where market forces are not sufficient to deliver a socially efficient allocation of resources (Evans, 1984; McGuire et al., 1988; Donaldson and Gerard, 2003). It leads to a situation which economists refer to as an outcome that is not Pareto optimal. Pareto optimality refers to a situation where you *cannot* make one person better off without making at least one other person worse off. It is an optimal situation. However, with market failure it *is* possible to make someone better off without making anyone else worse off—the market has failed to provide optimality (Sugden and Williams, 1978). It is assumed in markets for normal goods that the consumer is the best judge of his own welfare. This is not the case in the market for health care. In this type of situation governments may step in to provide the good or service in question in order that there is an optimal level of provision. Intervention entails governments purchasing health care on behalf of patients as well as providing that health care (Donaldson and Gerard, 2003).

2.3.1 Reasons for market failure

The main reason for market failure in the case of preventive goods and services is that these are often seen as public goods. These should not be confused with public health goods. A good is a public good if one cannot exclude anyone from enjoying it (non-excludability) and the consumption of it does not reduce the amount available for everyone else (non-rivalry in consumption). Examples of public goods include fresh air and the natural environment, national security, education, and street lighting. Information, as a good, has the properties of a public good in that it displays aspects of non-rivalry in consumption and non-excludability. The market will under-provide health information because there is not enough incentive to produce it since the producer does not gain enough of the benefits due to a 'free-rider' problem; people can consume the good without paying for it. There is, therefore, a case for government intervention in the provision and production of health information (Hale et al., 2012). Another reason for failure in the market for preventive goods and services is known as time inconsistent preferences (Donaldson and Gerard, 2003; Hale et al., 2012). This is the case where economic agents (i.e. those that make economic decisions) prefer instant satisfaction rather than thinking about the long term. This affects the market because individuals will not honour commitments made now to behave in a certain way in the future. In the present, people tend to be impulsive; costs seem large compared with perceived benefits. However, when we look to the future we are generally more rational and costs seem less compared to benefits. An example of this would be physical exercise (a well known public health-improving behavior). It is relatively easy to make a commitment today to start exercising tomorrow; the costs seem low compared to the benefits. However, when tomorrow arrives it becomes the present and the individual is again faced with high 'effort' costs relative to the benefits of exercising and can often be put off exercising. This concept is closely related to time discounting. Time discounting is when individuals value something more now than they would in the future. A pound is worth more now than it would be in ten years' time. These time-related issues affect the working of markets, rendering them inefficient, and allows for government intervention to provide socially optimal allocation of resources. Asymmetry of information can also lead to inefficient market outcomes. Clinicians are better informed than consumers about health care and so may promote excessive health care use if they have a financial incentive to do so. The market is not functioning properly in this case as there is an oversupply of health care. The last reason for market failure is that individuals violate some of the assumptions of rationality postulated in micro-economic theory. It is argued that this is especially true of children and young people who are not making decisions to maximize their utility over the long term but rather engage in sometimes health-harming behaviour that maximizes utility over the short term. Insofar as this is true, we may see preventive goods as a type of merit good. Merit goods are those where the benefit to society is greater than the benefit to the individual. There is an argument that society (through taxation) should provide and pay for these goods. We see, therefore, that economic theory shows that there is a strong case for intervention in preventive services within public health, as is true for medical care in general, based on the possibility that provision by the free market will be suboptimal and lead to inefficient outcomes—avoidable ill health, disability, and premature death with associated personal and societal costs.

2.3.2 **Market failure case study**

Let us demonstrate the ideas expressed thus far by employing a case study. Our case study is based on a paper by Watts and Segal, analysing the market for the management of chronic disease. The main finding in this paper is that,

> market failure from a preference of individuals for 'immediate gratification' in the form of health care and disease management, rather than preventive services, where benefits are delayed, has a major impact on achieving an efficient allocation of resources in markets for the management of chronic diseases. (Watts and Segal, 2009)

We return to this issue of time preference and its importance in the evaluation of HEIs in Chapter 3 of this book.

2.3.2.1 Background

Watts and Segal argue that although there is evidence of an increase in the prevalence of chronic disease, health care systems are reactive in their way of dealing with the problem rather than focusing on disease prevention. Although health care markets are often described as not adhering to the principles of economic theory, care must be taken in analysing features of separate markets within the health care system. These markets vary in their deviation away from the assumptions of competitive economic theory. These differences come about through differences in the asymmetry of information between producers and consumers, inter-temporal factors, and time discounting.

2.3.2.2 Discussion

As mentioned in section 2.3.1, asymmetry of information can lead to inefficient market outcomes. However, in the case of the market for the treatment of chronic diseases the consumer of health care is substantially better informed than is the case for acute care. Indeed, it is often the case that people with chronic disease have at least the same amount of knowledge about their condition as clinicians. These patients have to deal with their condition over the long term and hence they tend to want to gain as much knowledge as they can in order to manage their condition. In the literature they have been referred to as 'expert patients' and as such are able to engage in a 'partnership model' or 'co-production model' with their clinicians. This is where people with chronic diseases take an active role in making decisions about their own health care. It can be seen that funding models that do not take into account the specialized knowledge that these patients have do not support a partnership or co-production model and therefore may lead to treatment and management decisions that are not compatible with maximizing health outcomes.

Time-inconsistent preferences are another reason for market failure. An individual's time preference for their own health will depend on whether they are valuing an intervention that will provide an instant gain or one that will provide gains in the future. It can be seen that an individual is more likely to discount the downstream gains excessively that come from preventive services compared with the value they place on consumption that produces an immediate benefit. Further, social and private benefits of preventive care will differ. The benefits of preventing a health-threatening outcome will accrue to society in general as well as the individual concerned. This type of externality, a result of the definition of preventive goods as merit goods, will hinder the market for preventive services, and the individual's consumption of such services will not be at the socially optimal level if health behaviour does not take into account the effect consumption of preventive services will have on others. The main source of market failure that comes out of time-inconsistent preferences is the fact that, when considering future benefits, assumptions of economic rationality that underpin market economics do not necessarily hold.

2.3.2.3 Summary

Watts and Segal conclude their 2009 paper by stating that government subsidization of some public health preventive programmes over others without consulting the economic evidence is bound to lead to market inefficiencies. The management of chronic disease is especially affected by this. Governments, it is argued, favour subsidizing acute care over preventive programmes that offer a more cost-effective way of managing chronic disease. It is suggested that, with the increased prevalence of chronic disease, it is important that these issues are addressed.

2.3.3 Cohen's model of preventive behaviour

In 'Utility Model of Preventive Behaviour', David Cohen outlines an economic model that seeks to explain individual preferences over preventive goods and services (Cohen, 1984).

The utility model of preventive behaviour put forward by Cohen in his paper views preventive actions as economic 'goods' that are consumed. (For the full diagram of the utility model, see Cohen, 1984, p. 63) In his words, 'The utility model assumes that all preventive behaviour can be expressed as the consumption of risk-affecting economic goods' (Cohen, 1984, p. 63).

Cohen places prevention within the micro-economic theory of demand. Utility, it is suggested, can be gained from the consumption of these preventive or risk-affecting goods directly for their inherent worth (utility in use) or for the way they affect the risk of illness or injury (utility of anticipation). He gives an example of oatmeal bread, which is desired both for its taste, nourishment (use), and its health-promoting properties (anticipation). There is a continuum of utility here and a good may be anywhere on the scale between mainly utility in use and mainly utility in anticipation. It is suggested that the main motivating factor in preventive behaviour is the anxiety associated with the threat of ill health rather than ill-health itself (Cohen, 1984). Therefore, the benefits from consumption arise from the reduced anxiety that any preventive measure would instil. Assuming rationality in economic theory, a decision to consume a good is made by maximizing utility subject to a cost constraint. Consumption of preventive goods and services—that is, preventive behaviour—is affected by utility in use, utility in anticipation, and cost. At an individual consumer level, cost-effective prevention goods are therefore those that give the greatest increase in the quantity of the risk-affecting good consumed for any given expenditure. Further, when demand for risk-affecting products is highly elastic to cost (market price or other cost, e.g. time cost), then Cohen suggests that government intervention in terms of public provision, or taxes or subsidies, in a market is a more efficient way of altering consumption by individual consumers.

More recently, in an empirical analysis, Kenkel found that annual use of two preventive adult services decreases with age. This may be consistent with time preference shortening over the life course. Highest level of education was also found to be important in determining demand for preventive services. He also found that demand for preventive services was dependent on an individual's level of insurance cover (Kenkel, 2006).

2.4 An introduction to economic evaluation in the case for prevention: Why do we need economic evaluation?

Thus far we have discussed the demand for, and supply of, preventive goods and services in the light of market failure. This market failure in preventive activity, and the reasons behind it, lead to a requirement for government intervention as a means to allocate resources for this activity. As resources are finite with increasing demands for preventive goods or services, governments will need to know whether the preventive good or service is good value for money in order to decide which good or service to use. Therefore, the need for consideration of different forms of economic evaluation on behalf of the government or other payers for preventive goods and services. This section considers the main economic evaluation tools available to health economists in evaluating the case for prevention. This section also explains some of the basic ideas behind economic evaluation such as the fundamentals about the calculation of incremental cost-effectiveness ratios (ICER), quality-adjusted life years (QALYs), and consideration of uncertainty. Please also refer to Gray et al., the earlier handbook in the series entitled 'Applied Methods of Cost-effectiveness Analysis in health care' .

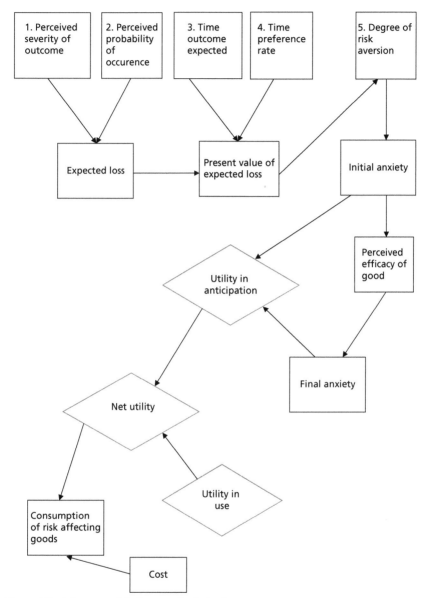

Figure 2.7 Cohen's model of preventive behaviour.
Source: data from Cohen, D. Utility model of preventive behaviour. *Journal of Epidemiological Community Health.* 38(1):61–5. Copyright © 1984 BMJ Group.

2.4.1 What is economic evaluation and why is it important?

Economic evaluation in health care settings has emerged as an important tool to determine the maximum value for money associated with new interventions or programmes. 'Value for money' simply implies achieving a predetermined objective at minimum cost or maximizing the outcome or benefit to the population of patients served from a limited amount of resources—an associated concept of efficiency in the field of health economics. To achieve this aim, the tools of economic evaluation are employed to select the most cost-effective options from a range of alternatives, that is, interventions or programmes. Cost-effectiveness analysis (CEA) is one of the types of economic evaluations, as are cost-minimization analysis (CMA), cost–utility analysis (CUA), and cost–benefit analysis (CBA) (Drummond et al., 2015). The differences between these methods become clear when considering the outcome measure, the number of health outcomes evaluated, the unit of health outcome, and the unit of measure (Table 2.1).

CMA considers which of the two or more competing alternatives is less costly when evidence proves that the outcomes for the competing alternatives are equivalent, the least costly alternative is then preferred. In CBA, many different outcomes can be considered and all outcomes are measured in monetary terms (see Chapter 9 for further discussion about cost–benefit analysis). Cost–effectiveness analysis (CEA) considers only one outcome and the outcome is measured purely in natural units, for example life years gained, the number of cases detected, or the number of events averted (see below 'Cost-effectiveness analysis' section 2.4.3 for further explanation). CUA is a type of cost-effectiveness analysis that measures health outcomes in terms of marginal gain to both quantity of life lived and health-related quality of life, for example using the quality-adjusted life year (QALY). Cost–utility analysis is the most commonly used method of health economic analysis as it allows comparisons to be made between interventions that have entirely different health outcomes (see below 'Cost-utility analysis' section 2.4.5 for further explanation). Cost–consequence analysis (CCA) considers a disaggregated range of relevant outcomes and costs which allows policy makers and commissioners to make decisions based on the relevance and relative importance to their decision-making context (Drummond et al., 2015).

2.4.2 **Allocative and technical efficiency**

The concepts of allocative and technical efficiency are central in economics. They are important because they provide context for benchmarking methods and evaluative frameworks in terms of what they can and can't address. Allocative efficiency refers to the way in which goods and services are allocated in an economy and an allocative efficient outcome is one where the level of production reflects consumer preferences. That is, it can be used to identify the impact of allocating resources across society. CBA is ideally placed to answer questions of allocative efficiency.

Technical efficiency explores how to maximize outputs for given inputs and doesn't offer guidance on how to distribute health gain across society. Resource allocation decisions can be made in terms of whether or not they lead to a net improvement in social welfare (Pearce and Nash, 1981) thus bolstering the welfarist paradigm. CEA addresses questions of technical efficiency. CEA does not allow for comparison across prevention programmes tackling different health problems across different populations because of the one-dimensional nature of how outcomes are measured and because of its reductivist basis in technical efficiency.

Table 2.1 Types of economic evaluation

Types	Outcome measure	Number of health outcomes	Unit of health outcome	Unit of measure
Cost-minimization analysis	Evidence proves that the outcome for competing alternatives are equivalent	None	None	Cost (£)
Cost-effectiveness analysis	Health outcomes are measured in natural units: e.g. life years gained, life saved, the number of cases detected, representing a main common goal for competing alternatives	One	Natural units: e.g. life years gained, life saved, the number of cases detected, etc.	Cost (£) per additional unit of the main common goal
Cost–utility analysis	Health outcome is measured in quality-adjusted life years (QALYs), a generic preference-based measure weighing the survival or the number of additional life years (quantity of life) by the quality of life (value) of the health state a person experienced in each year	One	QALYs	Cost (£) per QALY gained
Cost–benefit analysis	Both costs and benefits (e.g. lost productivity averted, disability-adjusted life year averted, case averted) are measured in monetary terms with the financial value of the costs compared with the financial value of the benefits	Many	Pound Sterling (£)	Cost (£)
Cost–consequence analysis	A disaggregated range of relevant outcomes and costs	Many	Varied	Not a ratio

2.4.3 Cost-effectiveness analysis

Cost-effectiveness analysis (CEA) is a form of economic evaluation that compares relative costs and outcomes (effects) of different alternatives for the same condition. These alternatives are mutually exclusive which means you can only choose one: A or B, but not both. This method has been used broadly in the field of health-related research to assess the extent to which alternatives can be regarded as providing good value for money. In this context, the currently available alternative, or treatment as usual, is normally used as a comparator to the new intervention or new programme. CEA plays an important role in facilitating decision-makers and health commissioners to make informed decisions on how, and where, to allocate limited health care resources within a disease area (Cohen and Reynolds, 2008).

2.4.4 How an incremental cost-effectiveness ratio is calculated

Cost-effectiveness of a new intervention, compared to a currently available alternative, is calculated as a ratio of the difference in mean costs to the difference in mean outcomes (effects) between two alternatives—this is known as the incremental cost-effectiveness ratio (ICER).

The ICER equation can be expressed as $\dfrac{\text{Costs2} - \text{Costs1}}{\text{Effects2} - \text{Effects1}}$, where

Costs2 = Mean costs of new intervention
Costs1 = Mean costs of currently available alternative
Effects2 = Mean effects of new intervention
Effects1 = Mean effects of currently available alternative

For example, if the chosen effect that related to the target outcome of a study is life years gained and the cost is measured in monetary units, for example, pounds Sterling (£), then the resulting incremental cost-effectiveness ratio (ICER) will be expressed as cost (£) per life year gained.

2.4.5 Cost–utility analysis

In health economics, a widely used unit in economic evaluation to assess effectiveness in units that are comparable across different health interventions or programmes, is the quality-adjusted life year (QALY). A QALY is a measure of utility combining survival (quantity of life lived) and quality of life (Morris et al., 2007).

QALYs are calculated by aggregating the number of years lived, weighted by the relative quality of life value attached to the given health state of an individual at the time (Morris et al., 2007; Drummond et al., 2015). A QALY is calculated by weighting survival (quantity of life lived) with quality of life (on a 0 to 1 scale) which can be measured using a preference-based measure, including the widely used European Quality of life-5 Dimension (EQ-5D) instrument. This is a generic preference-based health-related quality of life measure, developed by the EuroQol group (Morris et al., 2007; Drummond et al., 2015; EuroQoL, 2015). Figure 2.8a is an illustrative diagram

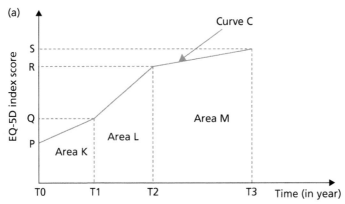

Figure 2.8a An illustrative graph showing how total QALYs are derived from a study with EQ-5D index scores: P, Q, R, and S collected at each study time-point: T0, T1, T2, and T3, respectively.

showing how QALYs are derived from a study with EQ-5D index scores, P, Q, R, and S (quality of life score values) collected at each of the study time points, T0, T1, T2, and T3 (time, measured in years) respectively.

Figure 2.8a, QALYs are calculated as the total areas under the curve (here in Curve C)—this means it is the sum of Area K, Area L, and Area M, where:

Area K = 0.5 × (P+Q) × (T1–T0)
Area L = 0.5 × (Q+R) × (T2–T1)
Area M = 0.5 × (R+S) × (T3–T2)

In a CUA study that compares a new intervention to a currently available alternative, QALY is used as a summary measure of health outcome and if the costs associated with the study to achieve that outcome, measured in monetary terms, can also be calculated, then an incremental cost–utility ratio (ICUR however, this is commonly refered to an 'effectiveness' ratio ICER) value can be derived (see below the equation of ICUR). Figure 2.8b is an illustrative diagram showing incremental QALYs (Area G) from the new intervention (Curve I) compared to currently available alternative (Curve C). The incremental QALY (Area G) is simply the area under the Curve I (QALYs of new intervention) less the area under the Curve C (QALYs of currently available alternative).

The equation of ICUR can be expressed as $\dfrac{\text{Costs2} - \text{Costs1}}{\text{QALYs2} - \text{QALYs1}}$, where

Costs2—Mean costs of new intervention
Costs1—Mean costs of currently available alternative
QALYs2—Mean QALYs of new intervention
QALYs1—Mean QALYs of currently available alternative

The incremental cost–utility ratio is expressed as the unit of cost (£) per QALY gained. It gives an estimate of how much extra a new intervention would cost to produce one additional QALY (one QALY equates to 1 year of life in perfect health) compared with

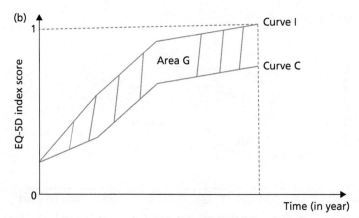

Figure 2.8b An illustrative graph showing incremental QALYs (Area G) from the new intervention (Curve I) compared to currently available alternative (Curve C).

the currently available alternative, for example, standard usual care or standard practice. Cost–utility analysis, using QALY as the health outcome, allows comparisons to be made across different interventions or disease areas on a single common scale. This allows allocative efficiency questions to be addressed. The National Institute for Health and Care Excellence (NICE), in the United Kingdom, has advocated the use of QALY, a common unit of effect, for cost–utility analysis (National Institute for Health and Care Excellence, 2013).

2.4.6 Illustrative case study: Examples of cost–utility ratio calculations for seven competing interventions for the same condition

In this section, we consider a situation where there are seven competing health care interventions (A–G) for the same condition that could be commissioned, and these interventions are mutually exclusive—that is, you can choose only one intervention amongst the seven interventions, but not all seven. These interventions are assumed to be fully defined by the QALYs and costs given in Table 2.2. The purpose of this illustrative example is to provide an overall picture of how the cost–utility ratio concept works in a situation where there are several competing interventions available for the same condition, though having seven interventions for the same condition may seem unrealistic in real-world settings. In this exercise, we will assess what are the additional benefits (QALYs) to be gained from alternative interventions, for example, and at how much greater cost?

(1) Step 1: First of all, rank the seven competing interventions according to their effectiveness (here in QALYs [Q]) in Table 2.2 in ascending order (see result in Table 2.3)—on the basis of securing maximum health benefit (here in QALYs [Q]) instead of considering cost at this stage.

(2) Step 2: Examine and exclude any interventions with smaller QALY and higher cost compared to an alternative intervention (dominated). (See Table 2.4)

Table 2.2 QALYs and costs for seven mutually exclusive interventions

Intervention	QALYs [Q]	Cost [C], £
A	16	56,350
B	71	1,150,500
C	5	110,500
D	76	1,615,500
E	41	155,800
F	51	750,000
G	44	130,800

Table 2.3 QALYs (rearranged) and costs for seven mutually exclusive interventions

Intervention	QALY [Q]	Cost [C], £
C	5	110,500
A	16	56,350
E	41	155,800
G	44	130,800
F	51	750,000
B	71	1,150,500
D	76	1,615,500

Table 2.4 QALYs and costs for seven mutually exclusive interventions

Intervention	QALY [Q]	Cost [C], £	Incremental QALY	Incremental Cost, £
C	5	110,500	—Dominated by A—	
A	16	56,350	—	—
E	41	155,800	—Dominated by G—	
G	44	130,800	28	74,450
F	51	750,000	7	619,200
B	71	1,150,500	20	400,500
D	76	1,615,500	5	465,000

(3) Step 3: Calculate the incremental QALY and incremental cost of each intervention in comparison with the prior (less effective) intervention. (See Table 2.4)

(4) Step 4: For a clearer view, remove rows C and E from this table. Then, calculate the incremental cost–utility ratio (ICUR) for each sequentially more effective intervention compared with the prior intervention. (See Table 2.5)

(5) Step 5: Identify and exclude any interventions that have a higher ICUR than more effective interventions (which this is known as extended dominated). For a clearer view, remove row F from this table. Then, recalculate the ICURs. (See result in Table 2.6)

(6) Step 6: Repeat Step 5 until all dominated interventions are removed and ICURs have been recalculated for all non-dominated interventions.

Results from this exercise show that the positive ICUR for G means that by adopting G rather than A there is a gain in QALY and an increase in cost. The ICUR for G works out to be 2,659, which means that it costs £2,659 to generate each additional QALY compared with A. Alternatives that are more costly and less effective are excluded. In Table 2.4, C and E are followed by interventions that have increased QALY and reduced cost. Therefore, C and E are excluded and removed from this table (as shown in Table 2.5). In Table 2.5, F has a higher ICUR than more effective intervention, which is

Table 2.5 QALYs and costs for the remaining five mutually exclusive interventions after excluding interventions C and E

Intervention	QALY [Q]	Cost [C], £	Incremental QALY	Incremental Cost, £	ICUR
A	16	56,350	—	—	—
G	44	130,800	28	74,450	2,659
F	51	750,000	7	619,200	88,457*
B	71	1,150,500	20	400,500	20,025
D	76	1,615,500	5	465,000	93,000

*Extended dominated.

Table 2.6 QALYs and costs for the remaining four mutually exclusive interventions after excluding interventions C, E, and F

Intervention	QALY [Q]	Cost [C], £	Incremental QALY	Incremental Cost, £	ICUR
A	16	56,350	—	—	—
G	44	130,800	28	74,450	2,659
B	71	1,150,500	27	1,019,700	37,767
D	76	1,615,500	5	465,000	93,000

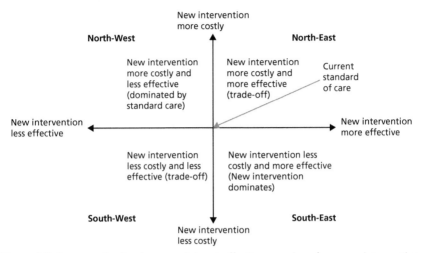

Figure 2.9 An example of an incremental cost-effectiveness plane for a new intervention and a current standard of care.

B. Intervention F is therefore further excluded and removed from this table (as shown in Table 2.6). Having further excluded F, ICUR is then recalculated for B and is as shown in Table 2.6.

2.4.7 **Introducing the concept of the cost-effectiveness plane**

In cost-effectiveness analysis, the incremental costs and effects for two mutually exclusive interventions (i.e. a new intervention versus a current standard of care for the same condition) can be illustrated graphically on a four quadrant diagram—often referred to as the 'cost-effectiveness plane' (Black, 1990; Drummond et al., 2015) (see Figure 2.9).

The plane is presented in a two-dimensional diagram by plotting the incremental costs (y axis) against the incremental effects (x axis) of two mutually exclusive interventions in which the current standard of care occupies the origin of the graph. The cost–effectiveness coordinates of the new intervention under the study will be placed either to the right or left of the origin if it is more or less effective compared to the current standard of care, and above or below the origin if it is more or less costly.

2.4.8 **Introducing the cost-effectiveness threshold**

When a new intervention is both more effective and cost-saving, compared to the current standard of care, it is denoted as a 'dominant' strategy (South-East quadrant) and so the new intervention should replace existing care. When a new intervention is both less effective and more costly than the current standard of care, it is then referred to as a 'dominated' strategy (North-West quadrant) and so the new intervention should not be used. The other two quadrants—North-East quadrant (new intervention more effective and more costly) and South-West quadrant (new intervention less effective and cost-saving)—are the trade-off quadrants.

When a new intervention falls into either of these quadrants, the adoption of the new intervention will be determined using a cost–effectiveness threshold (labelled as R_i in Figure 2.10) with regard to whether it is value for money compared to the current standard of care (i.e. the available alternative) (see Figure 2.10). The cost–effectiveness threshold, often referred to as the 'willingness-to-pay threshold' represents the maximum amount of money that the decision-maker (e.g. the NHS) is willing to spend in order to achieve one unit improvement in outcome, for example, gain 1 year of life (if life year gained is the outcome of the study) or to gain one QALY (if QALY is the outcome of the study). In the United Kingdom, NICE has recommended using the threshold range of £20,000–£30,000 per QALY as the standard reference to determine whether a new intervention is cost-effective compared to the alternative available, though not all the time as absolute standards (Williams et al., 2008).

Drummond and colleagues highlighted that a negative ICER needs to be interpreted with caution (Drummond et al., 2015). A negative ICER is yielded when the comparison is located in the North-West and South-East quadrants of the cost-effectiveness plane where one alternative is dominant. When the ICER is negative the magnitude of the ICER is meaningless (Drummond et al., 2015). Consider three different comparisons in the South-East quadrant:

(i) New intervention, P results in 2 quality-adjusted life years (QALYs) gained, a saving of £8,000, and hence an ICER of –£4,000;

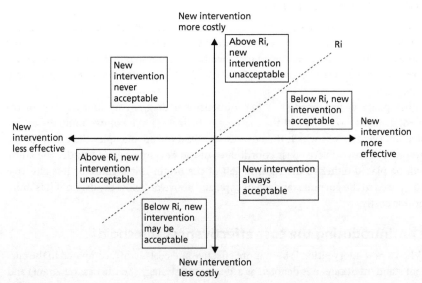

Figure 2.10 Cost-effectiveness plane with a cost-effectiveness threshold (Ri).

Adapted with permission from Black, W.C., The cost-effectiveness plane: a graphic representation of cost-effectiveness. *Medical Decision Making.* 10(3), 212–15. Copyright © 1990 Society for Medical Decision Making/SAGE.

(ii) New intervention, Q results in 4 QALYs gained, a saving of £8,000, and hence an ICER of –£2,000;

(iii) New intervention, R results in 4 QALYs gained, a saving of £4,000, and hence an ICER of –£1,000.

With regard to ICERs, amongst the three comparisons, R would be the most preferred option, followed by Q, and then P. However, in terms of joint changes in costs and QALYs, it is evident that Q would be preferred to P and R as it has the highest combination of QALY gain and cost saving.

Given the uncertainty surrounding the estimate of cost-effectiveness or cost-utility could span more than one quadrant of the cost-effectiveness plane, non-parametric bootstrapping is one method that has been widely adopted and used in cost-effectiveness and cost–utility studies for deriving confidence intervals (CIs) for the ICER (Briggs et al., 1997). Non-parametric bootstrapping is a re-sampling method where it involves simple random sampling with replacement from the original (observed) data to build an empirical estimate of the sampling distribution of the ICER (Drummond et al., 2015). This re-sampling is repeated a large number of times. For example, if the re-sampling is repeated, say, 5,000 times, the independent bootstrap of 5,000 replications can then be obtained which in this case is the empirical estimate of sampling distribution of the ICER. There are a few methods available to calculate CIs from this empirical estimate, one simple approach would be to base a 95 per cent CI on the 2.5 and 97.5 percentiles from the empirical sampling distribution (Drummond et al., 2015). Besides estimating the CIs for the ICER, non-parametric bootstrapping can construct a cost-effectiveness plane with the 5,000 bootstrapped replicates illustrated on the CE plane (see Figure 2.11 for an illustrative example of CE plane for a new intervention on 1-year follow up), and the corresponding cost-effectiveness acceptability curve (CEAC) can then be constructed (see Figure 2.12) based on the uncertainty in cost and effect differences shown in Figure 2.11. The CEAC shows the probability that an intervention is cost-effective, given the observed data, compared to its comparator at a range of willingness to pay thresholds (or cost-effectiveness thresholds) (Fenwick et al., 2001).

Figure 2.11 shows an illustrative example of the results of a non-parametric bootstrapping analysis with 5,000 replications (or iterations) based on the analysis of a new intervention versus its comparator (currently available alternative, i.e. current standard of care or current practice) based on 1-year follow-up. A number of lines are drawn on the CE plane in Figure 2.11 with each one passing through the origin. These lines (R_i) represent alternative values for the willingness-to-pay threshold for an additional QALY. There are two extreme values—one of the extreme values would be zero, which means there is no value attached to an additional QALY, this is presented by the horizontal line running along the x axis. The other extreme value would be the infinity (∞) which means there is no limit in terms of value (money) attached to an additional QALY. This is shown by the vertical line, running along the y axis, and corresponds with an infinite threshold willingness-to-pay for an additional QALY. Between these extremes, threshold values of £10,000, £20,000, and £30,000 per QALY are shown (see Figure 2.11).

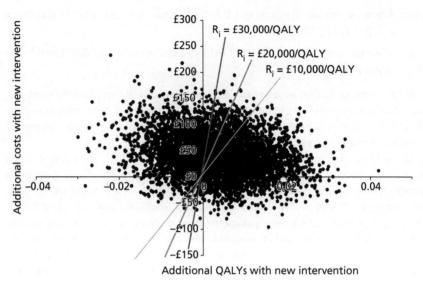

Figure 2.11 An illustrative example of cost-effectiveness plane with 5000 bootstrapped replicates for a new intervention compared to its comparator.

For a given threshold, all points on the cost-effectiveness plane below the threshold line would be considered cost-effective because the new intervention is either (1) dominant (i.e. in the South-East quadrant); (2) more costly and more effective but with an ICER below the threshold willingness-to-pay (i.e. below the threshold line in the North-East quadrant); or (3) less costly and less effective (i.e. below the threshold line in the South-West quadrant). When a threshold willingness-to-pay of £0 applies (the horizontal line running along x axis), all points on the cost-effectiveness plane below the x axis (i.e. all points in the South-East and South-West quadrants) would be considered cost-effective. The proportion of points on the cost-effectiveness plane below the threshold of £0 per QALY would be the corresponding point on the CEAC for a zero threshold. As the threshold gradually increases (swivels around the origin in an anticlockwise direction), the proportion of points on the cost-effectiveness plane below the threshold (i.e. these are points that can be described as cost-effective) changes and these proportions are shown on the corresponding CEAC. When the willingness-to-pay threshold reaches infinity (the vertical line running along y axis), the proportion of points to the right of the y axis (i.e. all points in the North-East and South-East quadrants) would be considered cost-effective and this is shown on the CEAC.

Thus, Figure 2.12 shows the CEAC for the new intervention. As the value of the willingness-to-pay threshold increases, the proportion of bootstrap replicates that fall in the cost-effective region of the plane changes. This can be interpreted as the probability that the new intervention is more cost-effective than its comparator. The shape of the CEAC will vary from one study to another depending on the joint uncertainty in cost and effect differences on the cost-effectiveness plane (Fenwick et al., 2004). In Figure 2.12, the ICER is shown on the CEAC as well as the UK NICE thresholds value

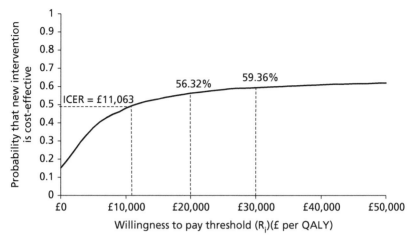

Figure 2.12 The corresponding cost-effectiveness acceptability curve (CEAC) for the new intervention based on the uncertainty in cost and effect differences shown in Figure 2.11.

of £20,000 and £30,000 per QALY. From the CEAC, the decision-maker would be able to decide whether to adopt the new intervention by assessing the probability that the new intervention is cost-effective at a particular willingness-to-pay threshold. For example, at the NICE threshold of £20,000 per QALY, the probability that the new intervention is cost-effective is 56.32 per cent (i.e. the proportion of bootstrap replicates on the cost-effectiveness plane below the threshold of £20,000 per QALY, as demonstrated in Figure 2.11).

2.4.9 **Net monetary benefit (NMB)**

The other approach to quantifying uncertainty around ICER estimates in a trial-based economic evaluation is to use net benefit (Willan, 2003; Drummond et al., 2015). The concept of net benefit was established as a way of placing both costs and effects on a single scale—either net monetary benefit (NMB) or net health benefit (NHB)—and this can be achieved by employing a simple rearrangement of the cost-effectiveness decision rule. Amongst those two net benefits, net monetary benefit is the most common and widely used version; it is defined as the difference in effects between two alternatives being evaluated and is rescaled into monetary value by multiplying it with the threshold willingness-to-pay for a unit of effect (R_i, the maximum amount the decision-maker is willing to pay for a unit of increased effectiveness), and then subtract the difference in costs between the alternatives from this value.

The net monetary benefit (NMB) can be expressed in mathematic formula:

$NMB = R_i \Delta E - \Delta C$, where
R_i—Threshold willingness-to-pay for a unit of effect
ΔE—Difference in effects between two alternatives
ΔC—Difference in costs between two alternatives

From the NMB formula above, it shows that the NMB is expressed as a function of the threshold willingness-to-pay (R_i). It is a linear expression and an illustrative linear graph, plotting the NMB of the new intervention versus its comparator (y axis) against the threshold willingness-to-pay for a unit of effect (R_i) , for example, for a QALY, can be performed using a parametric statistical analysis approach, namely regression analysis, that jointly considers costs and benefits (or effects, e.g. QALYs) (Briggs et al., 2002). An illustrative example of the presentation of NMB, together with its sampling uncertainty, as a function of the threshold willingness-to-pay for a unit of effect (R_i) is shown in Figure 2.13.

The use of NMB provides a statistically manageable way of presenting sampling uncertainty in cost-effectiveness measures. This approach also has another advantage. If we do not know what the threshold of willingness-to-pay is, it allows net monetary benefits to be calculated for any value of the threshold, as illustrated in Figure 2.13. However, it has not been extensively used in published cost-effectiveness and cost–utility studies compared to the cost-effectiveness acceptability curve (CEAC), and this is particularly the case in public health economics. A CEAC is produced based on the uncertainty in cost and effect differences exhibited in a cost-effectiveness plane resulting from non-parametric bootstrapping analysis (van Hout et al., 1994). This is because, in essence, the CEAC can facilitate the decision-making process showing a decision-maker, or commissioner, the probability that a new intervention is more cost-effective than its comparator (Fenwick et al., 2001; Drummond et al., 2015).

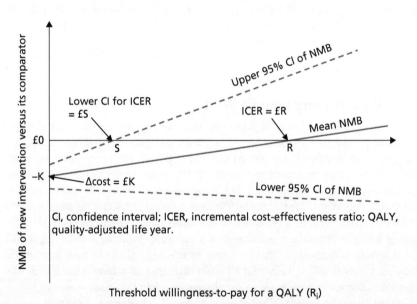

Figure 2.13 An illustrative example of the presentation of net monetary benefit (NMB), together with its sampling uncertainty, as a function of the threshold willingness-to-pay (Ri). The example is based on the comparison of a new intervention and its comparator based on 1-year follow-up

CI, confidence interval; ICER, incremental cost-effectiveness ratio; QALY, quality-adjusted life year.

Summary of Chapter 2

In this chapter:

♦ We have given a description of the theory and concepts behind the economics of public health programmes/interventions and, in particular, prevention.

♦ We have described how health care is different from normal goods and services and so needs to be provided by a third party payer (i.e. government) in order for allocation of health care resource use to be optimal. This idea is explored further in Chapter 12, where the business case for prevention is discussed.

♦ This chapter also introduces the different tools of economic evaluation which can be applied to public health interventions such as preventive goods and services. These techniques are further discussed in Chapters 7–10 where examples are given in the form of case studies.

♦ We discuss the measurement of costs and outcomes in this chapter with regard to how they are used in different economic evaluation methods; however, measuring and valuing costs and outcomes is discussed in more detail in Chapters 5 and 6.

♦ We have also highlighted how to deal with the uncertainty surrounding cost-effectiveness or cost-utility estimates.

♦ Last, we introduce an alternative approach (net monetary benefit (NMB)) to quantifying uncertainty around ICER estimates, though this has not been used extensively in public health economics.

References

Black, W.C., 1990. The CE plane: A graphic representation of cost-effectiveness. *Medical Decision Making, 10*(3): 212–14.

Briggs, A.H., Wonderling, D.E., and Mooney, C.Z., 1997. Pulling cost-effectiveness analysis up by its bootstraps: A non-parametric approach to confidence interval estimation. *Health Economics, 6*: 327–40.

Briggs, A.H., O'Brien, B.J., and Blackhouse, G., 2002. Thinking outside the box: Recent advances in the analysis and presentation of uncertainty in cost-effectiveness studies. *Annual Review of Public Health, 23*: 377–401.

Cohen, D., 1984. Utility model of preventive behaviour. *J Epidemiol Community Health*, 1984 Mar; *38*(1): 61–5.

Cohen, D.J. and Reynolds, M.R., 2008. Interpreting the results of cost-effectiveness studies. *Journal of the American College of Cardiology, 52*(25): 2119–26.

Donaldson, C. and Gerard, K., 2003. *The Economics of Health Care Financing: The Visible Hand*. Basingstoke: Palgrave Macmillan.

Drummond, M.F., Sculpher, M.J., Claxton, K., Stoddart, G.L., and Torrance, G.W., 2015. *Methods for the Economic Evaluation of Health Care Programmes* (4th edn). Oxford: Oxford University Press.

EuroQoL, 2015. *EQ-5D. User Guide version 5.0*. <https://euroqol.org/wp-content/uploads/2016/09/EQ-5D-3L_UserGuide_2015.pdf> (Accessed 2 November 2018).

Evans, R.G., 1984. *Strained Mercy: The Economics of Canadian Medical Care*. Toronto: Butterworths.

Fenwick, E., Claxton, K., and Sculpher, M., 2001. Representing uncertainty: The role of cost-effectiveness acceptability curves. *Health Economics*, *10*: 779–89.

Fenwick, E., O'Brien, B.J., and Briggs, A., 2004. Cost-effectiveness acceptability curves: Facts, fallacies and frequently asked questions. *Health Economics*, *13*: 405–15.

Gray, A., Clarke, P.M., Wolstenholme, J.L., and Wordsworth, S., 2011. *Applied Methods of Cost Effectiveness Analysis in health care*. Oxford: Oxford University Press.

Hale, J., Phillips, C.J., and Jewell, T., 2012 Making the economic case for prevention—a view from Wales. *BMC Public Health*, *12*: 460.

Kenkel, D.S., 2006. The demand for preventive medical care, *Applied Economics*, **26**:(4): 313–25.

Leavell, H.R. and Clark, E.G., 1979. *Preventive Medicine for the Doctor in his Community* (3rd edn). Huntington, NY: Robert E. Krieger Publishing Company.

Mankiw, G., 2011. *Principles of Economics* (6th edn). Stamford, CT: Southwestern Cengage Learning.

McGuire, A., Henderson, T., and Mooney, G., 1988. *The Economics of Health Care: An Introductory Text*. London, Routledge and Kegan Paul.

Morris, S., Devlin, N., and Parkin, D., 2007. *Economic Analysis in Health Care*. Chichester: John Wiley & Sons Ltd.

National Institute for Health and Clinical Excellence, (2013). *Process and Methods Guides: Guide to the Methods of Technology Appraisal 2013*. <http://www.nice.org.uk/article/pmg9/resources/non-guidance-guide-to-the-methods-of-technology-appraisal-2013-pdf (Last accessed 12th June 2015).

Pearce, D. and Nash, C., 1981. *The Social Appraisal of Projects: A Text in Cost–Benefit Analysis* (2nd edn). London: Macmillan.

Perucic, A., 2012. The demand for cigarettes and other tobacco products. Geneva: World Health Organization. Available at: <http://www.who.int/tobacco/economics/meetings/dublin_demand_for_tob_feb2012.pdf> (Accessed 13 October 2018).

Smith, A., 1776/1904. *An Inquiry into the Nature and Causes of the Wealth of Nations* (5th edn). London: Methuen & Co Ltd.

Sugden, R. and Williams, A., 1978. *The Principles of Practical Cost–Benefit Analysis*. New York, NY: Oxford University Press

van Hout, B.A., Al, M.J., Gordon, G.S., and Rutten, F.F.H., 1994. Costs, effects and c/e-ratios alongside a clinical trial. *Health Economics*, *3*: 309–19.

Wagstaff, A., 1986. The demand for health: Some new empirical evidence. *Journal of Health Economics*, **5**(3):195–233.

Watts, J.J. and Segal, L., 2009. Market failure, policy failure and other distortions in chronic disease markets. *BMC Health Services Research*, **9**: 102.

Willan, A., 2003. Analysing cost-effectiveness trials: Net benefits. In: A. Briggs (ed.), *Statistical Methods for Cost-Effectiveness Research: A Guide to Current Issues and Future Developments*. London: Office for Health Economics, pp. 8–23.

Williams, I., McIver, S., Moore, D., and Bryan, S., 2008. The use of economic evaluations in NHS decision-making: A review and empirical investigation. *Health Technology Assessment*, *12*: 1–196.

Chapter 3

Applying methods of economic evaluation to public health: Contemporary solutions to traditional challenges

Rhiannon T. Edwards and Emma McIntosh

Concepts, methodologies and practices within public health need further development if they are to be sufficient to allow us to develop, undertake and evaluate interventions in the twenty-first century.

Smith and Petticrew, 2010

3.1 Introduction

In Chapter 1 we noted that economic evaluation and the methods of economic evaluation in health care developed very much within a medical model of health care. In this chapter, as a starting point, we work from a paradigm of evidence-based medicine and we explore the challenges of applying the typically micro-economic evaluation toolbox to the evaluation of public health interventions. In section 3.66, we question the assumption of using the evidence-based medicine paradigm, which results in frequentist economic evaluation methods, to show readers the current methodological debates in action. A key feature of public health interventions is that they are largely preventive in nature and typically delivered outside the context of the traditional health care sector, for example, in schools, workplaces, and communities. Subsequent chapters in this book present a range of examples of economic evaluations of public health interventions delivered in these settings. This chapter introduces the concepts highlighted by Smith and Petticrew that economists and other evaluators of public health interventions need to move beyond primary and secondary health-related effects upon individuals and focus more on macro-economic evaluation of the wider range and distribution of direct and indirect effects upon individuals, communities, and populations (Smith and Pettigrew, 2010). Most recently, this has been discussed in a debate about whether or not spillover effects should be included in economic evaluation of health technology assessment, with associated implications for public health interventions (Brouwer, 2018; McCabe, 2018), we return to this issue in Chapter 15. As noted by Margaret Whitehead, 'the contemporary public health agenda continues the recent move away from the focus on infectious disease, and into behavioural, environmental and socio-economic factors influencing health' (Whitehead, 2007).

In his review of the UK NHS, Derek Wanless challenged health economists to apply their methods of analysis to public health and prevention (Wanless, 2004). This was reiterated by Kelly and colleagues in 2005 at the NHS Health Development Agency, which later became part of the National Institute for Health and Care Excellence (NICE) (Kelly et al., 2005). These authors viewed the application of economic evaluation methods to the appraisal of public health interventions as an under-explored area of health economics and as intrinsically challenging. This is broadly because of the differing perspective, time horizons involved, and typically much wider range of costs and effects pertinent in economic evaluation of public health interventions. In the evaluation of medical technologies within a health care setting the perspective of analysis is usually that of the health care payer (in the United Kingdom, it is the National Health Service (NHS)), hence the range of costs and outcomes to be measured is relatively straightforward, relating to health care inputs and patient-related outcomes, and these benefits are likely to be accrued within a relatively short period of time (Drummond et al., 2015). There are a number of excellent textbooks and sets of guidance on methods of economic evaluation of such health technologies (Ramsey et al., 2005; Glick et al., 2014; Drummond et al., 2015) as well as statements to increase consistency in the reporting and presenting of economic evaluations (Husereau, 2013), discussed in section 3.7.

3.2 Economic evaluation of medical technologies in a health care setting and the role of research study design

The main methods of economic evaluation introduced in Chapter 2 of this book (CBA, CCA, CEA, CMA, and CUA) were developed for application in the context of the evaluation of medical technologies in a health care setting (Drummond et al., 2015). Cost-minimization analysis (CMA) is widely thought to be of limited use outside of pharmacoeconomics (Briggs and O'Brien, 2001) and hence does not feature in this book. Cost–consequence analysis (CCA), however, does feature in the book (Chapter 10) and has been included in the UK's NICE guidance as being applicable to the economic evaluation of public health interventions (National Institute for Health and Care Excellence, 2012). These methods are well developed and have been applied across a wide range of clinical interventions with great success and have given rise to increased standardization in design, conduct, and reporting (Ramsey et al., 2005; Husereau, 2013). Economists need to strike a balance between the traditional research-led micro-economic evaluation methods as typically built in alongside funded trials or natural experiments with a need to increase the public health intervention economic evaluative space with the use of more contemporary systems approaches (Smith and Petticrew, 2010).

Conducting an economic evaluation requires a suitable 'vehicle' in which to identify, measure, and value the relevant costs and consequences of an intervention and comparator. To this end, there are a number of research study designs amenable to 'hosting' economic evaluation data collection. These research designs include randomized controlled trials (RCTs); cohort or longitudinal studies; cross-sectional studies; and natural experiments for the analysis of observational data. It is acknowledged that economic evaluation methods as they have been developed for health technology assessment (HTA) may not capture all the costs and benefits relevant to the assessment of public health interventions. Marsh and colleagues review the methods that could be employed to measure and value the broader set of benefits generated by public health interventions (Marsh et al., 2012). It is proposed that two key developments are required if this vision is to be achieved. First, there is a trend for modelling approaches that improve the capture of the effects of public health interventions (see Chapter 11 of this book). This trend needs to continue, and economists should also consider a broader range of modelling techniques than are currently employed to assess public health interventions (see e.g. sections 11.1.2 and 11.3 on agent-based models in Chapter 11 of this book). Second, economists are currently exploring a number of valuation paradigms that hold the promise of more appropriate valuation of public health intervention outcomes. These include the capabilities approach and the subjective well-being approach; both offer the possibility of broader measures of value than the approaches currently employed by health economists. Chapter 6 of this book explores outcomes in public health intervention evaluation in more depth.

Decision-makers are interested in the effectiveness and cost-effectiveness of clinical and public health interventions. RCTs are widely regarded as the 'gold standard' methodology for estimating the causal effects of public health interventions (Bonell et al., 2009). However, it has been recently argued that public health interventions are often not amenable to standard evaluation methodology such as RCTs; this is discussed further in relation to the precautionary principle in section 3.6. The specific role of alternative designs for the evaluation of public health interventions will be introduced in the following section.

3.2.1 Randomized controlled trials

A randomized controlled trial (RCT) is a type of scientific experiment which aims to reduce bias, for example, when testing a new medical treatment. Trial participants are allocated at random to either the treatment group or to a control group receiving standard treatment (or placebo) (Bowling, 2014). In brief, randomization minimizes selection bias so that it is possible to measure any effect attributable to a new intervention under investigation, relative to usual care and keeping all other factors constant. The RCT is often considered the gold standard for a clinical trial. The 'frequentist' approach to economic evaluation involves the collection of data on resource use alongside an RCT to enable the calculation of an incremental cost-effectiveness ratio (ICER) discussed in Chapter 2 of this book. Traditionally, RCTs were the domain of clinical interventions, however, there is a growing number of RCTs evaluating public health interventions which include economic evaluations, examples include McIntosh and colleagues (2009), Edwards and co-authors (2016), O'Brien and co-workers (2015), Clarkson and colleagues (2015), Hunter and colleagues (2016), and Minnis and co-workers (2017). Chapter 7 of this book reproduces an economic evaluation of a housing modification intervention to improve heating and ventilation in the homes of children with asthma (the CHARISMA trial; Edwards et al., 2011).

Randomized controlled trials have a long history of successful application in evaluating the effectiveness of social interventions, indeed cluster RCTs can accommodate communities, schools, or other 'clusters' as the unit of analysis and can cope with non-standard interventions (Rychetnik et al., 2002). Given the strength of the RCT study design, the use of a non-randomized study in settings where RCTs would have been feasible represents a lost opportunity in the opinion of Rychetnik and colleagues (2002). It is argued that a well-conducted RCT is the best (albeit sometimes impractical) study design for determining a causal relation between an intervention and its putative outcomes. However, study design alone cannot suffice as the main criterion for the credibility of evidence about public health interventions (Rychetnik et al., 2002).

Victora and colleagues argue that RCTs are often inappropriate for the scientific assessment of the performance and impact of large-scale interventions such as those required in public health (Victora et al., 2004). They note that although evidence-based public health is both possible and desirable, it must go well beyond RCTs. They agree that RCTs are essential for evaluating the efficacy of clinical interventions, where the causal chain between the agent and the outcome is relatively short and simple and where results may be safely extrapolated to other settings. However, they argue that the causal chains in public health interventions are much longer (and arguably more complex), making RCT results subject to effect modification in different populations. Both the internal and external validity of RCT findings can be greatly enhanced by observational studies using adequacy or plausibility designs (Habicht et al., 1999). For evaluating large-scale interventions, studies with plausibility designs may be the only feasible option and may provide valid evidence of impact.

The following sections outline alternative study designs and methodologies suitable for public health interventions (as well as public health economic evaluation). Chapters 4 and 11 of this book provide guidance on alternative methods of evidence synthesis and modelling which are also commonly used for generating economic evaluation evidence.

3.2.2 Observational studies: Cohort and case-control studies

Observational studies are those where analysts 'observe' the effect of a risk factor or diagnostic test, treatment, or other intervention. Unlike a RCT, researchers do not influence the design, nor those exposed to the risk factor or intervention. To address some investigative questions, RCTs are not always indicated or ethical to conduct (Song and Chung, 2010). Well-designed observational studies have been shown to provide results similar to RCTs, challenging the belief that observational studies are second-best. Cohort studies and case-control studies are two types of observational studies. For research purposes, a cohort is any group of people who are linked in some way (e.g. people who share a defining characteristic, typically who experienced a common event in a selected period). For instance, a 'birth cohort' includes all people born within a given time frame. Researchers can then compare what happens to members of the cohort that have been exposed to a particular variable with what happens to those who have not been exposed. Cohort studies are largely about the life histories of segments of populations and the individual people who constitute these segments. A cohort study can be useful in public health research as it is an analysis of risk factors, follows a group of people, and uses correlations to determine the absolute risk. For example, a recent study linked poor health in adult life to a range of adverse childhood events (Bellis et al., 2014), and Hyppönen and colleagues (2001) analysed data from a birth cohort in Finland to reveal that dietary vitamin D supplementation is associated with reduced risk of type 1 diabetes. Examples of full and partial economic evaluations alongside cohort studies evaluating public health interventions include the work of Merito and co-workers (2005) and Wolf and colleagues (2008).

3.2.3 Cross-sectional studies

A cross-sectional study or prevalence study is a type of observational study that analyses data collected from a population, or a representative subset, at a specific point in time. In economics, cross-sectional studies through the use of regression estimates the magnitude of causal effects of one or more independent variables upon a defined dependent variable at a given point in time. They differ from time series analysis, in which the behaviour of one or more economic aggregates is traced through time. Cross-sectional studies are different from case-control studies. These types of studies aim to provide data on the total population, whereas case-control studies concentrate on individuals with a specific characteristic (Bowling, 2014).

3.2.4 Natural experiments

Given the move away from RCTs in many evaluations of public health interventions, alternative methodologies to RCTs such as natural experiments can provide a valuable framework for public health intervention evaluation. Natural experiments can be defined as 'naturally occurring circumstances in which a subset of population have different level of exposure to a supposed causal factor, in a situation resembling an actual experiment where human subjects would be randomly allocated to groups' (Last, 1995). When researchers explicitly take into account the methodological approach used to evaluate the effect of that causal factor on health or other outcomes, this is referred to as a natural experiment evaluation (Craig et al., 2012). Craig and colleagues outline natural experiments in their MRC Guidance. Natural experiments refer to events, interventions, or policies which are not under the control of researchers but which are amenable to research which uses the variation in exposure that they generate to analyse their impact. Natural experimental studies refer to the methodological approaches to evaluating the impact on health or other outcomes of such events, interventions or policies. Craig and co-workers outline key features of these definitions as (i) the intervention is not undertaken for the purposes of research, and (ii) the variation in exposure and outcomes is analysed using methods that attempt to make causal inferences. Classic examples include the effect of famine on the subsequent health of children exposed *in utero*, or the effects of clean air legislation, indoor smoking bans, and changes in taxation of alcohol and tobacco (Craig et al., 2012). The key peculiarity of natural experiments is the existence of an 'intervention'—which represents an exogenous source of variation—determining assignment to treatment, so that any change in the outcome variables of interest can be attributed to the interventions and not to other confounding factors. Unlike RCTs, in a natural experiment the researcher cannot control assignment to treatment and control group, which might differ with respect to observable and unobservable factors that may be related to the outcome of interest (Deeks et al., 2003). Non-randomization represents a threat to internal validity, and a thorough investigation into the source of variation is needed in order to choose the appropriate methodology to reduce the selection bias that is inherent to non-randomized studies (Meyer, 1995). Despite a lower internal validity (ability to evidence causal relationships), natural experiments have the potential for a wider range of applicability and higher external validity (generalisability) than RCTs, and are increasingly used within public health intervention evaluations. Established guidelines such as STROBE (Von elm et al., 2014) or TREND (Des Jarlais and Lyles, 2004) should be followed when reporting natural experiment evaluation results, with particular attention to: clearly identifying the approach as a study of a natural experiment; providing a clear description of the intervention and the assignment process; and explicitly stating the methods used to estimate impact (Craig et al., 2012).

Using a natural experiment framework to conduct an economic evaluation can be challenging, especially in terms of dealing with data availability, non-normality of outcome and cost data, and correlation of cost and outcomes. Public health interventions are often not specifically designed for economic evaluation but are introduced to address social or political aims, and given that the researcher is only one of the stakeholders interested in the outcomes of the intervention, this might lead to a suboptimal design of the public health interventions for the economic evaluation purpose (Petticrew et al., 2005). To date, there has been little published comprehensive guidance on conducting an economic evaluation alongside a natural experiment. This is most likely in part due to their reliance on linked and routine data availability and typically without the economists' design control. Deidda and colleagues summarize a number of key challenges for specific consideration when conducting economic evaluations alongside natural experiments including: design of natural experiments; statistical and econometric methods for evaluating interventions using natural experiments; identifying, measuring, and valuing costs and outcomes; identifying the target population, subgroups, intervention, and control groups; data availability; relevant time horizon; type and perspective of economic evaluation and discounting (Deidda et al., 2017).

3.3 Why public health interventions are often 'complex' in nature

Since public health interventions are interventions often delivered outside of the health care setting, as Rychetnik and colleagues state 'public health interventions tend to be complex, programmatic, and context dependent' (Rychetnik et al., 2002, p. 119). Public health interventions often require behavioural change on the part of the individual and may have many outcomes, for example, for the individual, family, community, and wider society. In this way we may think of public health interventions as being 'complex' in nature. The Medical Research Council (MRC) produced a useful guide for the development, evaluation, and implementation of complex interventions. Complex health and social care interventions place additional challenges on the design, conduct, and reporting of these interventions, and fundamentally may require more health economics research resources (Byford and Sefton, 2003). Complex interventions are defined as interventions that have several interacting components. As outlined by the MRC Guidance (Craig et al., 2008), this complexity may take the form of:

◆ the number of and interactions between components within the experimental and control interventions (in an RCT).

◆ the number and difficulty of behaviours required by those delivering or receiving the intervention.

◆ the number of groups or organizational levels targeted by the intervention.

◆ the number and variability of outcomes.

◆ the degree of flexibility or tailoring of the intervention permitted.

This complexity has implications for the research methods required to evaluate public health intervention studies such as trials and other study designs, and also for the design of economic evaluation alongside such studies. From the MRC Guidance (Craig et al., 2008), these include:

◆ The need for a robust theoretical understanding of how the intervention causes change, so that weak links in the causal chain can be identified and strengthened.

◆ An awareness that a lack of impact of a public health intervention may reflect implementation failure (or teething problems) rather than genuine ineffectiveness; the inclusion in a trial or evaluative study of a 'process evaluation' in order to identify such implementation problems.

◆ Variability in individual level outcomes from public health interventions may reflect higher level processes; sample sizes for randomized controlled trials for public health interventions may need to be much larger in order to take account of the extra variability, and cluster rather than individually randomized designs adopted.

◆ Identification of a single public health primary outcome may not make best use of the data; a range of measures will be needed, and unintended consequences picked up where possible.

◆ The importance of fidelity (adhering to an evidence-based or specific public health intervention) may be difficult to disentangle. Fidelity may be necessary to demonstrate effectiveness of a particular evidence-based programme but, equally, the design and delivery mode of public health interventions may in fact need to be adaptable to different contexts or client groups.

The MRC Guidance stresses the need to understand the process by which complex interventions work, that is, to understand the process of causality (MRC, Craig et al., 2008). In terms of the evaluation of public health interventions, this means understanding what works, how it works, over what time period, in what setting, and in which population group. Here we are talking about the evaluation of effectiveness but these issues are equally relevant to the economic evaluation of the cost-effectiveness of public health interventions. Costs and benefits will vary for the delivery of public health interventions in different settings, over different time periods, and for different population groups.

3.3.1 The need for a 'systems' approach to economic evaluation of public health interventions

Due to the complexity of many public health issues, where numerous interacting variables need to be accounted for and multiple agencies and groups bring different values and concerns to bear, it is becoming increasingly common for stakeholders to call for a 'systems' approach to public health intervention delivery and evaluation (Best et al., 2003; Midgley, 2006; Smith and Petticrew, 2010). Anderson has proposed that the science of complex systems may be much more useful for the economic evaluation of public health interventions than the traditional clinical model of underpinning economic evaluation of health care interventions (Anderson, 2008). Smith and colleagues demonstrate the value of using a macroeconomic approach to modelling a major health problem, using the context of antimicrobial resistance (AMR) using a computable general equilibrium approach (Smith et al., 2005). Townshend and Turner present a useful exposition of the use of systems dynamic modelling to evaluate screening for chlamydia (Townshend and Turner, 2000). Their results not only suggest that the proposed screening programme would prevent significant numbers of infertility cases annually but also that the programme could be paying for itself after about 4 years and recouping the initial outlay after about 12 years.

The science of complex systems is the 'mathematical and philosophical investigation of the relationships between parts of a system, that give rise to the collective behaviours of a system and how the system interacts and forms relationships with its surrounding environment' (Yaneer, 2002). Complex systems models may be far more relevant to the evaluation of public health interventions such as behavioural-, community-, or population-level health programmes than more medical model-based evaluation framework (Anderson, 2008). Whilst this is likely to be the case, with many evaluations being driven by a 'health service' perspective as often recommended by government guidance, combined with a lack of methods guidance in contrast to traditional methods, it is likely that the move to routine use of the systems approach for economic evaluation will take some time.

Developments in the field of realist synthesis discussed in Chapter 4 have also improved our understanding of how we evaluate the effectiveness of public health interventions or what works for whom, in what setting, and why (Pawson and Tilley, 1997).

The 2008 MRC guidance (Craig et al., 2008) emphasizes a general shift in health services and health economics research in order to understand not only *what* interventions work but exactly *how* these interventions work, and why they work differently in different settings, and with different groups of the population. Likewise, in health economics research, not only *what* interventions are cost-effective but exactly *how* these interventions are cost-effective, and why cost-effectiveness may vary in different settings, and with different groups of the population. The MRC Guidance on economic evaluation of complex interventions currently provides little advice on how complexity affects how we should go about designing and undertaking economic evaluation of complex interventions (Craig et al., 2008).

In public health services research it is increasingly commonplace to include process evaluations in trials of complex public health interventions. Process evaluation may be explained in terms of the recognized need to understand the mechanisms of impact, for example, behaviour changes triggered, the context of delivery, in terms of how external factors influence the uptake of a public health programme, and what factors may influence the wider implementation or roll out of a programme (Moore et al., 2015). This is shown in Figure 3.1.

Such process evaluations tease out the mechanisms of how interventions work or do not work, barriers to uptake, reasons, for drop out, etc. (Anderson, 2008). Methods have emerged for process evaluation in health services research (Craig et al., 2008, Moore et al., 2015). Process evaluations alongside evaluations of complex interventions can also act as useful vehicles for the 'identification' and 'measurement' phases in economic evaluations of such complex interventions. In a feasibility study, tracking the process components can provide initial insights to the likely resource use and outcome impacts to be included within an economic evaluation. A health economic logic model layered onto an intervention logic model can also prove to be a useful aid for designing an economic evaluation and this approach is highly recommended in the early stages of an economic evaluation of a complex intervention (illustrated in a case study in Chapter 6). Section 3.4 now discusses the relevance of behavioural economics to the evaluation of public health interventions.

3.4 The relevance of behavioural economics to the evaluation of public health interventions

Part of the challenge of evaluating complex interventions are the behaviour changes required for many public health interventions to be effective. This takes us into the realms of 'behavioural economics'. Behavioural economics has become a dominant academic approach to understanding how decisions are made beyond those traditionally made by the 'rational economic man'. In the *Harvard Business Review*, Ariely writes: 'Drawing on aspects of both psychology and economics, the operating assumption of behavioural economics is that cognitive biases often prevent people from making rational decisions, despite their best efforts' (Ariely, 2009, p. 80). Practitioners of behavioural economics have had a major influence on business, government, and financial markets. Their books, including *Predictably Irrational* (Ariely, 2009), *Fast and Slow* (Kahneman, 2011), and *Nudge* (Sunstein and Thaler,

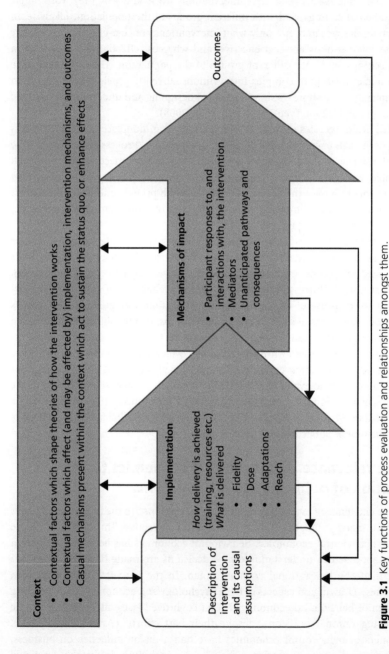

Figure 3.1 Key functions of process evaluation and relationships amongst them.

Context
- Contextual factors which shape theories of how the intervention works
- Contextual factors which affect (and may be affected by) implementation, intervention mechanisms, and outcomes
- Casual mechanisms present within the context which act to sustain the status quo, or enhance effects

Mechanisms of impact
- Participant responses to, and interactions with, the intervention
- Mediators
- Unanticipated pathways and consequences

Implementation
How delivery is achieved (training, resources etc.)
What is delivered
- Fidelity
- Dose
- Adaptations
- Reach

Description of intervention and its causal assumptions

Outcomes

2012), have become highly popular. The following section introduces the notion of behavioural economics and its relevance in the field of public health. In Chapter 1 of this book, we introduced the concepts of 'nudges' and 'choice architecture' in relation to behaviour change for the improvement of public health. There is a growing recognition and associated literature on the behavioural economics principles that are most relevant to public health. Behavioural economics can be employed to reduce health-harming behaviours, to reduce chances of developing diseases and addictions including obesity, smoking, risky sexual behaviour, and excessive alcohol consumption (Cohen et al., 2016). 'Behavioural nudges' are everywhere: nutritional advice on food products and menus, automated text reminders to encourage medication adherence, driver seatbelt noise alerts. Designed to help people make better health choices, these reminder 'nudges' have become commonplace (Cohen et al., 2016). The important evaluative matter for economists, however, is the extent to which these tools are effective in improving health outcomes and at what cost, namely are nudges cost-effective? Whilst behavioural science has swept the fields of economics and law through the study of nudges, cognitive biases, and decisional heuristics, it has only recently begun to impact how we design and evaluate health care, and the prevention of disease (Cohen et al., 2016). A number of questions are raised by Cohen and colleagues which reflect the contribution that behavioural economics can make to the evaluation of public health interventions: Does cost-sharing for health expenditures cause patients to make poor decisions? Is it right to make it difficult for people to opt out of having their organs harvested for donation when they die, as has been the policy change in Wales? Are behavioural nudges paternalistic? What is becoming clear is that health economists, working in the design and evaluation of public health interventions, will benefit from using methods from behavioural economics for more relevant models of how, what, and why some public health interventions work, and how to evaluate the cost-effectiveness of such interventions. Behavioural economics has been defined as the study of the boundaries of rationality (*homo-economicus*), as assumed in economic theory, and the influences of psychological, social, cognitive, and emotional factors on the economic decisions of individuals and institutions and, where relevant, the consequences for market prices, economic returns, and patterns of resource allocation. Clearly, this is relevant to lifestyle decisions made by individuals. For example, what lies behind an individual's decision to respond actively to an anti-smoking campaign or a campaign to reduce excessive alcohol consumption?

In Chapter 2 of this book we presented the Cohen model for the demand for prevention goods, suggesting that these goods have some utility in consumption (i.e. possibly enjoyment of attending the gym) and utility of knowing that consumption of a prevention good will produce benefits for the longer term (i.e. reduced risk factors resulting from regular attendance at the gym). In Chapter 2 we also introduced the idea of market failure for such prevention goods, where the government needs to intervene to allocate resources in this area. Governments are forced to legislate on the control and pricing of tobacco products, sugar content in beverages, alcohol, fatty foods, set speed limits, and set school curricula that introduce positive public health messages and create healthy environments.

Time preferences play an important role in understanding and designing behavioural economics-informed public health interventions and more broadly in developing public health policy. When we speak of time preferences and public policy, we must distinguish between individual time preferences and social time preferences (Lawless et al., 2013). Private time preferences refer to an individual's decisions, while societal time preferences refer to society's preferences for others' well-being. When making public policy decisions, the social discount rate is usually regarded as an appropriate measure to use.

3.4.1 The role of discounting in public health intervention evaluation

Economic considerations increasingly drive public investments in public health interventions. Vaccines are a perfect example of a preventive public health intervention provided up front which gives rise to cost savings and health outcomes at a later date. (Westra et al., 2012). Since vaccines prevent future disease from occurring, the costs and outcomes associated with vaccination usually fall at different time points. Economists regard present consumption as more valuable than future consumption, because (i) there is an opportunity cost to consuming now rather than in the future, since the money spent could have been invested elsewhere to generate some returns, and (ii) most people simply prefer to consume now rather than later, all other things being equal (Krahn and Gafni, 1993). This social discount rate discussion is distinct from the private discount rates referred to earlier.

The standard method of capturing these preferences for present over future consumption is by a technique termed discounting, which essentially reduces the value of future costs and benefits compared to those in the present. Discounting future costs and health benefits usually has a large effect on results of cost-effectiveness evaluations of vaccination programmes because of delays between the initial expenditure in the programme and the health benefits gained from averting disease (Jit and Mibei, 2015). Most guidelines currently recommend discounting both costs and health effects at a positive, constant, common rate back to a common point in time. A review of 84 published economic evaluations of vaccines found that most of them apply these recommendations (Jit and Mibei, 2015). Jit and Mibei provide both technical and normative arguments for discounting health at a different rate to consumption (differential discounting), discounting at a rate that changes over time (non-constant discounting), discounting intra-generational and inter-generational effects at a different rate (two-stage discounting), and discounting the health gains from an intervention to a different discount year from the time of intervention (delayed discounting). These considerations are particularly acute for vaccines because their effects can occur in a different generation from the one paying for them, and because the time of vaccination, of infection aversion, and of disease aversion usually differ. They conclude by noting that differential discounting appears to be technically sound, more equitable from an inter-generational perspective than equal discounting, and is already accepted in some countries as appropriate to all health economic evaluations.

Additional adjustments, such as decreasing rate of discounting or altering the time at which health is discounted, may also reflect a concern for inter-generational equity. Hence, it is argued that there are sound empirical, theoretical, and ethical justifications for considering other departures from standard discounting. For more detail on this topic of discounting as relevant to public health please refer to Bos et al., (2004, 2005) and Drummond et al., (2007).

Bonneux and Birnie (2001) discuss the role of the discount rate in prevention. They outline that when health care resources are scarce, trade-offs have to be made between investing in the care of existing disease and in the prevention of future disease. In the standard model of economic evaluation, costs and health outcomes are typically devalued by a constant discount rate. In line with Jit and Mibei (2015), they argue, however, that economic evaluation of prevention needs a more realistic model of time preference that reflects societal preferences. In the United Kingdom, the recommended discount rate for public health economic evaluations is 1.5 per cent (National Institute for Health and Care Excellence, 2012) as compared with 3.5 per cent HTA.

3.5 **Summary of challenges**

We referred to the work of Kelly and colleagues at the beginning of this chapter. They have discussed the key challenges of applying traditional methods of economic evaluation (as used in health technology appraisal in a clinical setting) to the evaluation of public health interventions (Kelly et al., 2005). Whilst there is an appreciation of the value of systems evaluation for economic evaluation of public health interventions, it is likely that, given the current precedent for economic evaluations from a health service perspective, the traditional approaches to economic evaluation will still retain a role. We have summarized these traditional economic evaluation challenges in Table 3.1.

In addition to these challenges, Shiell also comments on the role of social injustice and the broader factors that need to be considered: 'Public health evaluation in the 21st century is therefore not just about levels, sectors, methods, disciplines and stakeholders. It is also about political values' (Shiell, 2015; Shiell et al., 2008). The incorporation of political directives into economic evaluation in addition to the ability to 'equity-inform' economic evaluations is subject to much debate and the topic of the next book in the series (Cookson, 2018).

3.5.1 **The nature of many public health interventions is preventative, raising challenges relating to the measurement and valuation of costs and outcomes over time**

Most clinical interventions are delivered to patients at the time that they need them, that is, when they become ill or injured and are in need of drugs, surgery, or psychological therapies. One of the foremost goals of health improvement is to prevent ill health and injury 'downstream', by modifying risk factors, for example, by changing or influencing health harming behaviours and environments 'upstream'. This means that in the economic evaluation of clinical interventions, we can capture resource use at the

Table 3.1 Challenges of applying methods of economic evaluation to the evaluation of public health interventions

Challenges	Details	Examples
Determinants of health and inequalities in health	◆ Overall, in industrialized countries, life expectancy continues to increase. ◆ Inequalities in health between socio-economic groups are actually widening in many industrialized countries including the United Kingdom. ◆ There is little evidence across government sectors as to what interventions will be successful in reducing inequalities in health across the socio-economic gradient.	The 'back to sleep' campaign was successful in reduction of the total number of cot deaths but resulted in a widening of inequalities in the prevalence of deaths across the socio- economic gradient.
Relationship between upstream and downstream interventions	◆ Upstream interventions address environments in which adverse health behaviours can develop and aim to prevent these. ◆ Downstream interventions directly address adverse health behaviours often through individually or group-targeted interventions. ◆ Downstream interventions are almost inevitability mediated by upstream socio-economic circumstances and structures. ◆ Interventions to address upstream socio-economic structures may be a necessary precursor to successful downstream interventions aimed at tackling health-harming behaviours.	The effectiveness and cost- effectiveness of public health campaigns to raise awareness of the effects on the elderly and infirm of cold homes will be mitigated by the effects of fuel poverty across the socio-economic gradient.

Table 3.1 Continued

Challenges	Details	Examples
	◆ The cost-effectiveness of downstream interventions may vary across the socio-economic gradient requiring different delivery mechanisms where financial, transport, or other barriers to uptake may exist. ◆ Evaluation of single downstream interventions in isolation may miss outcomes from a synergy of upstream and downstream interventions.	
Mediating role of behaviour change	◆ There is particular need to understand what factors influence or determine behaviour change in the design or delivery of downstream individual- or population-focused public health interventions.	Understanding social and cultural attitudes and responses to pricing and advertising in the consumption of alcohol.
Separating cause and effect	◆ It is particularly difficult to isolate the relationship between cause and effect when public health interventions may occur against the backdrop of secular trends in health-harming behaviours.	Difficult to isolate the direct attributable impact of an anti-smoking campaign against the introduction of legislation of banning smoking in public places.
Biological and social variation	◆ The design and evaluation of public health interventions need to take into account vast biological and social variation which is less of a problem in the valuation of medical technologies which take place within a narrower spectrum of physiological response to treatment.	Stubborn socio-economic class differences in smoking and alcohol consumption.

(*continued*)

Table 3.1 Continued

Challenges	Details	Examples
Absence of 'D' in public health R&D	◆ Absence of development in R&D in public health. ◆ Many public health interventions evolve over time, and are not evaluated in a systematic way as is the case in pre-registration drug trials for new medicines. ◆ The issue of fidelity to a specific public health intervention—how it is delivered, where it is delivered, to whom and by whom—are all factors that need to be considered.	Evaluation of the effectiveness and cost-effectiveness of parenting programmes to reduce the impact of conduct disorder depend heavily on fidelity of original programmes, e.g. the Incredible Years Parenting Programme (Hutchins et al., 2007; Edwards et al., 2007).
When should effectiveness be measured?	◆ It is not clear when a public health intervention might or might not be judged to have had its desired effect, immediately, one year, or five years after implementation. ◆ It is not clear how we should handle the declining influence that a public health intervention may have on health-harming behaviour over time. ◆ The effects of some public health interventions may occur after many years or may be intergenerational. ◆ Need for collection of adequate data to allow for retrospective analysis for the effects over time of a single public health intervention or synergy of public health interventions.	The effectiveness and cost-effectiveness of a school-based campaign to reduce childhood obesity may have effects in the short term and longer term.

Table 3.1 Continued

Challenges	Details	Examples
How should effectiveness be measured?	◆ It is useful to benchmark the cost-effectiveness of public health interventions against health care interventions. ◆ The most common way of doing so is to use cost per quality-adjusted life year (QALY). ◆ The QALY undoubtedly does not capture all the benefits from a public health intervention as it has a focus on the physical functioning of the individual directly in receipt of the intervention. ◆ There is a growing body of evidence, however, that many public health interventions compare favourably with health care interventions in terms of cost per QALY. ◆ NICE is increasingly advocating the use of cost–benefit analysis and cost–consequence analysis to capture a wide range of costs and benefits. ◆ There is a growing interest in the use of capability-based measures as an alternative to QALYs as a measurement of outcomes in public health.	Owen and colleagues (2011), reproduced in full in Chapter 8 of this book, found 85 per cent of the 200 public health interventions they reviewed to have a cost per QALY ratio below the NICE threshold of £20,000 per QALY (Owen et al., 2011).
Individual versus population measures	◆ Here Rose's distinction between population versus targeted individual interventions is relevant. ◆ It may be useful to talk about 'shifting the curve' in terms of achieving population change in health-harming behaviours	Industry agreements to reduce salt content in bread have helped to reduce salt intake across the population. <http://www.actiononsalt.org.uk/>

Source: data from Kelly, M., et al. Evidence based public health: a review of the experience of the National Institute of Health and Clinical Excellence (NICE) of developing public health guidance in England. *Social Science & Medicine*. 71(6), 1056–1062. Copyright © 2010 Elsevier.

time of treatment (e.g. nights in hospital, staffing, and drugs), and measure health outcomes at the time of treatment. This is done by administering health-related quality of life (HRQoL) instruments such as the EQ-5D (introduced in section 2.4.5) in order to capture changes in self-reported HRQoL before and after treatment. In public health, however, we are often evaluating the cost-effectiveness of interventions delivered to essentially 'healthy' individuals. They may be currently undertaking health-harming behaviours such as smoking; consuming high sugar, fat, or salt diets; or drinking alcohol above recommended limits, but may still be, and feel, essentially 'healthy' thereby measuring short-term health outcomes will not capture the real long-term health impacts of 'prevention'. Chapters 5 and 6 of this book explore these cost and outcome challenges in more depth.

3.5.2 Delivery of public health interventions is outside the health sector

Two examples of settings where public health interventions are often delivered are workplaces and schools. Back pain is the leading cause of workplace absenteeism in the United Kingdom, accounting for more than 30.8 million sick days per annum (Office for National Statistics, 2016) at a cost of £5.6 billion (Confederation of British Industry, 2013) to the UK economy. Classes to improve musculoskeletal mobility have been shown to be cost-effective when delivered in an NHS setting (UK BEAM, 2004a and b). More recently, there has been growing interest in yoga-based programmes delivered in the workplace to prevent and manage back pain (Hartfiel et al., 2012, 2017).

There is also growing interest in delivering public health interventions in schools. Two examples of these are anti bullying programmes (KIVA Study; Clarkson et al., 2015) and programmes to encourage adolescent girls to exercise (Girls Active study (Edwardson et al., 2015). The design, delivery, and reporting of economic evaluations of such public health interventions in these settings pose a number of challenges relating to there being a range of stakeholders, the availability of information on resource use, the appropriateness of outcome measures, and the need to monitor outcomes over a long, extended period. Trials of interventions in schools need to be 'cluster randomized' in order to take account of the influence or interclass correlation of the delivery of an intervention across different schools (Cockcroft, 2017).

3.5.3 Identifying, measuring, and valuing costs and outcomes of public health interventions within the relevant time horizon

Economic evaluations often taken place alongside RCTs or non-randomized study designs of clinical interventions, described in section 3.2 of this chapter. Due to the high cost of running RCTs, they typically tend to have short follow-up periods of between one and three years. NICE guidance on health technology appraisal in the United Kingdom advocates the extrapolation of lifetime health gains beyond the end of such trials where possible (National Institute for Health and Care Excellence, 2012). However, many cost per QALY estimates in the literature are based on short follow-up periods of trials without such longer term extrapolation.

In section 3.5.2, we noted that many 'preventive' public health interventions are delivered to essentially 'healthy' individuals. The relevant time horizon in the evaluation of public health interventions is therefore ideally a lifetime such that the benefits of active prevention of ill-health can be realized. There may be some immediate and mid-term changes in health status or use of health services but there may be significant impact on life expectancy and quality-adjusted life expectancy from public health interventions that need modelling far into the future.

3.5.4 Attribution of health benefits, costs, and cost savings to public health interventions

This brings us to the challenge of establishing direct attribution of health benefits, costs, and cost savings to a specific public health intervention. If a person decides to try to stop smoking, perhaps for the second or third time, and they are successful, can this decision be directly or partially attributed to one or more public health interventions or a synergy of several? It may be that their decision has been influenced by a recent mass media television campaign showing the unseen harmful effects of smoke to children when parents smoke in or around the home; it may be a response to a price rise or change in packaging of tobacco products; their decision may be, in part, a response to the ban on smoking in public places. It is much simpler to attribute the health change effects of a new drug or surgery to a specific drug or surgical intervention than to attribute health outcomes, particularly in the long run, to specific public health interventions. This attribution problem extends to costs incurred and costs saved (Marteau et al., 2011).

3.5.5 Identifying the relevant perspective for economic evaluation

As noted in Chapter 2 of this book, the need for economic evaluation in health care in the first place links back to market failure in health care. Health care as an economic good does not fit with the conditions necessary for perfect competition. This means that the 'invisible hand' or price mechanism cannot function to signal to buyers and sellers the quantities of different types of health care that are demanded/needed (Donaldson and Gerard, 2005). All developed countries to a greater or lesser extent have chosen government intervention in the organization, finance, and delivery of health care systems. These governments and their health departments, or those delegated with the responsibility of organizing and delivering health care, need information on the relative value for money of devoting resources to different health care activities. Using a payer perspective in economic evaluation is therefore key. Traditionally we measure the range of costs and outcomes relevant from the payer's perspective.

As discussed in Chapter 1 of this book, with the movement from the fourth to a fifth wave of public health, a movement from individual behaviour-focused public health services, delivered within a traditional medical model, towards a 'health assets of communities' approach, the range of commissioners who potentially pay for and deliver services that impact on population health becomes wider than the NHS. One perspective that is increasingly used is what is referred to as a 'public sector multi-agency perspective' (Edwards et al., 2007; Edwards et al., 2013). This public sector multi-agency perspective is sometimes referred to as a health and personal social services perspective (PSS), and encompasses the NHS, social care, and local government depending on which are the most relevant stakeholders and payers in the delivery of specific public health interventions. The widest possible perspective is what is referred to as a 'societal perspective'. This is the perspective used in cost–benefit analysis (CBA) as discussed in Chapters 2 and 9 of this book (Mishan, 1971; McIntosh et al., 2010).

3.5.6 When is a micro or macro approach more effective in public health?

Earlier in this chapter, we alluded to the desire by economists (Smith and Petticrew, 2010) and public health practitioners (Midgley, 2006) to move beyond the micro-economic approach to economic evaluation and into a 'systems' or macro level approach. Economics, as a discipline, makes a distinction between 'micro' economics and 'macro' economics. Micro-economics is the study of individual elements in the economy—individuals, households, firms, etc. Macro-economics is the study of how the economy as a whole behaves—aggregated consumption, production, and savings. The traditional economic evaluation toolbox used in health economics has developed within a micro-economics paradigm. However, many public health interventions relate to government control over food and drink production, labelling, pricing, and retailing; packaging, and availability of, for example, tobacco products, and more recently high sugar foods, and as such require incorporation of a broader perspective for the evaluation. Economic evaluation of these kinds of government interventions requires a macro-economic approach to evaluation of likely consumer responses to price increases on health-harming goods. For example, in a meta-analysis of econometric studies of the relationship between alcohol pricing and tax levels and consumption, it was found that alcohol prices and taxes are inversely related to drinking levels, effects are large compared to other prevention policies and programmes, and more generally, public policies that raise prices of alcohol are an effective means to reduce drinking (Wagenaar et al., 2009).

3.5.7 The need for the inclusion of equity considerations in the evaluation of public health interventions

In Chapter 1 of this book we stressed that one of the key tenets of public health is the goal of reducing inequalities in health. This has led to a focus in local public health strategies on targeting 'hard-to-reach' groups in society; for example, providing contraceptive services to reduce the number of unplanned or unwanted repeat teenage pregnancies or delivering free toothpaste and toothbrushes into children's pre-school nurseries. In Chapter 2 of this book, we briefly discussed, the concept of the quality-adjusted life year (QALY). The saying 'a QALY is a QALY is a QALY' embodies the idea that it does not matter who receives a QALY or at what age or from what clinical or public health intervention. At the heart of economic evaluation of medical interventions is the concept of 'efficiency', to be precise, 'allocative efficiency', of maximizing the total number of QALYs that can be gained from available health care resources in society. This is the Benthamite utilitarian goal that implicitly underpins the role of NICE in the United Kingdom in evaluating the clinical and cost-effectiveness of new drugs and health technologies. Research is underway to find out whether the public think QALYs should be weighted differently for end-of-life care and people with extremely rare conditions, to reflect societal values about the relative value of a healthy year of life to different individuals or groups of individuals in society (Linley and Hughes, 2013).

NICE has adopted a higher threshold of £50,000 per incremental QALY for end-of-life drugs to reflect the different valuation for this patient group. What this means for the economic evaluation of public health interventions is that as well as calculating an incremental cost-effectiveness ratio for a specific public health intervention (as discussed in Chapter 2 and Chapter 8 of this book), it may be helpful to undertake sub-group analyses to explore the costs and outcomes of achieving a health gain in those facing greatest socio-economic challenges or those hardest to reach in society. Such sub-group analyses may be under-powered to detect changes but may highlight important barriers to uptake, or reasons why public health interventions are effective in some groups and not in others. General econometric advice on this is found in Espinoza and colleagues (2014). Cookson and colleagues outline four approaches to explicit incorporation of equity considerations into economic evaluation in public health: (i) review of background information on equity, (ii) health inequality impact assessment, (iii) analysis of the opportunity cost of equity, and (iv) equity weighting of health outcomes (Cookson et al., 2009).

3.5.8 The importance of context in economic evaluation of public health interventions

The context in which public health interventions are delivered will have an impact on the potential effectiveness and cost-effectiveness of the intervention in question. An example of this has been the relatively strong evidence base for the cost-effectiveness of the Incredible Years Parenting Programme developed by Caroline Webster-Stratton in Seattle (Webster-Stratton, 2000). This was delivered, with attention paid to reduce all potential financial and practical effectiveness barriers, to parents attending parenting groups. Groups were held at various times of the day to offer choice, offered meals and crèche facilities for younger siblings and even subsidized travel to parenting groups. Evidence from the United Kingdom has shown this to be one of the most repeatedly cost-effective interventions for ameliorating the longer-term impact of conduct disorder in pre-school children (Edwards et al., 2007; Hutchings et al., 2007; Bywater et al., 2009, Edwards et al., 2016).

3.5.9 Implications of the 'rule of rescue' for public health

Jonsen coined the term 'rule of rescue' to describe the imperative people feel to rescue identifiable individuals facing avoidable death (Jonsen, 1986). McKie and Richardson draw a more detailed picture of the rule of rescue, identifying its conflict with cost-effectiveness analysis, the preference it entails for identifiable over statistical lives, the response it elicits, the preference it entails for lifesaving over non-lifesaving measures, its extension to non-life-threatening conditions, and whether it is motivated by duty or sympathy (McKie and Richardson, 2003). They also outline how the rule of rescue induces complex measurement problems for economic evaluation. The rule of rescue means that when resources are limited there will always be pressure to put the claims of those ill or injured today ahead of the claims of those for whom, through prevention upstream, it may be possible to reduce the probability of future illness or injury by devoting resources to prevention today. In the United Kingdom, it has been estimated that the NHS spends between 1 per cent and 4 per cent on prevention (Marmot et al., 2010). This is not the whole picture of spending on prevention, it is the contribution that the UK NHS makes, through often traditional models of one-to-one or group interventions such as smoking cessation motivational interviewing. Sometimes this is through hospitals or primary care in the form of brief interventions; sometimes in the community, for example, pharmacy-led smoking cessation initiatives. Maintaining spending on prevention in times of financial constraint, or arguing for transfer of resources from curative medicine to prevention requires evidence of the short-term as long as the longer-term cost-effectiveness or return on investment.

3.5.10 The available published guidance on the application of economic evaluation methods to the appraisal of public health interventions

In 2013, Edwards and co-authors published a systematic review of available published guidance for the evaluation of public health interventions. We have reproduced and updated this as a resource in the OUP Electronic Resource of this book. We have distinguished between guidance available specifically for the United Kingdom and international guidance. We suggest that when selecting guidance for the design of an economic evaluation of a public health intervention, the following checklist could be helpful.

3.5.11 Theoretical roots of potential analytical frameworks for applying economic evaluation methods to the appraisal of public health interventions

In the OUP Electronic Resource to this book we reproduce and update the available published guidance on techniques for the economic evaluation of public health interventions (Edwards et al., 2013). We note the theoretical basis for these sets of guidance. It is worth pausing to acknowledge that all established methods of economic evaluation of health care technologies have their roots in cost–benefit analysis, which in turn has its theoretical roots in neoclassical welfare economics. In cost–benefit analysis, all costs and outcomes are measured in monetary terms. The difficulty of doing this led to what Culyer referred to as 'extra-welfarism', with health as a goal in itself in the societal welfare function (Culyer, 1989). CEA, CUA, and CBA have their theoretical roots in extra-welfarism. Methods of social return on investment (SROI), discussed in Chapter 12 later in this book, has its roots in welfare economics. Debate over this issue continues.

Box 3.1 Checklist of considerations when considering published guidance for the economic evaluation of public health interventions

1   What is the appropriate theoretical framework for analysis: e.g. welfarist, extra-welfarist, capability theory?

2   What is the setting of the public health intervention under evaluation: e.g. environmental change; infectious disease control; screening; supporting behaviour change; supporting government legislation or policy?

3   Is this best described as a primary, secondary, or tertiary prevention intervention: i.e. upstream or downstream, and has it been evaluated on the basis of an RCT, natural experiment, or other research design?

4   What is the main agency (government; health service; local government; voluntary sector; employer) responsible for implementation and who are the key stakeholders?

     If this is an intervention aimed at behaviour change, what are the key levers of change: legislation; price; changing social norms; choice architecture; and nudging?

6   What is the appropriate time horizon of analysis and what is the most appropriate discount rate for costs and outcomes? Can we record intermediate costs and benefits in the first year as well as over a longer time horizon to meet the needs of policy-makers within a political cycle of government?

7   If the public health intervention aims to 'shift the curve', are we most interested in the centre or tails of the distribution?

8   How is this public health intervention likely to impact on inequalities in health?

9   Will subgroup analysis help identify the range of cost-effectiveness estimates across different settings, delivery methods, and population groups?

10 What are the main final outcome measures of interest, e.g. QALYs/DALYs/capabilities?

11 How important is it to value costs, benefits, and returns in monetary terms? Is it reasonable to expect the intervention to be cost saving in the short, medium, or long term?

12 How relevant will it be to compare an ICER for the public health intervention with the NICE threshold of £20,000–£30,000 or an international equivalent, or are there other sources of relevant societal payer thresholds?

Source: data from Edwards, R.T., et al. 2013. Public health economics: a systematic review of guidance for the economic evaluation of public health interventions and discussion of key methodological issues. *BMC Public Health*, 13(1), 1001–1004. Copyright © Edwards et al.; licensee BioMed Central Ltd. 2013

3.5.12 Spotlight on UK guidance on conducting economic evaluations alongside PHIs

Current guidance from the UK's NICE on conducting economic evaluations of PHIs has re-invigorated interest in methods of CBA for these evaluations. The main change to NICE's previous approach (pre-2013) to economic evaluation is now to place more emphasis on CCA and CBA than has been the case in previous economic evaluation methods manuals. CEA and CUA will still be required routinely, for several reasons:

◆ CUA provides a single yardstick or 'currency' for measuring the impact of interventions on health. This form of analysis should be maintained wherever health is the sole or predominant benefit or influence.

◆ CUA allows interventions in health care to be compared so that resources may be allocated more efficiently.

◆ It should continue to be possible to compare estimates of cost effectiveness in the new institutional environment (mainly local government) with previous estimates of similar interventions made for use in the UK's NHS.

◆ All NICE programmes should include the use of a common method of CEA that allows comparisons between programmes.

◆ In some circumstances, almost all benefits are health benefits. In that case, where there is a clear indication of cost effectiveness or ineffectiveness, further analysis (such as use of CCA and/or CBA) that is unlikely to change a decision about an intervention would not be required.

The suite of methods of economic evaluation techniques typically applied routinely to health technologies in a clinical setting by health economists all have their roots in CBA (see Chapter 9) CBA was developed as the operationalization of welfare economics and requires the measurement of all costs and outcomes in monetary terms (McIntosh et al., 2010). With very little consensus on suitable evaluation methods in public health (Mathes et al., 2017), CBA arguably provides a very useful framework for consideration of the broad-ranging costs and outcomes pertinent to the economic evaluation of public health interventions. The difficulty of, in particular, measuring and valuing health outcomes in monetary terms led to the development of CEA, CUA, and CCA methods that measure outcomes in non-monetary terms (Drummond et al., 2015). Current guidance from NICE Centre for Public Health Excellence has re-invigorated interest in methods of CBA as it allows for the capture of a wide range of benefits across health and other sectors of the economy in a common currency: money.

3.6 Exploring the precautionary principle of if and when RCTs are necessary in public health

Fischer and colleagues (2013) have argued that the traditional approach to economic evaluation is aligned and has its roots in evidence-based medicine and the principles of randomized controlled trial methodology (Fischer et al., 2012, 2013) aligned with frequentist economic evaluation methods. These authors argue that this approach may not be appropriate when the objective of public health interventions is to deliver programmes that aim to achieve small individual level benefit, such as in reducing health-harming behaviour, across large numbers of people (e.g. daily salt intake across the whole population). They argue that very large RCTs with sufficient power to detect a statistically significant difference in the primary outcome measure are impractical and prohibitively expensive. They argue that, in fact, these kind of population-level public health interventions should be assumed to be effective, and the question then becomes how they can be delivered at a reasonable cost. Instead of relying on the gold standard RCT, they argue for the use of decision theory when prior beliefs are sufficiently strong and well-grounded to support decision-making. In contrast to evidence-based medicine, frequentist approach to cost-effectiveness analysis, Fischer and co-workers support the use of Bayesian decision theory which makes use of prior knowledge and beliefs to inform policy. These authors argue that in Bayesian theory, the most appropriate estimate of the health effect of an intervention need not come exclusively from evidence gleaned from RCTs but could alternatively depend on prior beliefs based on theory, observation, and experience. In essence they are proposing a paradigm shift away from the use of RCTs to justify evidence-based policy in public health, towards the use of Bayesian analysis to support policy which could, they argue, achieve large gains at no additional cost. Looking at Figure 3.2 showing effect size against probability, the middle curve shows an increased effect size by the incorporation of prior beliefs and current knowledge with results from RCTs.

The point made here is that public health interventions are intended to provide health benefits to the population, and if possible do no harm. Fischer and colleagues give the example of the introduction of a 20 mile-per-hour speed limit in residential areas, which is unlikely to have health-harming effects but does limit individual freedom. They also give the example that seatbelts on average have saved lives, but that seatbelts have occasionally resulted in chest injuries, though this may have been a more desirable outcome than enduring those injuries sustained without a seat belt. We do not know who are the individuals affected adversely by public health policies. In the same way we do not know who will have an adverse reaction to a drug. Bayesian decision theory requires policy-makers to be risk-neutral or to spread risk across a large number of decisions. Going a step further, Fischer and Ghelardi argue that the

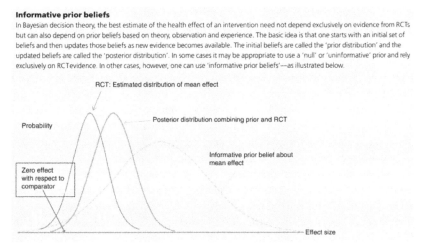

Informative prior beliefs
In Bayesian decision theory, the best estimate of the health effect of an intervention need not depend exclusively on evidence from RCTs but can also depend on prior beliefs based on theory, observation and experience. The basic idea is that one starts with an initial set of beliefs and then updates those beliefs as new evidence becomes available. The initial beliefs are called the 'prior distribution' and the updated beliefs are called the 'posterior distribution'. In some cases it may be appropriate to use a 'null' or 'uninformative' prior and rely exclusively on RCT evidence. In other cases, however, one can use 'informative prior beliefs'—as illustrated below.

Figure 3.2 Effect size against probability.
Reproduced with permission from Fischer, A.J., et al. The appraisal of PHIs: An overview. *Journal of Public Health*, 35(4), 488–494. Copyright © The Author 2013. Published by Oxford University Press on behalf of Faculty of Public Health. All rights reserved.

precautionary principle used previously in environmental science can be applied to the evaluation of public health interventions with respect to the societal goal of reducing harm (Fischer and Ghelardi, 2016).

Evidence-based medicine places the onus of proof on showing that a new drug or, in the case of this book, a new public health intervention, is superior to current practice with a sufficient level of certainty. In contrast, application of the precautionary principle to the evaluation of public health interventions would use prior knowledge to assume their effectiveness, explore their cost-effectiveness, or the reasonableness of their costs of delivery. This would in essence reverse the onus of proof. They argue that this is particularly relevant to potential catastrophic health events. In the face of potential catastrophic events, policy-makers will be willing to pay more. For example, an outbreak of Ebola in the United Kingdom would force policy-makers to challenge the current NICE threshold of £20,000–£30,000 were sufficient supply of an effective treatment to be available. Presumably this is because the consequences of not spending public money to avert a catastrophe are so great.

3.7 Reporting and publishing the findings of economic evaluation of public health interventions

In 2007, McDaid and Needle published a systematic review of economic evaluations of public health interventions undertaken over the previous 40 years. They used English- and non-English-language search terms, scientific databases, and grey literature. They found 7,000 unique references of which 1,700 were included. What is interesting is that 75 per cent were cost-effectiveness studies, 13 per cent calculated QALYs, and only 5 per cent were cost–benefit analyses. Since then, and particularly since the 2012 guidance from NICE, there is a renewed interest in the application of cost–benefit analysis and cost–consequence analysis as the method of choice in the economic evaluation of public health interventions (McDaid and Needle, 2007; National Institute for Health and Care Excellence, 2012).

It is interesting to think about how well reporting guidance for economic evaluation studies in general works for the reporting of the economic evaluation of public health interventions. The Consolidated Health Economic Evaluation Reporting Standards (CHEERS) statement published in 2013 was an attempt to bring together previous sets of guidance for the reporting and publication of the findings of economic evaluation studies and to aid transparency (Husereau et al., 2013; Sanghera et al., 2015). This guidance was prepared for editors of journals that publish economic evaluation studies and for the researchers producing them. A systematic review of these guidance generated a potential list of items to be included in the CHEERS checklist. A 24-item checklist was distilled down from an original 44-item list through a Delphi process with representatives from pharmaceutical industry, clinical practice, government, the editorial community, and academia.

Sanghera and colleagues have argued that the CHEERS checklist is less appropriate for the reporting of cost–benefit analysis than for the reporting of cost-effectiveness analysis and cost–utility analysis. They identify a number of gaps such as information on willingness to pay elicitation formats and payment vehicles necessary for the transparent reporting of CBA (Smith et al., 2003; McIntosh et al., 2010; Sanghera et al., 2015). It is important that methods for the reporting of CBA studies are standardized (Sanghera et al., 2015), this will most likely encourage a greater uptake of CBA methods for public health intervention economic evaluation.

Summary of Chapter 3

This chapter:

- Described public health interventions as often being complex interventions, hence economic evaluation will benefit from taking this complexity into account.
- Stressed the need for process evaluation in evaluations of public health interventions to understand mechanisms of change and barriers to the effectiveness of public health interventions as well as providing a useful framework for identification of key economic evaluation parameters.
- Summarized methodological challenges to the application of traditional methods of economic evaluation to the evaluation of public health interventions.
- Identified the use of systems modelling as highly relevant for economic evaluation of public health interventions.
- Discussed the increasing and important role of behavioural economics in the design, implementation and evaluation of complex public health interventions.
- Referred to available published guidance on techniques of economic evaluation of public health interventions set out in full in the OUP Electronic Resource to this book.
- Discussed, in particular, NICE guidance on supporting the wider use of CBA and CCA in order to capture the wider societal cost and benefits associated with public health interventions.
- Discussed the extent to which published guidance on the reporting of economic evaluation studies in general are applicable to, and suitable for, the reporting of CBA and CCA. An alternative suggested checklist is provided in Chapter 15.

References

Anderson, R., 2008. New MRC guidance on evaluating complex interventions. *BMJ (Clinical Research edn)*, *337*: a1937.

Ariely, D., 2009. *Predictably Irrational*. London: Harper Collins.

Ariely, D., 2009. The end of rational economics. *Harvard Business Review*, *87*(7–8): 78–84.

Bellis, M.A., Lowey, H., Leckenby, N., Hughes, K., and Harrison, D., 2014. Adverse childhood experiences: Retrospective study to determine their impact on adult health behaviours and health outcomes in a UK population. *Journal of Public Health*, *36*(1): 81–91.

Best, A., Moor, G., Holmes, B., Clark, P.I., Bruce, T., Leischow, S., Buchholz, K., et al., 2003. Health promotion dissemination and systems thinking: Towards an integrative model. *American Journal of Health Behavior*, *27*(1): S206–S216.

Bonell, C.P., Hargreaves, J.R., Cousens, S.N., Ross, D.A., Hayes, R.J., Petticrew, M., and Kirkwood, B., 2009. Alternatives to randomisation in the evaluation of public health interventions: Design challenges and solutions. *Journal of Epidemiology & Community Health*, 65: 582–87.

Bonneux, L. and Birnie, E., 2001. The discount rate in the economic evaluation of prevention: A thought experiment. *Journal of Epidemiology & Community Health*, 55(2): 123–5.

Bos, J.M., Beutels, P., Annemans, L., and Postma, M.J., 2004. Valuing prevention through economic evaluation. *Pharmacoeconomics*, 22(18): 1171–9.

Bos, J.M., Postma, M.J., and Annemans, L., 2005. Discounting health effects in pharmacoeconomic evaluations. *Pharmacoeconomics*, 23(7): 639–49.

Bowling, A., 2014. *Research Methods in Health: Investigating Health and Health Services*. London: McGraw-Hill Education.

Brenzel, L.E., 1993. *Selecting an Essential Package of Health Services Using Cost-Effectiveness Analysis: A Manual for Professionals in Developing Countries*. The Project. Available from: <http://pdf.usaid.gov/pdf_docs/PNACJ346.pdf> (Accessed 13 October 2018).

Briggs, A.H. and O'Brien, B.J., 2001. The death of cost-minimization analysis? *Health Economics*, 10(2): 179–84.

Brouwer, W.B., 2018. The inclusion of spillover effects in economic evaluations: Not an optional extra. *Pharmacoeconomics*, 1–6.

Brouwer, W.B., Culyer, A.J., van Exel, N.J.A., and Rutten, F.F., 2008. Welfarism vs. extra-welfarism. *Journal of Health Economics*, 27(2):325–38.

Byford, S. and Sefton, T., 2003. Economic evaluation of complex health and social care interventions. *National Institute Economic Review*, 186(1): 98–108.

Bywater, T., Hutchings, J., Daley, D., Whitaker, C., Yeo, S.T., Jones, K., Eames, C., et al., 2009. Long-term effectiveness of a parenting intervention for children at risk of developing conduct disorder. *British Journal of Psychiatry*, 195(4): 318–24.

Cheraghi-Sohi, S., Hole, A.R., Mead, N., McDonald, R., Whalley, D., Bower, P., and Roland, M., 2008. What patients want from primary care consultations: A discrete choice experiment to identify patients' priorities. *Annals of Family Medicine*, 6(2): 107–15.

Clarkson, S., Axford, N., Berry, V., Edwards, R.T., Bjornstad, G., Wrigley, Z., Charles, J., et al., 2015. Effectiveness and micro-costing of the KiVa school-based bullying prevention programme in Wales: Study protocol for a pragmatic definitive parallel group cluster randomised controlled trial. *BMC Public Health*, 16(1): 104. doi:10.1186/s12889-016-2746-1 [JIF:2.26] (B).

Cockcroft, A., 2017. Randomised controlled trials and changing public health practice. *BMC Public Health*, 17(1) :409. doi:10.1186/s12889-017-4287-7©

Cohen, D., 1984. Utility model of preventive behaviour. *Journal of Epidemiology and Community Health*, 38(1): 61–5.

Cohen, J.D., Ericson, K.M., Laibson, D., and White, J.M., 2016. Measuring time preferences. NBER Working Papers 22455, National Bureau of Economic Research, Inc.

Confederation of British Industry, 2013. *Fit for Purpose: Absence and Workplace Health Survey*. Available at: <http://www.kmghp.com/assets/cbi-pfizer_absence___workplace_health_2013-(1).pdf> (Accessed 1 November 2018).

Cookson, R., 2018. *Does Contract Enforcement Mitigate Holdup?*. Oxford: Oxford University Press.

Cookson, R., Drummond, M., and Weatherly, H., 2009. Explicit incorporation of equity considerations into economic evaluation of public health interventions. *Health Economics, Policy and Law*, 4(2): 231–45.

Craig, P., Cooper, C., Gunnell, D., Haw, S., Lawson, K., Macintyre, S., Ogilvie, D., et al., 2012. Using natural experiments to evaluate population health interventions: New Medical Research Council guidance. *Journal of Epidemiology and Community Health, 66*(12): 1182–6 jech-2011.

Craig, P., Dieppe, P., Macintyre, S., Michie, S., Nazareth, I. and Petticrew, M., 2008. Developing and evaluating complex interventions: the new Medical Research Council guidance. *British Medical Journal, 337*: a1655.

Culyer, A.J., 1989. The normative economics of health care finance and provision. *Oxford Review of Economic Policy, 5*(1):34–58.

Deeks, J.J., Dinnes, J., D'amico, R., Sowden, A.J., Sakarovitch, C., Song, F., Petticrew, M., et al., 2003. Evaluating non-randomised intervention studies. *Health Technology Assessment (Winchester, England), 7*(27): iii–x.

Deidda, M., Geue, C., Kreif, N., Dundas, R., and McIntosh, E., 2017. *Conducting economic evaluations alongside natural experiments: A practical guide.* Paper presented at the Health Economists Study Group, Birmingham, 4–6 January 2017.

Deidda M., Geue C., Kreif N., Dundas R., and McIntosh E., 2019. A framework for conducting economic evaluations alongside natural experiments. *Social Science and Medicine*, 220:353–61.

Des Jarlais, D.C., Lyles, C., Crepaz, N., and TREND Group, 2004. Improving the reporting quality of nonrandomized evaluations of behavioral and public health interventions: The TREND statement. *American Journal of Public Health*, 94(3):361–6.

Donaldson, C. and Gerard, K., 2005. *The Economics of Health Care Financing: The Visible Hand.* Basingstoke: Palgrave Macmillan.

Drummond, M., Chevat, C., and Lothgren, M., 2007. Do we fully understand the economic value of vaccines? *Vaccine, 25*(32): 5945–57.

Drummond, M., Sculpher, M., Claxton, K., Stoddart, G., and Torrance, G., 2015. *Assessing the Challenge of Applying Standard Methods of Economic Evaluation to PHIs.* Available at: <http://phrc.lshtm.ac.uk/papers/PHRC_D1-05_Final_Report.pdf> (Accessed 1 November 2018).

Edejer, T.T., 2003. *Making Choices in Health: WHO Guide to Cost-Effectiveness Analysis.* Geneva: World Health Organization.

Edwards, R.T., Céilleachair, A., Bywater, T., Hughes, D.A., and Hutchings, J., 2007. Parenting programme for parents of children at risk of developing conduct disorder: Cost effectiveness analysis. *British Medical Journal, 334*(7595): 682–7.

Edwards, R.T., Charles, J.M., and Lloyd-Williams, H., 2013. Public health economics: A systematic review of guidance for the economic evaluation of public health interventions and discussion of key methodological issues. *BMC Public Health, 13*(1): 1001.

Edwards, R.T., Jones, C., Berry, V., Charles, J., Linck, P., Bywater, T., and Hutchings, J., 2016. Incredible Years parenting programme: Cost-effectiveness and implementation. *Journal of Children's Services, 11*(1): 54–72.

Edwards, R.T., Neal, R.D., Linck, P., Bruce, N., Mullock, L., Nelhans, N., Pasterfield, D., et al., 2011. Enhancing ventilation in homes of children with asthma: Cost-effectiveness study alongside randomised controlled trial. *British Journal of General Practice, 61*(592): e733–e741.

Edwardson, C.L., Harrington, D.M., Yates, T., Bodicoat, D.H., Khunti, K., Gorely, T., Sherar, L.B., et al., 2015. A cluster randomised controlled trial to investigate the effectiveness and cost effectiveness of the 'Girls Active' intervention: A study protocol. *BMC Public Health, 15*(1): 526.

Espinoza, M.A., Manca, A., Claxton, K., and Sculpher, M.J., 2014. The value of heterogeneity for cost-effectiveness subgroup analysis: Conceptual framework and application. *Medical Decision Making*, 34(8): 951–64.

Fischer, A.J. and Ghelardi, G., 2016. The precautionary principle, evidence-based medicine, and decision theory in public health evaluation. *Frontiers in Public Health*, 4: 107.

Fischer, A.J., Threlfall, A., Meah, S., Cookson, R., Rutter, H., and Kelly, M.P., 2013. The appraisal of PHIs: An overview. *Journal of Public Health*, 35(4): 488–94.

Fischer, A., Threlfall, A., Cookson, R., Meah, S., Rutter, H., and Kelly, M., 2012. The appraisal of PHIs. *The Lancet*, 380: S17.

Glick, H.A., Doshi, J.A., Sonnad, S.S., and Polsky, D., 2014. *Economic Evaluation in Clinical Trials*. Oxford: Oxford University Press.

Graham, H. and Kelly, M.P., 2004. *Health Inequalities: Concepts, Frameworks and Policy*. London: Health Development Agency.

Grossman, M., 1972. *The Demand for Health: A Theoretical and Empirical Investigation*. New York, NY: NBER Books.

Habicht, J.P., Victora, C.G., and Vaughan, J.P., 1999. Evaluation designs for adequacy, plausibility and probability of public health programme performance and impact. *International Journal of Epidemiology*, 28(1): 10–18.

Hartfiel, N., Burton, C., Rycroft-Malone, J., Clarke, G., Havenhand, J., Khalsa, S.B., and Edwards, R.T., 2012. Yoga for reducing perceived stress and back pain at work. *Occupational Medicine*, 62(8): 606–12.

Hartfiel, N., Clarke, G., Havenhand, J., Phillips, C. and Edwards, R.T., 2017. Cost-effectiveness of yoga for managing musculoskeletal conditions in the workplace. *Occupational Medicine*, 67(9):687–95.

Honeycutt, A.A., Clayton, L., Khavjou, O., Finkelstein, E.A., Prabhu, M., Blitstein, J.L., Evans, W.D., et al., 2006. Guide to analyzing the cost-effectiveness of community public health prevention approaches. Available from: <http://aspe.hhs.gov/health/reports/06/cphpa/report.pdf> (Accessed 13 October 2018).

Hunter, R.F., Brennan, S.F., Tang, J., Smith, O.J., Murray, J., Tully, M.A., Patterson, C., et al., 2016. Effectiveness and cost-effectiveness of a physical activity loyalty scheme for behaviour change maintenance: A cluster randomised controlled trial. *BMC Public Health*, 16(1): 618.

Husereau, D., Drummond, M., Petrou, S., Carswell, C., Moher, D., Greenberg, D., Augustovski, F., et al., 2013. Consolidated health economic evaluation reporting standards (CHEERS) statement. *BMC Medicine*, 11: 80-7015-11-80.

Hutchings, J., Bywater, T., Daley, D., Gardner, F., Whitaker, C., Jones, K., Eames, C., et al., 2007. Parenting intervention in Sure Start services for children at risk of developing conduct disorder: Pragmatic randomised controlled trial. *BMJ (Clinical research)*, 334(7595): 678.

Hyppönen, E., Läärä, E., Reunanen, A., Järvelin, M.R., and Virtanen, S.M., 2001. Intake of vitamin D and risk of type 1 diabetes: A birth-cohort study. *Lancet*, 358(9292): 1500–3.

Jit, M. and Mibei, W., 2015. Discounting in the evaluation of the cost-effectiveness of a vaccination programme: A critical review. *Vaccine*, 33(32): 3788–94.

Jonsen, A.R., 1986. 3. Bentham in a box: Technology assessment and health care allocation. *Law, Medicine and Health Care*, 14(3-4): 172–4.

Kahneman, D. and Egan, P., 2011. *Thinking, Fast and Slow*, vol. 1. New York, NY: Farrar, Straus and Giroux.

Kelly, M.P., McDaid, D., Ludbrook, A., and Powell, J., 2005. *Economic Appraisal of PHIs*. London: Health Development Agency London.

Kelly, M., Morgan, A., Ellis, S., Younger, T., Huntley, J., and Swann, C., 2010. Evidence-based public health: a review of the experience of the National Institute of Health and Care Excellence (NICE) of developing public health guidance in England. *Social Science & Medicine*, *71*(6): 1056–62.

Kim, S.Y. and Goldie, S.J., 2008. Cost-effectiveness analyses of vaccination programmes. *Pharmacoeconomics*, *26*(3): 191–215.

Krahn, M. and Gafni, A., 1993. Discounting in the economic evaluation of health care interventions. *Medical Care*, *31*(5): 403–18.

Lawless, L., Drichoutis, A.C., and Nayga, R.M., 2013. Time preferences and health behaviour: A review. *Agricultural and Food Economics*, *1*(1): 1–19.

Linley, W.G. and Hughes, D.A., 2013. Societal views on NICE, cancer drugs fund and value-based pricing criteria for prioritising medicines: A cross-sectional survey of 4118 adults in Great Britain. *Health Economics*, *22*(8): 948–64.

Marmot, M.G., Allen, J., Goldblatt, P., Boyce, T., McNeish, D., Grady, M., and Geddes, I., 2010. Fair society, healthy lives: Strategic review of health inequalities in England post-2010. London: The Marmot Review.

Marsh, K., Phillips, C.J., Fordham, R., Bertranou, E., and Hale, J., 2012. Estimating cost-effectiveness in public health: A summary of modelling and valuation methods. *Health Economics Review*, *2*(1): 1–6.

Marteau, T.M., Ogilvie, D., Roland, M., Suhrcke, M., and Kelly, M.P., 2011. Judging nudging: Can nudging improve population health? *British Medical Journal*.

Mathes, T., Antoine, S.L., Prengel, P., Bühn, S., Polus, S., and Pieper, D., 2017. Health Technology assessment of public health interventions: A synthesis of methodological guidance. *International Journal of Technology Assessment in Health Care*, *33*(2): 135–46.

McCabe, C., 2018. Expanding the scope of costs and benefits for economic evaluations in health: Some words of caution. *Pharmacoeconomics*, 1–4.

McDaid, D., Byford, S., and Sefton, T., 2003. *Because It's Worth It: A Practical Guide to Conducting Economic Evaluations in the Social Welfare Field*. Joseph Rowntree Foundation. Available from: <https://www.researchgate.net/profile/Sarah_Byford/publication/237868089_Because_It's_Worth_It_A_Practical_Guide_to_Conducting_Economic_Evaluations_in_the_Social_Welfare_Field/links/0c96051bef05a57fd1000000/Because-Its-Worth-It-A-Practical-Guide-to-Conducting-Economic-Evaluations-in-the-Social-Welfare-Field.pdf> (Accessed 1 November 2018).

McDaid, D. and Needle, J., 2007. The Use of Economic Evaluation for PHIs: Desert or Oasis? A Systematic Review of the Literature. iHEA 2007 6th World Congress: Explorations in Health Economics Paper. Available from: <http://ssrn.com/abstract=994702> (Accessed 13 October 2018).

McGregor, G., Nichols, S., Hamborg, T., Bryning, L., Tudor-Edwards, R., Markland, D., Mercer, J., et al., 2016. High-intensity interval training versus moderate-intensity steady-state training in UK cardiac rehabilitation programmes (HIIT or MISS UK): Study protocol for a multicentre randomised controlled trial and economic evaluation. *British Medical Journal Open*, *6*(11): e012843.

McIntosh, E., Barlow, J., Davis, H., and Stewart-Brown, S., 2009. Economic evaluation of an intensive home visiting programme for vulnerable families: A cost-effectiveness analysis of a public health intervention. *Journal of Public Health*, *31*(3): 423–33.

McIntosh, E., Clarke, P.M., Frew, E.J., and Louviere, J.J., 2010. *Applied Methods of Cost–Benefit Analysis in Health Care*. Oxford: Oxford University Press.

McKie, J. and Richardson, J., 2003. The rule of rescue. *Social Science & Medicine*, 56(12): 2407–19.

Merito, M., Bonaccorsi, A., Pammolli, F., Riccaboni, M., Baio, G., Arici, C., Monforte, A.D.A., et al., 2005. Economic evaluation of HIV treatments: The I. CO. NA cohort study. *Health Policy*, 74(3): 304–13.

Midgley, G., 2006. Systemic intervention for public health. *American Journal of Public Health*, 96(3): 466–72.

Midgley, G., 2000. *Systemic Intervention: Philosophy, Methodology, and Practice*. New York, NY: Kluwer Academic/Plenum Publishers.

Minnis, H., Fitzpatrick, B., Wilson, P., Boyd, K., McIntosh, E., McConnachie, A., Messow M., et al., 2017. Protocol for the Best Services Trial (BeST?): Effectiveness and cost-effectiveness of the New Orleans Intervention Model for Infant Mental Health. *The Lancet*.

Mishan, E. J., 1971. *Cost–Benefit Analysis: An Introduction*. New York, NY: Praeger Publishers.

Moore, G.F., Audrey, S., Barker, M., Bond, L., Bonell, C., Hardeman, W., Moore, L., et al., 2015. Process evaluation of complex interventions: Medical Research Council guidance. *British Medical Journal*, 350: h1258.

National Institute for Health and Care Excellence, 2012. *Methods for the Development of NICE Public Health Guidance* (3rd edn). Available from: <http://www.nice.org.uk/article/pmg4/chapter/1%20Introduction> (Accessed 13 October 2018).

National Institute for Health and Care Excellence, 2011. *Supporting Investment in Public Health: Review of Methods for Assessing Cost Effectiveness, Cost Impact and Return on Investment*. Available from: <https://www.nice.org.uk/media/default/About/what-we-do/NICE-guidance/NICE-guidelines/Public-health-guidelines/Additional-publications/Cost-impact-proof-of-concept.pdf> (Accessed 1 November 2018).

O'Brien, T.D., Noyes, J., Spencer, L.H., Kubis, H.P., Edwards, R.T., Bray, N., and Whitaker, R., 2015. Well-being, health and fitness of children who use wheelchairs: Feasibility study protocol to develop child-centred 'keep-fit' exercise interventions. *Journal of Advanced Nursing*, 71(2): 430–40. DOI: 10.1111/jan.12482.

Office for National Statistics, 2016. *Sickness absence in the UK labour market: 2016*. London: Office of National Statistics.

Pawson, R. and Tilley, N., 1997. *Realistic Evaluation*. London: Sage.

Owen, L., Morgan, A., Fischer, A., Ellis, S., Hoy, A., and Kelly, M.P., 2011. The cost-effectiveness of public health interventions. *Journal of Public Health*, 34(1): 37–45.

Ramsey, S., Willke, R., Briggs, A., Brown, R., Buxton, M., Chawla, A., Cook, J., et al., 2005. Good research practices for cost-effectiveness analysis alongside clinical trials: the ISPOR RCT-CEA task force report. *Value in Health*, 8(5): 521–33.

Rychetnik, L., Frommer, M., Hawe, P., and Shiell, A., 2002. Criteria for evaluating evidence on public health interventions. *Journal of Epidemiology & Community Health*, 56(2): 119–27.

Sanghera, S., Frew, E., and Roberts, T., 2015. Adapting the CHEERS statement for reporting cost–benefit analysis. *Pharmacoeconomics*, 33(5): 533–4

Shiell, A., Hawe, P., and Gold, L., 2008. Complex interventions or complex systems? Implications for health economic evaluation. *British Medical Journal*, *336*(7656): 1281–3

Shiell, A., 2010. Market failure is bad for your health but social injustice is worse. *Journal of Public Health*, *32*(1): 12–13.

Smith, R.D., 2003. Construction of the contingent valuation market in health care: A critical assessment. *Health Economics*, *12*(8): 609–28.

Smith, R.D. and Petticrew, M., 2010. Public health evaluation in the twenty-first century: Time to see the wood as well as the trees. *Journal of Public Health*, *32*(1): 2–7.

Smith, R.D., Yago, M., Millar, M., and Coast, J., 2005. Assessing the macroeconomic impact of a health care problem: The application of computable general equilibrium analysis to antimicrobial resistance. *Journal of Health Economics*, *24*(6): 1055–75.

Song, J.W. and Chung, K.C., 2010. Observational studies: Cohort and case-control studies. *Plastic and Reconstructive Surgery*, *126*(6): 2234–42.

Sunstein, C.R. and Thaler, R.H., 2012. *Nudge: Improving Decisions About Health, Wealth and Happiness*. London: Penguin.

Townshend, J.R.P. and Turner, H.S., 2000. Analysing the effectiveness of Chlamydia screening. *Journal of the Operational Research Society*, *51*(7): 812–24.

UK BEAM Trial Team, 2004a. United Kingdom back pain exercise and manipulation (UK BEAM) randomised trial: Cost effectiveness of physical treatments for back pain in primary care. *British Medical Journal*, *329*(7479): 1381–5.

UK BEAM Trial Team, 2004b. United Kingdom back pain exercise and manipulation (UK BEAM) randomised trial: Effectiveness of physical treatments for back pain in primary care. *British Medical Journal*, *329*(7479): 1377.

Victora, C.G., Habicht, J.P., and Bryce, J., 2004. Evidence-based public health: Moving beyond randomized trials. *American Journal of Public Health*, *94*(3): 400–5.

Von Elm, E., Altman, D.G., Egger, M., Pocock, S.J., Gøtzsche, P.C., and Vandenbroucke, J.P., 2014. Strengthening the reporting of observational studies in epidemiology (STROBE) statement: Guidelines for reporting observational studies. *International Journal of Surgery*, *12*(12): 1495–9.

Wagenaar, A.C., Salois, M.J., and Komro, K.A., 2009. Effects of beverage alcohol price and tax levels on drinking: A meta-analysis of 1003 estimates from 112 studies. *Addiction*, *104*(2): 179–90.

Wanless, D., 2004. Securing Good Health for the Whole Population. London: HM Treasury. Available at: <https://www.southampton.gov.uk/moderngov/documents/s19272/prevention-appx%201%20wanless%20summary.pdf> (Accessed 1 November 2018).

Weatherly, H., Drummond, M., Claxton, K., Cookson, R., Ferguson, B., Godfrey, C., Rice, N., et al., 2009. Methods for assessing the cost-effectiveness of public health interventions: Key challenges and recommendations. *Health Policy*, *93*(2): 85–92.

Webster-Stratton, C., 2000. *The Incredible Years Training Series*. Washington, DC: US Department of Justice, Office of Justice Programs, Office of Juvenile Justice and Delinquency Prevention.

Westra, T.A., Parouty, M., Brouwer, W.B., Beutels, P.H., Rogoza, R.M., Rozenbaum, M.H., Daemen, T., et al., 2012. On discounting of health gains from human papillomavirus vaccination: effects of different approaches. *Value in Health*, *15*(3): 562–7.

Whitehead, M., 2007. A typology of actions to tackle social inequalities in health. *Journal of Epidemiology and Community Health*, *61*(6): 473–8.

Wolf, A.M., Finer, N., Allshouse, A.A., Pendergast, K.B., Sherrill, B.H., Caterson, I., Hill, J.O., et al., 2008. PROCEED: Prospective Obesity Cohort of Economic Evaluation and Determinants: baseline health and health care utilization of the US sample. *Diabetes, Obesity and Metabolism*, *10*(12): 1248–60.

Yaneer, B-Y., 2002. *General Features of Complex Systems*. Oxford: Encyclopedia of Life Support Systems (EOLSS), UNESCO Publishers.

Chapter 4

Synthesizing evidence for economic evaluations of public health interventions

Olivia Wu, Joanna M. Charles, and
Nathan Bray

4.1 Introduction

Decisions on the adoption of health care interventions need to be underpinned by best available evidence. Evidence synthesis, including systematic review and meta-analysis, and economic evaluations are tools used typically in a decision-analytical framework to inform such decisions. Systematic reviews are useful for mapping, summarizing, and identifying gaps in the existing evidence base. Meta-analysis provides a quantitative approach to synthesizing multiple data sources to generate an overall estimate of the effect of interest and the associated uncertainty surrounding this measure. These estimates are subsequently used to inform economic evaluations to derive estimates of cost-effectiveness.

Approaches to synthesizing evidence from randomized controlled trials (RCTs) of pharmacological interventions have been well established. For instance, the step-by-step guidance produced by the Cochrane Collaboration has been widely adopted (Higgins and Green, 2011), and the Preferred Reporting Items for Systematic Reviews and Meta-Analysis (PRISMA) statement is considered the gold standard in reporting systematic reviews and meta-analysis (Moher et al., 2009). However, in the context of PHIs, there are unique challenges, outlined in Chapter 3 of this book. PHIs are considered to be 'complex'—in comparison to pharmacological interventions, they often consist of multiple interacting components and non-linear causal pathways (Craig et al., 2008). There is a paucity of evidence from high-quality RCTs due to the inherent difficulties related to methodological, ethical, and/or pragmatic issues in conducting such studies. Therefore, evidence synthesis of PHIs relies on inclusion of diverse data types and sources, making synthesis challenging—quantitative synthesis is rarely possible or appropriate, while narrative (non-quantitative) synthesis often fails to draw clear conclusions.

Evidence synthesis of complex interventions is an active area of methodological development. Some guidance does exist. The Cochrane Public Health Review Group has produced an overview of issues specific to conducting systematic reviews of public health and health promotion interventions (Higgins and Green, 2011); and subsequently, the National Institute of Health and Care Excellence (NICE) has updated their Methods for the development of NICE Public Health Guidance (National Institute of Health and Care Excellence, 2012). These are useful references and provide a good summary of the challenges in evidence synthesis of PHIs. In this chapter, we highlight the key issues and discuss novel methodological approaches in synthesizing evidence on PHIs, in the context of economic evaluation and the decision-analytical framework.

4.2 Clarifying the question and defining relevant evidence

As a principle, economic evaluations of interventions require 'a systematic evaluation of the relevant evidence' (National Institute for Health and Care Excellence, 2013). How we determine 'relevance', and how relevant evidence should be identified and summarized requires value judgements. Typically, in the evaluation of pharmacological or clinical interventions, we aim to estimate the clinical benefits associated with these interventions in order to inform subsequent cost-effectiveness analysis. We seek evidence from RCTs, which test the hypothesis of whether an intervention works and estimate relative treatment effects. However, PHIs are typically 'complex' due to varying intervention components, characteristics of participants, contextual factors, and multiple causal pathways. In this context, relying solely on evidence that seeks to accept or reject hypothesis on whether something works or not is not always adequate or appropriate. In the evaluation of PHIs, there is now a general movement for a systematic review of PHIs to move from addressing the question of 'what works' to 'what happens'. Evidence synthesis of PHIs should follow three key steps: (i) clarification of the review question; (ii) identification of the sources of complexity; and (iii) determination of relevant evidence related to those aspects of complexity to be sought (Petticrew et al., 2015).

The first step to evidence synthesis is to frame the review question(s). Far too often, systematic reviewers fail to dedicate sufficient attention to this crucial step. It is important that we develop review questions that are relevant to addressing the health care decision, and that we maximize the value from our review efforts. In the context of PHIs, there is also a need to understand and describe the various aspects of complexity; these could then be mapped onto the study selection criteria (Box 4.1). Ultimately, this would lead to a need to adopt broader inclusion criteria, to consider the totality of the evidence, and to incorporate relevant randomized, non-randomized, and qualitative evidence.

Contrary to evaluation of pharmacological interventions, the use of RCTs to determine health benefits of PHIs is not always feasible. There are methodological and pragmatic challenges to evaluating the health benefits of PHIs using RCTs (Sanson-Fisher et al., 2007). Many PHIs are associated with modest benefits to individuals (but can lead to substantial impact when delivered to extremely large populations). As a result, large sample sizes are required to achieve the appropriate statistical power for detecting the predefined treatment effect (Fischer et al., 2013). This is further complicated by many PHIs that are designed to be delivered to groups or communities

Box 4.1 An example of framing questions for a systematic review of a complex intervention (Flowers et al., 2017)

A systematic review of evidence to determine the clinical effectiveness of individual behaviour change interventions to reduce risky sexual behavior after a negative human immunodeficiency virus test in men who have sex with men.

What works?

♦ Do individual behavioural change interventions reduce behaviours of high-risk HIV transmission?

♦ If the interventions are effective, how well do they work?

What happens?

♦ How do we define behavioural change interventions?

♦ How do we define high-risk behaviours?

♦ Through what mechanisms do the interventions work?

♦ Given the heterogeneity of the data, for whom and in what context do they work?

Source: data from Flowers, P. et al. "The Clinical Effectiveness of Individual Behaviour Change Interventions to Reduce Risky Sexual Behaviour after a Negative Human Immunodeficiency Virus Test in Men Who Have Sex with Men: Systematic and Realist Reviews and Intervention Development. *Health Technology Assessment* 21(5). Copyright © 2017 NHS.

instead of individuals. In evaluating these interventions, cluster RCTs are needed, which require large numbers of participating groups or communities to be followed over time. Such trials are costly and difficult to deliver.

Another issue relates to the ability to generalize findings. Although RCTs generally have high internal validity, they tend to have limited external validity. Unlike pharmacological interventions, which target specific indications and patient populations with strict inclusion/exclusion criteria, PHIs are intended to be adopted at a population level consisting of a heterogeneous mix of individual characteristics. Finally, in some circumstances, the RCT design is not feasible, such as evaluation of the effectiveness of smoking cessation policies or the introduction of green space to communities, where the implementation of intervention is on a large scale and where randomization is not feasible.

Therefore, non-randomized comparative study designs such as natural experiments are highly relevant in evaluating PHIs. For some questions relating to the effectiveness and cost-effectiveness of PHIs and whether they should be adopted, non-randomized studies may represent the best source of evidence. Approaches such as controlled before/after studies design (with interrupted time-series analyses), and natural experiments (with difference-in-differences and regression discontinuity analyses) are increasingly being used (Craig et al., 2012). Deidda et al. (2019) provide useful guidance on conducting economic evaluations alongside natural experiments. However, these studies are susceptible to high risk of bias due to confounding issues.

Synthesizing data from randomized and non-randomized evidence requires complex methodological approaches.

Qualitative evidence also has a role in the evaluation of complex PHIs. However, there is currently a lack of consensus on the best approach to synthesizing qualitative evidence.

4.3 **Searching for evidence**

A good search strategy to identify relevant evidence requires a balance of sensitivity and precision. Essentially, it is a trade-off between searching broadly to ensure all relevant studies are captured and dealing with a large volume of potential irrelevant studies. This is particularly relevant to complex review questions such as those related to PHIs. An effective search may require the use of multifaceted search techniques that involve combinations of concepts to capture a review topic. Further, searching beyond the commonly used electronic biomedical databases are also important. One example is the inclusion of grey literature. These are sources of literature which may be considered unpublished or non-standard academic literature (e.g. working papers, technical reports, and reports from government agencies).

Search algorithms for 'traditional' systematic reviews are usually built upon search terms that reflect the review question, and structured according to the Population–Intervention–Comparator–Outcomes (PICO) framework (Schardt et al., 2007). However, summarizing complex review questions according to few distinct keywords can be intrinsically difficult. Pearl growing (also known as snowballing or citation mining) is a useful approach to searching by building on citations (Booth et al., 2012). This involves starting with one key relevant citation based on a very precise and specific search, and expanding the search terms based on the additional search terms that the key relevant citation may introduce. This is then repeated as additional relevant citations are identified.

In recent years, there has also been a rise in interests in the use of text-mining software. Searches are based on the meaning of words and concepts within a set of records, rather than simply the presence of these terms or concepts. Sematic analysis has the capacity to interrogate a large volume of search results to retrieve records based on the probability of relevance (Lefebvre et al., 2013). Such searches are based on the meaning of words or concepts instead of the presence of keywords. For qualitative studies, the potential of purposive searching and saturation has been discussed in recent literature (Booth, 2016). This is the process in which individual studies are sought and included on the basis that they can add conceptually to the review. This poses a trade-off between the minimization of publication bias as a result of a comprehensive search and the incremental value of additional studies to answering the review question beyond saturation.

4.4 **Quality assessment**

Economic evaluations should be informed by the best available evidence. Therefore, we need to have a clear understanding of the strength of the evidence that we are using to inform such evaluations. Various tools exist to assess the internal validity (the quality or the potential risk of bias) of specific study types. The Risk of Bias tool is arguable the most consistently used tool for evaluating RCTs (Higgins et al., 2011). For evaluating evidence from non-RCT design, a mix of different tools has been used in the literature (Table 4.1).

According to the Cochrane Handbook, '[i]t is not helpful to include evidence from which there is a high risk of bias in a review, even if there is no better evidence' (Higgins and Green, 2011). There is an ongoing debate on whether 'weak evidence' should be excluded from systematic review and meta-analysis (Petticrew, 2015). While inclusion of 'weak evidence' may introduce heterogeneity and uncertainty, especially

Table 4.1 Quality assessment tools

Study Type	Tool
All	Hierarchy of evidence
	GRADE (Grading of Recommendations Assessment, Development and Evaluation)
Randomized controlled trials	ISPOR AMCP Task force on ITC Network Meta-Analysis
	Cochrane Risk of Bias tool for RCTs
	JADAD
	CASP (RCTs)
	CONSORT
Observational studies	ISPOR AMCP Task force on Real World Evidence
	ACROBAT-NRSI (A Cochrane Risk of Bias Assessment Tool: for Non-Randomized Studies of Interventions)
	CASP (cohort)
	CASP (case control)
	MOOSE
	STROBE
	GRACE
	Newcastle–Ottawa (case control)
	Newcastle–Ottawa (cohort)
	NICE (cohort)
	NICE (case control)
	MERGE (Method for Reviewing Research Guideline Evidence)
Systematic review/ meta-analysis	CASP (systematic review)
	NICE (systematic review/meta-analysis)
	EVAT (External validity assessment tool)
	PRISMA

in the case of meta-analysis, there are issues with applying a blanket rule of excluding such evidence. In situations where evidence is sparse, these studies may be the only source of available evidence. This would result in a trade-off between obtaining an estimate of effect with large uncertainty or not being able to derive an estimate at all. Furthermore, the definition of study quality is dependent on the tool or the criteria that have been used to form the judgement. For instance, assessment tools that are designed to address internal validity would ultimately rate RCTs to be of superior quality as compared with observational studies. In the context of complex PHIs, these different study types are useful in addressing different questions. Therefore, exclusion of 'weak evidence' here may lead to misleading results.

4.5 **Synthesis**

There is currently a general lack of consistency in the approach to synthesizing data on PHIs. Generally, the most commonly adopted approach to synthesizing evidence is quantitative synthesis of pairwise comparisons between the intervention of interest and a common comparator. Pairwise meta-analysis is effective at estimating a pooled relative treatment effect based on data from multiple RCTs that have made comparisons between the same intervention of interest and the same comparator. However, given the diverse sources and the potential complex structure of the data required to evaluate a complex PHI, this approach is restrictive and limited. Therefore, in synthesizing evidence related to PHIs, studies are often summarized using narrative (non-quantitative) synthesis methods.

In a review of NICE public health appraisals between 2006 and 2012, Achana and colleagues found 29 of 39 appraisals presented narrative synthesis only (Achana et al., 2014). Nine appraisals performed pairwise meta-analyses, while one did not present any review of effectiveness and cost-effectiveness. The primary reason for lack of quantitative synthesis was heterogeneity—of outcomes, methods, and interventions, and meta-analysis was deemed inappropriate in these cases. However, not being able to undertake a quantitative analysis severely restricted the utility of the review for decision making. In summary, Achana and colleagues highlighted the following methodological challenges to synthesizing data from PHIs: (i) increased methodological heterogeneity and risk of bias as a result of including different study designs; (ii) interventions (or programmes) being evaluated is often described in little detail; (iii) wide range of outcomes often used and variously defined across studies; and (iv) use of intermediate and/or surrogate outcomes.

Synthesizing evidence of complex PHIs, particularly in the context of economic evaluations will typically require a mixed-methods approach. In order to fully inform an economic evaluation, evidence synthesis is often required to inform the structure the model and to derive estimates for parameters of the model. Inevitably, this involves synthesis of different types of data structure and a mixed-method approach is required.

4.5.1 **Quantitative synthesis**

Regardless of complexity, there is value in understanding whether a PHI is effective and the magnitude of the related 'treatment effect'. Pairwise meta-analysis can only compare one type of intervention with a single comparator. In the context of PHIs, this would require some level of 'lumping' of interventions and comparators to conform with the requisite data structure. For instance, if we were interested in 'individual behavioural interventions', we would need to 'lump together' various individual behavioural interventions—for example, interventions that are delivered in person and online; and varying frequency and intensity of delivery. Similarly, if these interventions were compared with 'usual care' in individual studies, this could be a heterogeneous mix of varying practices. The issue is that a statistically significant benefit from a meta-analysis of 'lumping' these studies together simply suggests that at least one format of the intervention is 'better' than at least one form of usual care being evaluated. This masks important and relevant heterogeneity across intervention types, and is useful for decision-makers, especially in making recommendations on implementation.

Network meta-analysis has been widely used to compare treatment effects across multiple clinical treatment comparisons. Generally used in pharmacological, 'non-complex' interventions, it is less well-adopted in public health. There are clear advantages to network meta-analysis. In considering complex interventions, network meta-analysis has the capacity to present a more complete picture of evidence than either 'lumping' or 'splitting' according to multiple subgroups (e.g. by intervention types) which is often underpowered and difficult to hypothesize *a priori*. The complexity and heterogeneity of complex interventions can be modelled within a network meta-analysis approach, using clinically meaningful units and components and dismantling (Melendez-Torres et al., 2015). Clinically meaningful units group interventions by similarity of modality or into groups that are relevant according a theoretical standpoint (e.g. supported by 'theory of change'). These groups can then be evaluated using a multiple treatment comparison approach through a network meta-analysis. For example, Cooper and colleagues extended a pairwise meta-analysis to a network meta-analysis to evaluate the effectiveness of educational initiatives to increase the uptake of smoke alarms (Cooper et al., 2012). The definitions of educational initiatives were further refined to reflect the increasing intensity of the interventions, ranging from education alone to a combined initiative of education, equipment fitting, and home inspection. The network meta-analysis simultaneously compared the relative treatment effects and provided probability ranking of their relative effectiveness between all comparisons (six distinct intervention initiatives and usual care).

In components and dismantling, complex interventions are viewed as systems of components. These interventions are grouped according to the combination of components (i.e. aspects of interventions) of which they are composed. Welton and colleagues demonstrated this in the context of psychological interventions in coronary heart disease (Welton et al., 2009). Psychological interventions were classified into six types: usual care, educational, behavioural, cognitive, relaxation, and support. Through a network meta-analysis, they were able to show that interventions with either behavioural or cognitive components were more likely to be effective than interventions without these components. However, understanding and dismantling complexity is not always straightforward. This is an evolving field and there are tools that have been developed to help dismantle and assess the complexity of interventions. For instance, the intervention Complex Assessment Tool for Systematic Reviews (iCAT_SR) is a tool that has been developed 'to assess and categorize levels of intervention complexity in systematic reviews' (Lewin et al., 2017). The tool consists of core dimensions relating to the intervention (number of components, organizational levels), recipients (number of behviours, skills required for receiving the intervention), implementation (tailored intended or flexibility, skills required for delivery), and optional dimensions relating to interaction between components, effects change according to context, recipients and providers, and nature of causal pathway between intervention and outcome. This tool is potentially useful in systematic disaggregation of complex interventions but has yet to be tested extensively.

4.5.2 **Narrative synthesis**

When synthesizing multiple sources of data together, heterogeneity is a key issue and is particularly problematic in synthesizing PHIs. Although statistical approaches to adjusting for heterogeneity exist (e.g. meta-regression, hierarchical modelling), it is not unusual that the presence of substantial heterogeneity would lead to any pooled estimates being meaningless. Narrative synthesis has become a key focus in synthesizing complex PHIs. However, there is a lack of consistency and clarity in the way these analyses are performed, and the results presented are often opaque. In a review of systematic reviews published between 2010 and 2015 from the McMaster Health Evidence database (a comprehensive database of systematic reviews of PHIs), narrative synthesis was used in 53 per cent of all reviews (Campbell et al., 2016). However, there were deficiencies in how the methods were applied and reported, and clear up-to-date guidance in this area is still lacking.

Narrative synthesis, especially of quantitative data, aims to describe textually the overall treatment effect while noting variations due to potential heterogeneity. This goes beyond summarizing findings of studies individually, and explores relationships in the data using cross-study analysis and graphical tools. Cross-study analysis consists of examination of themes or patterns that may emerge from the data, or use of vote counting to describe groups of studies reporting similar findings. Graphical tools can be used to summarize and present quantitative data, such as harvest plots, which present complex and diverse data within easily interpreted graphical formats (Ogilvie et al., 2008). These plots illustrate the extent to which specific interventions are effective at improving at least one relevant outcome, and are primarily used to synthesize narrative evidence from complex and heterogeneous interventions (Turley et al., 2013). An example of a harvest plot is presented in Figure 4.1.

Another useful tool in narrative synthesis is the use of logic (conceptual) models. Consistent with systems thinking in evaluating complex interventions and policies, logic models are a means of presenting the processes by which an intervention has an effect on an individual or a group, and can be used to highlight the factors which influence a given outcome (Kneale et al., 2015). They are useful for describing relationships between determinants of outcomes. Anderson and colleagues highlighted the utility of logic models in guiding systematic reviews (Anderson et al., 2011).

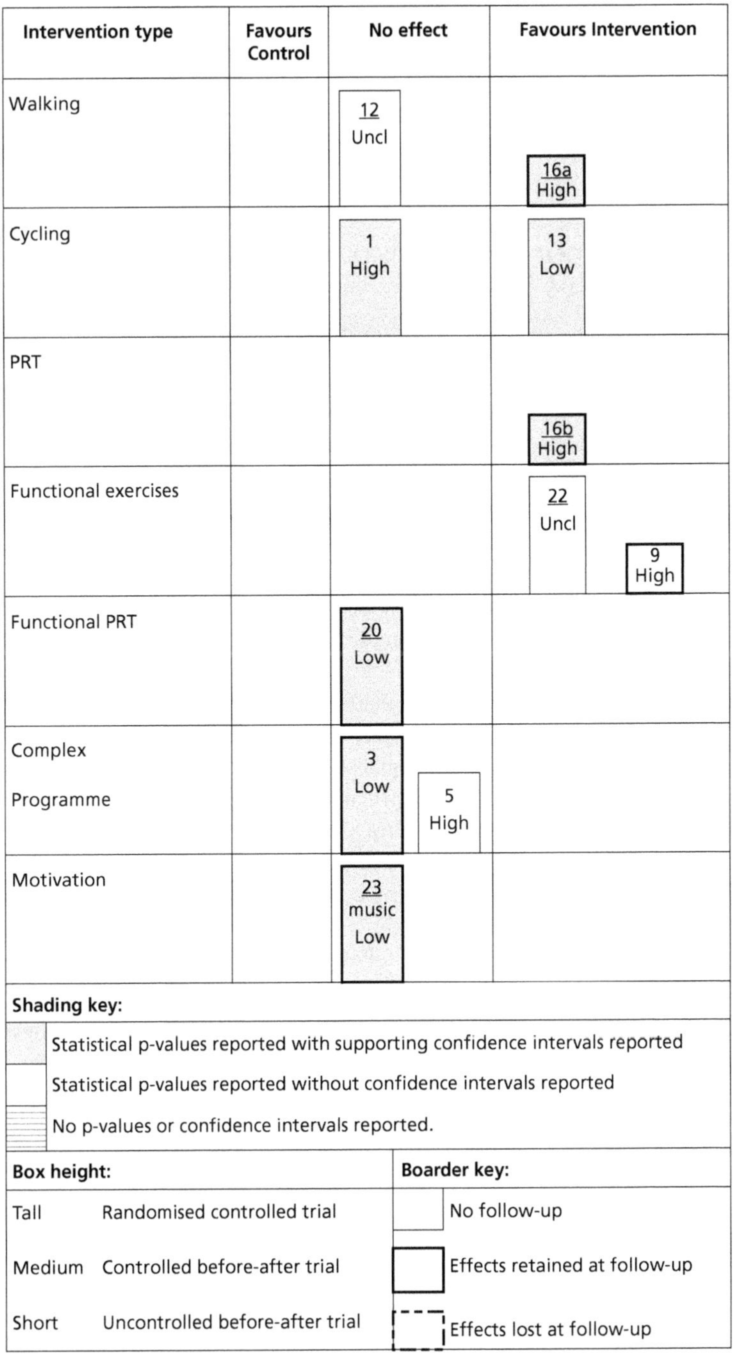

Intervention type	Favours Control	No effect	Favours Intervention
Walking		12 Uncl	16a High
Cycling		1 High	13 Low
PRT			16b High
Functional exercises			22 Uncl / 9 High
Functional PRT		20 Low	
Complex Programme		3 Low / 5 High	
Motivation		23 music Low	

Shading key:

Statistical p-values reported with supporting confidence intervals reported

Statistical p-values reported without confidence intervals reported

No p-values or confidence intervals reported.

Box height:		Boarder key:	
Tall	Randomised controlled trial		No follow-up
Medium	Controlled before-after trial		Effects retained at follow-up
Short	Uncontrolled before-after trial		Effects lost at follow-up

Figure 4.1 Harvest plot of intervention effects on quality of life and attitudes. Each box represents the findings of a single article, and contains the article number, which is underlined for studies with undefined intervention attributes (i.e. wheelchair use), and the risk of bias rating (high, unclear or low).

4.5.3 **Mixed-method systematic reviews**

Systematic reviews are traditionally structured around the collation and synthesis of quantitative data, particularly with regards to meta-analysis. Structuring a systematic review around one type of evidence can have a number of benefits, including focused search strategies and clear research questions, but conversely this can lead to a narrow understanding of a given topic or phenomenon. For this reason, mixed-method systematic reviews have become increasingly popular, particularly for complex interventions where statistical data only reveal part of the story. PHIs are rarely simple and their effects are often difficult to quantify fully, thus by examining qualitative evidence alongside quantitative evidence, it will be possible to understand how various personal, social, and environmental factors influence the effectiveness and cost-effectiveness of a given PHI. By identifying and synthesizing all the relevant quantitative and qualitative evidence for a given condition or intervention, mixed-method systematic reviews make it easier for commissioners, policy-makers, and clinicians to make evidence-based decisions (Pearson et al., 2015).

The inclusion of qualitative evidence within a systematic review allows the experiences of the target population to be accounted for and understood, which in turn can help to improve the applicability and effectiveness of the intervention (Thomas et al., 2004). For instance, incorporating qualitative evidence alongside quantitative evidence allows an understanding of the relationship between intervention effectiveness and service-user experience. Although qualitative evidence alone cannot tell us about the effectiveness of interventions, it can help us to understand how interventions affect individuals and the service-user experience. Quantitative data can be used to extrapolate and generalize results from a specific study cohort to the wider population, while qualitative data can be used to reveal why certain groups within that population are more or less responsive to an intervention.

There are three general frameworks, following Sandelowski and colleagues' work (2006), for conducting a mixed-method systematic review:

1. Segregated: explicitly differentiating different types of evidence (i.e. quantitative and qualitative) and conducting separate syntheses.
2. Integrated: combining all forms of evidence into a single synthesis.
3. Contingent: sequential syntheses which are contingent on the results of each separate synthesis.

Although all of these frameworks utilize quantitative and qualitative evidence, only segregated methodologies present evidence as both individual and aggregative syntheses (Pearson et al., 2015). Segregated mixed-method reviews commonly consist of three stages: first, examining and synthesizing the different types of evidence as independent streams of evidence; second, examining the relationships between the different types of evidence; and finally, examining and synthesizing all the evidence as a whole in an aggregated synthesis (Pearson et al., 2015).

Bayesian approaches to mixed-method reviewing can also be used to generate summative statements and meta-aggregation of data (Pearson et al., 2015). This approach can be conducted by either giving all qualitative data a numerical value or by attributing a thematic descriptor to all quantitative data, thereby permitting a translation from one type of evidence to another. The downside is that this approach risks reducing the richness of the qualitative data in order to increase uniformity with the quantitative data (Harden and Thomas, 2005)

When including qualitative evidence in a systematic review, thematic approaches to analysis and synthesis may be used to identify key themes within the qualitative data (Thomas and Harden, 2008). This process includes three stages; line-by-line coding of text, development of descriptive themes, and generation of analytical themes. The output is a thematic summary of the main analytical themes emerging from the data. The aim of this analytical technique is to go beyond the results with an inductive approach to analysis and synthesis of data, which in turn allows grounding of theory within the qualitative evidence (Thomas and Harden, 2008). Along with data extraction and analysis, assessment of quality, risk of bias, and rigour should also be tailored to the types of evidence included in the review.

The types of evidence included in a mixed-method review do not need to be limited to published quantitative and qualitative data; for instance, government and policy literature can be used to understand if policy intentions reflect actual practice and patient experience. Furthermore, economic data can also be synthesized separately to quantitative effectiveness data in order to differentiate economic and clinical outcomes.

4.5.4 Realist synthesis

Realist review or synthesis has developed from the philosophical traditions of critical realism, which questions and addresses the perceived or assumed interrelationship between science, knowledge, and reality (Collier, 1994). The realist research question is often summarized as: 'what works for whom, under what circumstances, how, and why?' (Pawson et al., 2005). The aim of realist inquiry is to understand and describe causality using a configuration of context + mechanism = outcome (Pawson and Tilley, 1997). According to Pawson and colleagues, context often refers to the 'backdrop' of programmes and research (Pawson et al., 2005). This could be cultural norms or the environment in which the programme or research takes place. In the field of realist research, context is broadly understood as any condition that triggers and/or modifies the behaviour of a mechanism (Pawson et al., 2005). A mechanism is the generative force that leads to or triggers outcomes. This could be the programme's strategy (e.g. delivering a programme in a group setting), or the way in which the participant responds to the programme (Pawson et al., 2005). The identification of mechanisms is integral to understanding and theorizing not only what happened but *why* it happened, for whom, and under what circumstances. Outcomes can be intended, unintended, proximal, intermediate, or final. Examples of outcomes could range from improved health, greater education, or knowledge. These outcomes could also include personal outcomes such as improved self-efficacy or development of coping strategies.

It is also worth noting that some contexts and mechanisms can be latent or dormant. Ray Pawson, a prominent figure in the field of realist synthesis, uses a cricket analogy to explain this concept of latent or dormant contexts and/or mechanisms. Pawson states that every player has the latent power to hit a six; however, whether or not a player does so is dependent upon the rest of the game and the actions of the other players. Justin Jagosh, another prominent figure in the field of realist synthesis, prefers to use an iceberg as a metaphor for this concept of latent or dormant contexts and/or mechanisms. Stating that the tip of the iceberg above the surface of the water is at the level of the observable or experienced, the remainder of the iceberg, which is under the surface of the water, is considered the level of the actual. At this level, these contexts and/or mechanisms can be seen but one may need specialist equipment to do so. Until specialized equipment is used, these contexts and/or mechanisms may be latent or dormant. In the depths of the ocean, under the iceberg, is the level of the real where contexts and/or mechanisms may lie hidden, and depending upon how well these are hidden, they may not be uncovered as part of the research. The process of a realist review adapted from Pawson and colleagues (2005) and Rycroft-Malone and co-workers (2012) is summarized in Figure 4.2.

Researchers should be aware that there is no right or wrong way to go through the process of realist synthesis. What matters is what is appropriate for the field of research or intervention in question. Pawson and colleagues make this point by stating that a realist review should be viewed as producing a highway code to programme building or evaluation, warning decision-makers of the dangers or possible problems that may arise, but also highlighting the best methods to confront these issues (Pawson et al., 2005). Though there is no right or wrong way to conduct a realist review, publication standards are available through the Realist And MEta-narrative Evidence Syntheses: Evolving Standards (RAMESES) (Wong et al., 2013). RAMESES was developed to provide a standard of reporting of realist reviews in order to improve the reporting of realist syntheses as a relatively new method in research inquiry. Researchers undertaking realist reviews should consult these standards when reporting their research.

4.5.4.1 Strengths of realist synthesis

The method is pluralist and flexible, embracing both the qualitative and quantitative, formative and summative, and prospective and retrospective. It seeks to explain rather than to judge. Realist review learns from (rather than controls for) real-world phenomena such as diversity, change, and adaptation (Wong et al., 2013; Jagosh et al., 2012). It can assist programme developers to adapt their programmes to work effectively in different settings. Pawson and colleagues believe realist review also has the potential to maximize learning across policy, disciplinary, and organizational boundaries (Pawson et al., 2005). Realist review can also help decision-makers interpret and utilize findings regarding why a programme worked better in one context than another, rather than relying on understanding and interpretation of statistics from mediators and moderator analysis.

4.5.4.2 Limitations of realist synthesis

Realist review cannot be used as a formulaic, protocol-driven approach; it is considered iterative (Rycroft-Malone et al., 2012). Realist review findings are based on

Stage	Key Activities

1. Clarify the scope of the review	• Identify the review question
	• Consult widely with relevant stakeholders and conduct exploratory searches
	• Key questions at this stage to get a feel for the literature include:
	  o What is the nature and content of the intervention?
	  o Is it based on a particular strategy, programme theory or school of thought?
	  What are the circumstances or context for the intervention's use?
	  What are the policy intentions or objectives?

2. Refine the purpose of the review	• Theory integrity – does the intervention work as predicted? • Theory adjudication – which theories fit best? • Comparison – how does the intervention work in different settings, for different groups? • Reality testing – how does the policy intent of the intervention translate into practice?
3. Articulate key theories to be explored	• Draw up a 'long list' of relevant programme theories by exploratory searching. • Theory development can be top down (i.e. read high-level literature and develop a list of overarching theories) or bottom-up (i.e. speak to practitioners and other stakeholders as well as search through high-level literature). • Group, categorize or synthesize theories • Design a theoretically based evaluative framework to be 'populated' with evidence

4. Search the evidence	• Define your strategy
	  o E.g. will you use databases and search terms? OR use key references from the exploratory search and then use snowballing techniques from these key references to further understanding OR a mixture of both.
	  o Will there be any cut-off with regards to the date of relevance for literature? How will this be decided?
	• Define what the term saturation means and how this will be used by the researchers conducting the search.

5. Test these theories in the evidence	• Develop bespoke data extraction forms to gather all information. Extracts should be directly taken from the evidence with particular reference to explanations of how an intervention is supposed to work.

Figure 4.2 Stages and key activities for a realist review

Adapted from Rycroft-Malone, J., et al. Realist synthesis: illustrating the method for implementation research. *Implementation Science*. (7):33. Copyright © Rycroft-Malone et al.; licensee BioMed Central Ltd 2012. Open Access.

the judgements and interpretation of the reviewer, therefore they are individualistic. The same set of evidence and theories to test when given to different researchers would yield different findings. Realist review will never produce generalizable effect sizes since all its conclusions are contextual. A further potential limitation of realist review is its relative newness, though the RAMESES publication standards should ensure a consistent standard of reporting as use of this method increases (Wong et al., 2013).

4.5.4.3 Applications of realist synthesis within health economics

Realist methods of evidence synthesis are beginning to be applied to health economic questions and problems (Anderson, 2010; Charles et al., 2013; Hardwick et al., 2013; Pearson et al., 2013; Anderson and Hardwick, 2016). The inclusion of economic evidence in realist synthesis can provide a further dimension to realist studies, alerting decision-makers to the potential of effects on resources such as monetary budgets, beds available on a ward, staff required to meet demand, the types of staff that may be most effectively employed, cost-effective interventions that may be more meaningful to individuals depending on settings, population groups, or other contexts and mechanisms. Taking this more holistic view can inform decision-makers not only what works for whom, how, and under what circumstances but also of the implications for required resources. Resources are also important for decision-makers to consider, as they are charged with making the best use of them. This is especially important when they wish to roll out a different or new programme/service in their locality.

4.6 Value of information

In public health, as in all other disciplines, evidence is constantly being generated. In areas where existing evidence is sparse, timely updating of systematic reviews and meta-analyses to incorporate relevant and emerging evidence is extremely useful. In 2016, the Cochrane Collaboration launched the concept of 'living systematic reviews'—'systematic review which is continually updated, incorporating relevant new evidence as it becomes available' (Elliot et al., 2014). Living systematic reviews draw on the increasing number of open and shared data initiatives and the promising developments in data-mining technologies to keep reviews current and useful.

However, as systematic review questions become more complex and the volume of literature expands, 'the perennial question of when enough is enough' is increasingly relevant (Lefebvre et al., 2013). In economic evaluations, health economists have been assessing the Value Of Information (VOI) to determine whether it is cost-effective to seek further data to reduce uncertainty associated with individual parameter estimates within an economic model (Minelli and Baio, 2015). This approach can also be used in evidence synthesis (Welton et al., 2012; Petticrew, 2015). The VOI approach can be used to inform the value of further evidence to the estimation of the pooled treatment effect, and judge whether a future study would be likely to have an important impact on the direction and magnitude of the effect.

4.7 **Evidence synthesis and equity considerations**

There are highly likely to be specific equity considerations to be taken into account when synthesizing evidence in the context of PHIs. In particular, when estimating the health benefits of PHIs through meta-analysis, we estimate an average treatment effect for the whole population. Such an approach does not address distribution of benefits and potential health inequality across equity-relevant characteristics such as socio-economic status, ethnicity, and sex. It is also possible that the estimated average treatment effects mask difference in effects between groups. Interventions that are effective among those in mid to high socio-economic status may not be as effective for those who are of low socio-economic status (Higgins and Green, 2011). This is particularly relevant to the implementation of effective interventions from the perspective of high-income countries, to the context of low- and middle-income countries.

One reason for what seems to be an oversight of reviewers is the absence of, or the difficulty in, accessing relevant data. In general, there is limited participation in research, from hard-to-reach and disadvantaged groups. The Cochrane Public Health Group recommends the PROGRESS-Plus framework to identify population and individual characteristics that may contribute to health inequity (Box 4.2).

Reviews of effectiveness in relation to health inequalities require three components for calculations: valid measure of health status (change in status); measure of socio-economic status (disadvantage); and statistical method for pooling size of health differences between people in different groups (Higgins and Green, 2011). Guidance now exists for equity-focused systematic reviews (Welch et al., 2013), such as the Cochrane Equity checklist (Equity Checklist for Systematic Review Authors, 2012) and the PRISMA-Equity guidance (Welch et al., 2012).

Box 4.2 **PROGRESS acronym (Evans and Brown, 2003)**

PROGRESS

- Place of residence
- Race/ethnicity/culture/language
- Occupation
- Gender/sex
- Religion
- Education
- Socio-economic status
- Social capital
- Plus other characteristics that may indicate a disadvantage (e.g. age and disability)

Source: data from Evans, T. & Brown, H. Road traffic crashes: Operationalizing equity in the context of health sector reform. *Injury Control Safety Promotion.* 10(1–2), 11–12. Copyright © 2003 Taylor & Francis.

4.8 **Discussion**

Evidence synthesis requires a systematic and transparent approach to evaluating relevant evidence. For the purpose of informing economic evaluations, evidence synthesis seeks to assemble different types of relevant evidence for decision-making. For pharmacological interventions, clear and consistent approaches to synthesizing evidence exist. However, in the context of PHIs, there are unique challenges. PHIs are complex in nature, consisting of multiple interacting components. These interventions are intended to be delivered to large heterogenous populations. Therefore, in synthesizing evidence in this context, there is a need to disentangle intervention effects from the influence of the context in which the intervention is implemented.

This requires broader and more iterative consideration of evidence, and a more flexible and pragmatic approach to synthesizing evidence (beyond traditional pairwise meta-analysis). However, for a robust assessment of evidence, the core principles of evidence synthesis must be maintained—the process of systematic review and synthesizing evidence need to be systematic and transparent. There is ongoing rapid development of more sophisticated and complex quantitative and qualitative methodologies in synthesizing evidence for complex interventions. Ultimately, we should heed the advice from Petticrew and colleagues—'to consider not only just complexity but also logic and the use of Occam's razor ... and that systematic reviews should be as complex as they need to be' (Petticrew et al., 2015).

Summary of Chapter 4

This chapter has highlighted the key challenges and discussed novel methodological approaches in synthesizing evidence on PHIs. In the context of PHIs, there is a need to go beyond 'what works' to 'what happens'. In order to achieve this, careful framing of the review question and consideration of evidence beyond randomized controlled trials are warranted. Synthesizing complex public health evidence for the economic evaluations would ultimately require a mixed-method approach. Quantitative methods such as component network meta-analysis is useful in understanding the effects of specific components of complex interventions. Non-quantitative methods such as narrative synthesis, mixed methods reviews, and realist synthesis are particularly useful in exploring heterogeneity and understanding potential mechanisms of action. Ultimately, judgement is required on a case-by-case basis to select the appropriate tool to address the review question at hand.

References

Achana, F., Hubbard, S., Sutton A., Kendrick, D., and Cooper, N., 2014. An exploration of synthesis methods in public health evaluations of interventions concludes that the use of modern statistical methods would be beneficial. *Journal of Clinical Epidemiology*, 67(4): 376–90. <http://dx.doi.org/10.1016/j.jclinepi.2013.09.018> (Accessed 13 October 2018).

Anderson, L.M., Petticrew, M., Rehfuess, E., Armstrong, R., Ueffing, E., Baker P, Francis, D., et al. 2011. Using logic models to capture complexity in systematic reviews. *Research Synthesis Methods*, *2*(1): 33–42.

Anderson, R., 2010. Systematic reviews of economic evaluations: utility or futility? *Health Economics*, *19*(3): 350–4.

Anderson, R. and Hardwick, R., 2016. Realism and resources: Towards more explanatory economic evaluation. *Evaluation*, *22*(3): 323–41.

Booth, A., Papaioannou, D., and Sutton, A., eds. 2012. *Systematic Approaches to a Successful Literature Review*. London: SAGE Publications.

Booth, A., 2016. Searching for Qualitative Research for Inclusion in Systematic Reviews: A Structured Methodological Review. *Systematic Reviews*, *5*(1): 1–23.

Campbell, M., Thomson, H., Katikireddi, S.V., and Sowden, A., 2016. Reporting of Narrative Synthesis in Systematic Reviews of PHIs: A Methodological Assessment. *Lancet*, *388*: S34. <http://linkinghub.elsevier.com/retrieve/pii/S014067361632270X> (Accessed 13 October 2018).

Charles, J.M., Edwards, R.T., Williams, N., Din, N., on behalf of the FEMuR Realist Review Study Group, 2013. The application of realist synthesis review methods in public health economics. *Lancet*, *382*(3): S28 (published abstract).

Collier, A., 1994. *Critical Realism: An Introduction to Roy Bhaskar's Philosophy*. Verso, London

Cooper, N.J., Kendrick, D., Achana, F., Dhiman, P., He, Z., and Wynn, P., 2012. 'Network meta-analysis to evaluate the effectiveness of interventions to increase the uptake of smoke alarms'. *Epidemiologic Reviews*, *34*(1): 32–45.

Craig, P., Dieppe, P., Macintyre, S., Michie, S., Nazareth, I., and Petticrew, M., 2008. Developing and Evaluating Complex Interventions: New Guidance. *Science*, *337*(a1655): a1655. <http://discovery.ucl.ac.uk/103060/> (Accessed 13 October 2018).

Craig, P., Cooper, C., Gunnell, D., Haw, S., Lawson, K., Macintyre, S., Olgilvie, D., et al., 2012. Using natural experiments to evaluate population health interventions: New medical research council guidance. *Journal of Epidemiology and Community Health*, *66*(12): 1182–6.

Deidda, M., Geue, C., Kreif, N., Dundas, R., and McIntosh, E., 2019. A framework for conducting economic evaluations alongside natural experiments. *Social Science and Medicine*, 220: 353-61.

Elliot, J.H., Turner, T., Clavisi, O., Thomas, J., Higgins, J.P.T., Mavergames, C., and Gruen, R.L., 2014. Living systematic reviews: An emerging opportunity to narrow the evidence–practice gap. *PLoS Medicine*, *11*(2): e1001603. doi:10.1371-journal.pmed.1001603. papers3://publication/doi/10.1371/journal.pmed.1001603.g001.

Equity Checklist for Systematic Review Authors. 2012. <http://methods.cochrane.org/sites/methods.cochrane.org.equity/files/public/uploads/EquityChecklist2012.pdf> (Accessed 14 October 2018).

Fischer, A.J., Threlfall, A., Meah, S., Cookson, R., Rutter, H., and Kelly, M.P., 2013. The appraisal of PHIs: An overview. *Journal of Public Health*, *35*(4): 488–94.

Flowers, P., Wu, O., Lorimer, K., Ahmed, B., Hesselgreaves, H., MacDonald, J., Cayless, S., et al., 2017. The clinical effectiveness of individual behaviour change interventions to reduce risky sexual behaviour after a negative human immunodeficiency virus test in men who have sex with men: Systematic and realist reviews and intervention development. *Health Technology Assessment*, *21*(5): 1–164.

Greenhalgh, T., Kristjansson, E., and Robinson, V., 2007. Realist review to understand the efficacy of school feeding programmes. *British Medical Journal*, *335*(7625): 858–61.

Harden, A. and Thomas, J., 2005. Methodological issues in combining diverse study types in systematic reviews. *International Journal of Social Research Methodology*, 8(3): 257–71.

Hardwick, R.1., Pearson, M., Byng, R., and Anderson, R., 2013. The effectiveness and cost-effectiveness of shared care: protocol for a realist review. *Systematic Reviews*, 2(12). doi:10.1186/2046-4053-2-12.

Higgins, J.P.T., Altman, D.G., Gotzsche, P.C., Juni, P., Moher, D., Oxman, A.D., Savovic, J., et al., 2011. The Cochrane Collaboration's Tool for Assessing Risk of Bias in Randomised Trials. *British Medical Journal*, 343(Oct18 2): d5928–d5928. <http://www.bmj.com/cgi/doi/10.1136/bmj.d5928> (Accessed 14 October 2018).

Higgins, J.P.T., and Green, S. (eds), 2011. *Cochrane Handbook for Systematic Reviews of Interventions Version 5.1.0 (Updated March 2011)*. Available from <http://handbook.cochrane.org: The Cochrane Collaboration>.

Jagosh, J., Macaulay, A.C., Pluye, P., Salsberg, J., Bush, P.L., Henderson, J., Sirett, E., Wong, G., e al., 2012. Uncovering the benefits of participatory research: Implications of a realist review for health research and practice. *Milbank Quarterly*, 90(2): 311–46.

Kneale, D., Thomas, J., and Harris, K., 2015. Developing and optimising the use of logic models in systematic reviews: Exploring practice and good practice in the use of programme theory in reviews. *PLoS ONE*, 10(11): 1–26. <http://dx.doi.org/10.1371/journal.pone.0142187> (Accessed 14 October 2018).

Lefebvre, C., Glanville, J., Wieland, L.S., Coles, B., and Weightman, A.L., 2013. Methodological developments in searching for studies for systematic reviews: Past, present and future? *Systematic Reviews*, 2: 78. <https://www.scopus.com/inward/record.uri?eid=2-s2.0-84888333320&partnerID=40&md5=1bfa7344c017a96b16aa52a856b510cc> (Accessed 14 October 2018).

Lewin, S., Hendry, M., Chandler, J., Oxman, A.D., Michie, S., Shepperd, S., Reeves, B.C., et al., 2017. Assessing the complexity of interventions within systematic reviews: Development, content and use of a new tool (ICAT-SR). *BMC Medical Research Methodology*, 17(1): 1–13.

Melendez-Torres, G.J., Bonell, C., and Thomas, J., 2015. Emergent approaches to the meta-analysis of multiple heterogeneous complex interventions data collection, quality, and reporting. *BMC Medical Research Methodology*, 15(1): 1–7. <http://dx.doi.org/10.1186/s12874-015-0040-z> (Accessed 14 October 2018).

Minelli, C. and Baio, G., 2015. Value of information: A tool to improve research prioritization and reduce waste. *PLoS Medicine*, **12**(9): 1–5.

Moher, D., Liberati, A., Tetzlaff, J., Altman, D.G., the PRISMA Group, 2009. Preferred Reporting Items for Systematic Reviews and Meta-Analyses: The PRISMA Statement. *PLoS Medicine*, **6**(7): e1000097. papers3://publication/uuid/B4EE4872-54E8-4846-B947-949E3AE1855B.

National Institute for Health and Care Excellence. 2013. Guide to the Methods of Technology Appraisal 2013. *National Institute for Health and Care Excellence*, (April): 1–93. <https://www.nice.org.uk/process/pmg9/resources/guide-to-the-methods-of-technology-appraisal-2013-pdf-2007975843781> (Accessed 12 November 2018).

National Institute for Health and Care Excellence. 2012. Methods for the development of NICE Public Health Guidance (3rd edn). *National Institute of Health and Clinical Excellence*, (September): 284. <https://www.nice.org.uk/process/pmg4/resources/methods-for-the-development-of-nice-public-health-guidance-third-edition-pdf-2007967445701> (Accessed 14 October 2018).

O'Brien, T.D., Noyes, J., Spencer, L.H., Kubis, H.-P., Hastings, R.P., and **Whitaker, R.**, 2016. Systematic review of physical activity and exercise interventions to improve health, fitness and well-being of children and young people who use wheelchairs. *British Medical Journal Open: Sport & Exercise Medicine*, **2**(1): e000109.

Ogilvie, D., Fayter, D., Petticrew, M., Sowden, A., Thomas, S., Whitehead, M., and **Worthy, G.**, 2008. The harvest plot: A method for synthesising evidence about the differential effects of interventions. *BMC Medical Research Methodology*, **8**(8):1–7.

Pawson, R. and Tilley, N., 1997. *Realistic Evaluation*. London: Sage.

Pawson, R., Greenhalgh, T., Harvey, G., and Walshe, K., 2005. Realist review: A new method of systematic review designed for complex policy interventions. *Journal of Health Services Research and Policy*, **10**(Suppl 1): 21–34.

Pearson, M., Hunt, H., Cooper, C., Shepperd, S., Pawson, R., and Anderson, R., 2013. Intermediate care: A realist review and conceptual framework. <http://www.netscc.ac.uk/hsdr/files/project/SDO_FR_10-1012-07_V01.pdf> (Accessed 12 November 2018).

Pearson, A., White, H., Bath-Hextall, F., Salmond, S., Apostolo, J., and Kirkpatrick, P., 2015. A mixed-methods approach to systematic reviews. *International Journal of Evidence Based health care*, **13**(3): 121–31. doi:10.1097/XEB.0000000000000052.

Petticrew, M., Anderson, L., Elder, R., Grimshaw, J., Hopkins, D., Hahn, R., Krause, L., et al., 2015. Complex interventions and their implications for systematic Reviews: A pragmatic approach. *International Journal of Nursing Studies*, **52**(7): 1211–16. <http://dx.doi.org/10.1016/j.jclinepi.2013.06.004> (Accessed 114 October 2018).

Petticrew, M. 2015. Time to rethink the systematic review catechism? Moving from 'what works' to 'what happens'. *Systematic Reviews*, **4**(1): 1–6.

Rycroft-Malone, J., McCormack, B., Hutchinson, A.M., DeCorby, K., Bucknall, T.K., Kent, B., Schultz, A., et al., 2012. Realist synthesis: Illustrating the method for implementation research. *Implementation Science*, **19**(7): 33. doi:10.1186/1748-5908-7-33.

Sandelowski, M., Voils, C.I., and Barroso, J., 2006. Defining and designing mixed research synthesis studies. *Research Scholarship*, **13**(1): 29

Sanson-Fisher, R.W., Bonevski, B., Green, L.W., and D'Este, C., 2007. Limitations of the randomized controlled trial in evaluating population-based health interventions. *American Journal of Preventive Medicine*, **33**(2): 155–61.

Schardt, C., Adams, M.B., Owens, T., Keitz, S., and Fontelo, P., 2007. Utilization of the PICO framework to improve searching PubMed for clinical questions. *BMC Medical Informatics and Decision Making*, **7**: 1–6.

Thomas, J. and Harden, A., 2008. Methods for the thematic synthesis of qualitative research in systematic reviews. *BMC Medical Research Methodol*, **8**: 45.

Thomas, J., Harden, A., Oakley, A., Oliver, S., Sutcliffe, K., Rees, R., Brunton, G., et al., 2004. Integrating qualitative research with trials in systematic reviews. *British Medical Journal*, **328**: 1010–12

Turley, R., Saith, R., Bhan, N., Doyle, J., Jones, K., and Waters, E., 2013. Slum upgrading review: Methodological challenges that arise in systematic reviews of complex interventions. *Journal of Public Health*, **35**(1): 171–5.

Welch, V., Petticrew, M., Tugwell, P., Moher, D., O'Neill, J., Waters, E., White, H., the PRISMA-Equity Bellagio group, 2012. PRISMA-Equity 2012 Extension: Reporting guidelines for systematic reviews with a focus on health equity. *PLoS Medicine*, **9**(10).

Welch, V.A., Petticrew, M., O'Neill, J., Waters, E., Armstrong, R., Bhutta, Z.A., Francis, D., et al., 2013. Health equity: Evidence synthesis and knowledge translation methods. *Systematic Reviews*, 2(1): 43.

Welton, N.J., Sutton, A.J., Copper, N.J., and Abrams, K., 2012. Expected value of information for research prioritization and study design. In: *Evidence Synthesis for Decision Making in health care* (Welton, N.J., Sutton, A.J., Copper, N.J., and Abrams, K., eds) Wiley, pp. 251–69.

Welton, N.J., Caldwell, D.M., Adamopoulos, E., and Vedhara, K., 2009. Mixed treatment comparison meta-analysis of complex interventions: Psychological interventions in coronary heart disease. *American Journal of Epidemiology*, 169(9): 1158–65.

Wong, G., Greenhalgh, T., Westhorp, G., Buckingham, J., and Pawson, R., 2013. RAMESES publication standards: Realist syntheses. *BMC Medicine*, 11(1): 21. doi:10.1186/1741-7015-11-21.

Chapter 5

Identification, measurement, and valuation of resource use in economic evaluations of public health interventions

Carys Jones, Joanna M. Charles, and Rhiannon T. Edwards

5.1 Introduction

To support fully informed resource allocation decision-making, the costs and benefits of competing options need to be evaluated. Identifying and measuring the resources used for each option is one of the first steps that needs to be carried out before an economic evaluation of a public health intervention (PHI) can take place.

This chapter outlines approaches to the identification, measurement, and valuation of resource use alongside trials and other study designs. As outlined in Chapter 3 in this book, PHIs are often complex in nature, which has implications for the methods used to identify, measure, and value resource use as well as the breadth of coverage (e.g. health and social care, education, and judicial sectors) (Weatherly et al., 2009). The methods described are relevant for interventions in National Health Service (NHS) settings, workplace, school, and other settings. The identification of resource-use parameters for inclusion in modelling studies, often used to extrapolate findings over a longer time period or different population group (Squires et al., 2016), is discussed in Chapter 11 of this book.

Accounting costs and economic costs differ. Whilst accountants are interested in the monetary cost of resources, health economists are interested in the opportunity cost (Russell, 1992). The opportunity cost is the true value of using resources and can be thought of as the value of 'benefits forgone' by not using resources for their next best alternative use. Putting it another way, the opportunity cost of investing in a health care intervention is best measured by the health benefits (life years saved, quality-adjusted life years (QALYs) gained) that could have been achieved had the money been spent on the next best alternative intervention or health care programme (Palmer and Raftery, 1999; Russell, 1992). Pragmatically however, it is easier to measure monetary cost than opportunity cost, which is why researchers seeking to estimate the cost of setting up and delivering a PHI will typically calculate the monetary cost rather than opportunity cost (Morris et al., 2007; Drummond et al., 2015).

We begin this chapter by discussing the types of costs used in economic evaluation, before moving on to discuss elements of costing of particular importance to the economic evaluation of PHIs including: choice of perspective; multi-sectoral costing; sources of unit costs; time horizon; discounting, and incorporating uncertainty. A micro-costing case study within a PHI economic evaluation is presented later in this chapter. There are excellent existing texts which also cover the principles of costing in economic evaluation more generally (e.g. Drummond et al., 2015).

5.2 Types of costs used in economic evaluation

A summary of the categories of cost with examples from a clinical setting and a non-clinical (school) setting are summarized in Table 5.1.

Table 5.1 Summary of the categories of cost with examples from a clinical setting and a non-clinical (school) setting

Type of cost	Description	Clinical setting example (GP clinic)	Non-clinical setting example (school)
Direct	Costs that are directly associated with the programme under evaluation (e.g. equipment)	Staff costs (both monetary and opportunity costs) for a nurse to deliver a smoking cessation service	Teacher time (both monetary and opportunity costs) to deliver an anti-bullying intervention
Indirect	Costs that are associated with the programme under evaluation, but are not directly attributable	Loss of earnings for the individual to attend the smoking cessation service appointment during working hours	Parental loss of wages to meet with school to discuss bullying incidents
Intangible	Costs that are associated with concepts that are difficult to quantify and measure (e.g. pain and anxiety)	Cravings during first few days of nicotine withdrawal	Emotional distress of child who is being bullied
Marginal	Costs of providing one more unit of a good or service	Treating one additional person at the smoking cessation service	Rolling out the anti-bullying intervention to an additional year group in the school
Incremental	Additional costs incurred by one service compared to another	The additional cost of providing the smoking cessation service by a nurse compared to providing the service through a smoking cessation leaflet service	The additional cost of providing the anti-bullying intervention by a school teacher compared to providing the intervention through a mobile phone app or other online service

5.2.1 **Direct costs**

Direct costs are directly associated with the programme under evaluation, such as staff salaries, equipment, capital and overhead costs of running a public health initiative. Direct costs can be either medical (e.g. drugs) or non-medical (e.g. transportation costs for attending a clinic). Direct costs are often incurred by the service provider, but can also be incurred by the person receiving treatment through out-of-pocket expenses such as paying for parking tickets.

Within direct costs, we can further categorize by fixed, semi-fixed, and variable costs. Fixed costs are usually the capital and overhead costs for a service; these costs do not depend on the level of activity and will be incurred whether a person attends their appointment or not (e.g. heating and lighting for the building). Semi-fixed costs include staffing costs; they are fixed to a certain degree, but if extra staff are employed to deal with higher than expected attendance rates the cost of providing the service increases. Variable costs vary by the amount of activity at an appointment; for example, some people attending an asthma clinic may be offered an allergy test while others will not. For an example of the types of direct costs associated with obesity, see the systematic review by Withrow and Alter (2011). Further detail on the estimation of overhead costs and superannuation is available in Curtis and Burns (2017).

5.2.2 **Indirect costs**

Indirect costs are the costs associated with lost productivity, such as a person's lost wages due to missing work, or their income forgone due to a premature death. Indirect costs can also fall on people other than the person receiving treatment; for example, other members of the family may take time off work to provide childcare so that a patient is able to attend a clinic for treatment. Importantly, productivity 'costs' can also be positive and be measured in the form of productivity 'gains' arising through improved health and subsequent return to work.

5.2.3 **Intangible costs**

Intangible costs are the costs associated with the pain, anxiety or distress of receiving treatment. Quantifying subjective feelings is possible using an appropriate outcome measure (see Younger et al., 2009 for a review of instruments for measuring pain); however, assigning a monetary value to intangible costs, which would be required for a cost–benefit analysis (CBA) (see Chapter 9 of this book) or social return on investment (SROI) analysis (see Chapter 12 of this book), can be challenging. Contingent valuation methods are often used to value intangible outcomes, for example willingness to pay (WTP) to avoid or achieve an outcome, or willingness to accept (WTA) monetary compensation to forego a positive outcome or to accept a negative outcome. Caution needs to be taken when employing contingent valuation methods. Bayoumi notes that bias may be introduced through the way that questions are framed, the way that extreme responses are interpreted, the way that respondents are selected (general population or affected individuals), and the way that individuals understand and interpret gains relative to losses (Bayoumi, 2004).

5.2.4 **Marginal costs**

The marginal cost is the cost of producing one more unit of a good or service, for example treating one additional person at a smoking cessation clinic. Due to diminishing returns, the marginal cost of producing an additional unit increases at higher levels of output; for example, the smoking cessation clinic may have a relatively low marginal cost for treating each of the first 50 people attending it, but for the 51st person onwards the clinic may need to increase their staffing levels, resulting in higher marginal costs to treat person 51 onwards. In economics, the optimal level to produce a good or service occurs at the point where the marginal cost is equal to the marginal revenue/benefit (the additional revenue/benefit generated by producing/consuming one more unit of output), as this is where the total profit is maximized.

5.2.5 **Incremental costs**

Incremental costs are the additional costs incurred in providing one service compared to another service (Drummond et al., 2015). For example, the incremental cost of replacing 'standard care' with a new health care initiative is the cost differential between the new initiative and the current practice. Analysis of incremental costs and benefits through the calculation of an incremental cost-effectiveness ratio (ICER) [see Chapter 2] is central to cost-effectiveness analysis (CEA) and cost-utility analysis (CUA); see Chapters 7 and 8 for further detail.

5.3 **Choice of perspective in economic evaluation**

Before starting an economic evaluation, it is important to consider which perspective will be used. The perspective is the point of view that will be used when measuring resources and evaluating costs and outcomes. It is often selected based depending upon the purpose of the evaluation and which costs and outcomes are relevant.

PHIs can be complex, targeting a number of different stakeholders and outcomes. The National Institute for Health and Care Excellence (NICE) recommend a public sector perspective for such PHI econonomic evalautions, this perspective includes the NHS, personal social services, and local government (National Institute for Health and Care Excellence, 2012). In comparison, for technology appraisals NICE recommends the use of an NHS and personal social services-only perspective (National Institute for Health and Care Excellence, 2013). The choice of a broader perspective for PHIs reflects the wider remit of PHIs and breadth of sectors likely to bear costs and receive benefits (Weatherly et al., 2009). A societal perspective may also be used in economic evaluations of PHIs. The societal perspective encompasses direct, indirect, and intangible costs and is even broader than the public sector perspective, which is apt as PHIs typically seek to improve health and well-being at a population level.

Employer and patient/client perspectives are less commonly used in economic evaluations of PHIs. The employer perspective includes direct costs and indirect costs such as loss of productivity due to illness. A recent PHI evaluation of a employee physical activity card scheme revealed that indeed the only scenario to be cost-beneficial was that from the employer perspective, namely when impacts on absenteeism were included (Hunter et al., 2018). The patient/client perspective includes direct, indirect, and intangible costs but is focused more narrowly on the individuals directly affected by an intervention rather than on population-level effects.

The broader the perspective used, the more challenging the task of identifying and measuring resource use across multiple agencies (see Table 5.2). One benefit of a wider prespective is transparency, as costs cannot be 'shifted' into other sectors to make an initiative appear more favourable. On the other hand, time and funding constraints may prevent a broad perspective being used (Byford and Raftery, 1998). McCabe argues economic evaluations should endeavour to capture all credible related costs and outcomes (McCabe, 2018). For resource allocation decisions, the appropriate scope for costs and benefits should be informed by the decision-maker. However, when the budget is fixed, care should be taken not to extend the scope beyond direct costs and benefits resulting from the intervention under consideration. McCabe argues the inclusion of wider costs and benefits may lead to unintended effects on the distribution of health and access to health care for which the decision-maker is responsible. When the scope is required to be extended, the economic evaluation should endeavour to identify those individuals or households who will bear the opportunity cost, so decision-makers can assess the impact of their decision (McCabe, 2018).

There are also wider considerations such as spillover effects to be aware of when identifying, measuring, and valuing resource use to be included in an economic evaluation of a PHI. Spillover effects refer to a secondary effect that follows from a primary effect; for example, a lifestyle and diet intervention to improve health aimed at one family member may improve the health of all family members as their living situation causes them to adopt changes to their diet and lifestyle. Brouwer argues that spillover effects should be taken into consideration when undertaking economic evaluations, as they may provide large health and wellbeing effects in caregivers and family members (Brouwer, 2018). Brouwer states that ignoring such effects in economic evaluations may result in decisions being made that do not improve health or welfare (Brouwer, 2018). In contrast to Brouwer, McCabe (2018) argues that spillover effects should not be routinely included in economic evaluations, as they increase inequity in the value and voice of those who bear the cost of funding decisions. Brouwer notes that more work is needed in this area, as the more we learn about spillover effects, the better we will be in estimating them to assist decision-making (Brouwer, 2018).

The economic evaluation framework used may also influence the choice of perspective; CEAs generally take a public sector perspective, whereas CBAs generally take a societal perspective. Cost–consequence analyses (CCAs) also take a societal perspective

Table 5.2 Common perspectives and types of costs used in economic evaluation

	NHS and personal social services	Public sector	Societal	Employer	Patient
Direct costs	Y	Y	Y	Y	Y
Indirect costs	N	N	Y	Y	Y
Intangible costs	N	N	Y	N	Y

typically and are useful for complex PHI interventions because they present costs and consequences in a disaggregated form, allowing readers and decision-makers to assess the impact of an intervention on health and non-health outcomes across sectors. CCA is discussed further in Chapter 10.

5.4 **Identifying and measuring resource-use data**

Once the perspective of the evaluation has been chosen, and therefore the relevant costs and outcomes to measure have been identified, data collection can begin. The costs of setting up and delivering an intervention need to be identified, as well as the costs of resource use by participants in a study; for example GP visits, nights in hospital, and contacts with social care services.

A top-down or bottom-up approach can be used for costing. A top-down approach uses total costs generated through information about budgets for the delivery of a programme (e.g. overheads, administration, staff costs, and consumables) to produce an average cost per person. The advantage of taking a top-down approach is that it requires less resource-intensive data collection. The disadvantage of a top-down approach is that it does not consider variation; a top-down costing of participants' resource use would assume that all people have used resources equally.

A bottom-up approach uses individual-level data to calculate total costs. Bottom-up costing is also known as micro-costing. Identifying and measuring data for a bottom-up/micro-costing approach are more resource-intensive on the part of the researcher; however, the richer data allow analyses to take into account the variation between individuals and settings. A worked example of a micro-costing exercise of setting up and delivering a parenting programme (Charles et al., 2013) is presented in section 5.10.

There are two main methods for measuring individual level resource-use data:

1. Asking the person (or their carer if relevant) to recall their frequency and duration of contacts with relevant health and social care services during a given period.

2. Extracting routinely collected information from health and social care databases, and the use of linked databases.

Asking people to recall their resource use over previous months can be challenging, especially when individuals are too young to be interviewed or have a cognitive impairment such as dementia or learning difficulties (Thorn et al., 2013). The optimal patient recall period is uncertain (Clarke et al., 2008); however, a survey of resource-use measures found six months or less to be the most commonly asked recall period (Ridyard et al., 2012).

An alternative to asking people to recall their own service use is asking family or staff carers to report as a proxy on the individuals' resource use. In trials, researchers can give participants a diary at the start of the study to keep a record of their resource use as and when it happens, which avoids the need for them to attempt to recall resource use over the previous months at the end of the trial. The Database of Instruments for Resource Use Measurement (DIRUM; <http://www.dirum.org/>) has been developed as an online repository for researchers to share resource-use measures that have been used for trial-based economic evaluations. However, resource-use measures are equally important for cohort and other study designs, the DIRUM repository and lessons from previous research may be appropriate in these other types of research design.

Figure 5.1 shows an extract of the resource-use questionnaire that was used in the Depression in Visual Impairment (DEPVIT) trial (Margrain et al., 2012). DEPVIT was a trial of a preventative intervention, which evaluated problem-solving therapy or GP referral for people with depression and visual impairment compared to a waiting list control (Margrain et al., 2012). The prevalence of depression in patients accessing vision rehabilitation services has been estimated to be approximately 30 per cent (Brody et al., 2001); however, depression screening and referral for treatment is not routinely embedded in vision rehabilitation services. In DEPVIT, a researcher conducted telephone interviews with both control group and intervention group participants at the start of the trial (baseline) and six months later to collect information about their service use over the previous months. Participants were asked whether their contacts with key health and social care services were related to depression, vision, or other reasons. Information on community-based resource use, hospital services, and prescribed medication was collected.

When measuring individual level resource-use data, a balance between the quantity of information requested and the burden on participants of completing questionnaires should be considered. This will vary between trials depending on the nature of the trial population (e.g. cognitively impaired or not), the number of other outcome measures that people are expected to complete, and the number of assessment points in the trial. The longer a questionnaire takes to complete, the more likely it is that a participant will stop part way through, resulting in missing data. In trials taking place in a workplace or school setting, it may be possible to obtain certain routine data, such as sickness absence, through organization records.

Obtaining resource-use information from routinely collected health and social care data removes the burden from participants. Participants' consent is required to access their personal data if researchers choose to use this method for data collection. In cases where resource-use records are held centrally and the research team have ethics approval and participants' consent, data for the relevant participants can be extracted and sent to the researcher in a spreadsheet format. Under new General Data Protection Regulations (GDPR), which came into force in May 2018; researchers should ensure they have informed consent from participants, including consent to access digital information, if applicable. Under GDPR regulations, researchers should also ensure they provide participants with information about how their data will be used and stored (Information Commissioner's Office, 2018). The Hospital Episode Statistics (HES) database (<http://www.hscic.gov.uk/hes>) is an example of centrally held information; it contains records on all hospital stays for patients in England. HES data cover hospital activity relating to in-patient, out-patient, and accident and emergency. The Health & Social Care Information Centre (HSCIC) runs the HES service. The Secure Anonymized Information Linkage (SAIL) Databank (<http://www.saildatabank.com/>) in Wales and the Scottish Informatics System (SHIP) (<http://www.scot-ship.ac.uk/>) in Scotland also contain datasets on health service use. When centrally held records of routinely collected data are not available, the study research team have the more

1.1 Community Based Service

Use Interviewer instructions: Please complete the table to show the community based services that the participant has used over the last 6 months.

Service [Used by participant]	No. of home visits (see key)			No. of visits to surgery or clinic (see key)			Provider agency (please tick)				Average duration of contact (minutes)
	E	D	O	E	D	O	NHS	Local authority	Voluntary organi sation	Private organi sation	
General practitioner [GP]											
Practice nurse (GP Clinic)											
District Nurse											
Health Visitor											
Community Psychiatrist											
Psychologist											
Therapist /Counsellor											
Community Psychiatric Nurse / Mental Health Nurse											
Mental health worker (unknown)											
Physiotherapist											
Occupational therapist											

Key:
E: eyesight
D: depression
O: other

Figure 5.1 Extract from the resource use questionnaire used in the DEPVIT trial.

time-consuming task of requesting physical access to participants' records and manually copying down the required information. It is important to build a good relationship between the research team and staff at sites where information is being collected and stored in this manner.

A disadvantage of using electronic records to measure resource-use data is that at present, information about health and social care records are stored separately. However, there are efforts to link health and social care records, for example the SAIL Databank in Wales and the SHIP Databank in Scotland.

5.5 Multi-sectoral costing in public health economic evaluation

PHIs often require the measurement of multi-sectoral impacts, as they may have benefits that are felt across many sectors, including health care, social care, education, and justice. Collecting information on resource use across sectors poses challenges. When using patient report questionnaires or proxies, questions can be included to obtain the impact across many sectors. However, if the research team is extracting individual-level resource-use data from the centrally held records of multiple agencies there is the challenge of linking the datasets. If the research team intends to copy data manually from patient records, access to the data may need to be negotiated separately with each agency and the logistics of visiting multiple sites should be considered. Linking large electronic datasets will become increasingly important in public health research.

5.6 Valuation of resource use: sources of unit costs for public health economic evaluation

Once the resource use has been identified and measured, the next step is to apply unit costs to the trial or other study design data i.e. to 'value' these resources. As mentioned at the start of this chapter, opportunity cost is often difficult to measure in reality and consequently economists typically use monetary costs as a proxy for opportunity cost.

As discussed in Chapter 2 of this book, when the market for a good or service is functioning efficiently and without distortion, the monetary cost is the market price of the good or service. In economic costing it is usual practice to take the market price of a good or service and multiply it by the quantity of the good or service used to calculate the total cost (Morris et al., 2007; Drummond et al., 2015).

Where available, national unit costs are the preferred source of unit costs (National Institute for Health and Care Excellence, 2013; Glick et al., 2014). Using national unit costs allows for consistency and comparability across evaluations. The Personal Social Services Research Unit (PSSRU) at the University of Kent publishes updated UK unit costs for a range of health and social care professionals annually (Curtis and Burns, 2017). The data is collated from a number of sources and presented broken down by key components; for example, for a practice nurse the costs are broken down into wages, salary on-costs, qualifications, and overheads. Workload information, such as the average length of a consultation and the average number of working hours per week are also given. Researchers can then choose between different units of measurement (e.g. the hourly cost or the average appointment cost) for their costing analysis as appropriate.

National unit costs for medications are available for England, Wales, Scotland, and Northern Ireland separately (see <https://digital.nhs.uk/data-and-information/publications/statistical/prescription-cost-analysis> for links to the national sites). The prescription cost analysis sheets hold information on the number of thousands of prescriptions made for each medication annually, as well as the unit cost per item of medication.

National unit costs for secondary health care services, such as hospital procedures, are available at <https://improvement.nhs.uk/resources/reference-costs/>. The UK's Department of Health collects the cost data from NHS providers in England annually to produce the average unit cost of services such as day cases, elective inpatient stays, surgical procedures, and rehabilitation. Groupings of treatments that use common levels of health care resources are called Health Resource Groups (HRGs), and these can also be used as a source of costs. HRG currencies cover a spell of care from admission to discharge. When a patient is discharged, clinical coders categorize their care into codes using the ICD-10 and OPCS-4 classification systems. Patient data is then submitted to a national database called the Secondary Uses Service, and clinical codes are grouped into HRGs to calculate the payment to the hospital.

In cases where there are no monetary transactions for a good or service, for example informal care time, assumptions need to be made about the value of the good or service. For informal carers, the opportunity cost of their time may be lost wages if they are in employment, or leisure time foregone if they are not in employment. Shadow prices can be estimated through identifying a similar good or service that does have a market price; for example, the market price of employing a home care assistant may be used as a shadow price for informal care.

5.7 **Time horizon and discounting**

It is recommended that resource-use data be measured for as long as effects relating to the intervention are present (Elliott and Payne, 2005; National Institute for Health and Care Excellence, 2012). However, this is not always practical for PHIs that are expected to accrue benefits over a long-term time period. NICE guidance suggests that a time horizon of less than a lifetime can be justified if there is no differential mortality effect between the intervention and control groups, and if the differences in costs and other outcomes relate to a shorter period (National Institute for Health and Care Excellence, 2012). For infectious disease modelling a time horizon of greater than the individual lifetime may be appropriate; see Chapter 11 of this book for further details.

When costs are incurred over a period of longer than one year, adjustment for differential timing is needed (Glick et al., 2014). Inflation and time preference need to be considered for this. Inflation refers to the general trend for prices to increase over time. Adjustment for inflation is only needed when unit costs from different price years are used within the same evaluation. Time preference refers to consumers' valuation of a good or service differing depending on when it is consumed. Time preferences can be related to individual decisions, or societal preferences for the well-being of others; see

Chapter 3 of this book for more detail. As a society we tend to have a positive rate of time preference; being given £100 today is valued more highly than being given £100 in five years' time. Discounting is used to express costs occurring in the future (FV) in present day values. The formula for discounting costs is:

$$\mathrm{Present\ value} = FV \times \frac{1}{(1+r)^t}$$

Where r is the discount rate and t is the time period. In the United Kingdom, 3.5 per cent is commonly used as the discount rate (H.M. Treasury, 2018). A discount rate of 3.5% is also the rate recommended in the NICE reference case for technology appraisals (National Institute for Health and Care Excellence, 2013), with a suggested sensitivity analysis using a discount rate of 1.5 per cent for both costs and health effects. Conversely, as the effects of PHIs typically last over a longer time horizon, the recommended discount rate in the NICE reference case for PHIs is 1.5 per cent for the base case analysis and 3.5 per cent for the sensitivity analysis (National Institute for Health and Care Excellence, 2012).

5.8 Incorporating uncertainty

All economic evaluations will have a degree of uncertainty; however, explicitly stating all of the assumptions underpinning the costing and the sources of the unit costs used allows readers to assess the degree of uncertainty present in the costing.

Conducting a sensitivity analysis, where key parameters are varied one at a time while holding all others constant, is one method of assessing how sensitive the results of an evaluation are to the assumptions made. Sensitivity analyses can be deterministic or probabilistic. In deterministic sensitivity analysis, parameters and their associated values are varied manually one at a time (e.g. varying the cost of the intervention based on differing staffing levels or salary bands) (Briggs et al., 2012). Conversely, in probabilistic sensitivity analysis all parameters are varied simultaneously, using parameter values sampled from *a priori*-defined probability distributions, for example, using boot-strapping techniques or Monte Carlo simulation (Briggs et al., 2012).

Resource-use cost data is typically positively skewed; more people tend to be at the lower end of the resource-use scale, with fewer high-cost outliers. Presenting the range of costs is more informative than presenting the standard deviation for a skewed distribution. Skewed data violate the assumptions of a normal distribution; therefore, consideration needs to be given as to whether to use parametric or non-parametric statistical tests when analysing the data. Parametric tests may still be used with skewed data when the sample size is large.

5.9 Reporting cost information in published economic studies

The Consolidated Health Economic Evaluation Reporting Standards (CHEERS) statement (Husereau et al., 2013) was developed to promote transparency and structure

---

Box 5.1 Highlighted items from the CHEERS checklist relating to reporting costs

- Study perspective: this affects the range of costs included in the evaluation
- Time horizon over which costs and outcomes are being evaluated
- Discount rate used for costs and outcomes
- Estimating resources and costs: describing the approach used to estimate resource use
- Currency, price rate, and conversion: describing methods for converting costs into a common currency and price year
- Incremental costs and outcomes
- Characterising heterogeneity: reporting differences in costs and outcomes that can be explained by variations between subgroups of patients with different baseline characteristics

---

in the reporting of health economic evaluations. A task force consisting of editors of health economic journals and content experts from around the world were involved with the process, and the resulting guidance was co-published in ten journals to ensure wide dissemination. The 24-item CHEERS checklist contains 7 items relating to reporting costs, described in Box 5.1.

Concerns have been raised about the completeness of the CHEERS checklist for reporting cost–benefit analysis (Sanghera et al., 2015), specifically around the lack of information required to be reported on preference elicitation formats and payment vehicles. However, the authors of the CHEERS statement have acknowledged that the checklist reflects the current emphasis on cost-effectiveness analysis in published literature, and it is still appropriate for reporting cost–benefit analyses (Husereau et al., 2015). The CHEERS checklist is due to be reviewed every five years and a document elaborating how cost–benefit analyses can be reported using CHEERS may be an output of the next guidance revision.

5.10 Micro-costing of an intervention: A worked example of costing a parenting programme

Adverse Childhood Experiences (ACEs) such as neglect, abuse, and exposure to a harmful living environment contribute to poorer health and social prospects in later life (Ford et al., 2016). Behavioural and emotional problems in childhood that are not addressed can have long-term consequences on the health and socio-economic status of individuals. The societal costs of conduct disorder are large; it has been estimated that preventing conduct disorder in children could save £150,000 per child with conduct disorder over the course of their lifetime (Friedli and Parsonage, 2009). A review of early intervention initiatives found that there was the potential to make long-term savings in public spending by investing in programmes that promote strong social and emotional foundations for children, particularly the most vulnerable (Allen, 2011).

In this section we present a trial based example of a micro-costing, or bottom-up costing, of setting up and delivering the Incredible Years (IY) parenting programme (Charles et al., 2013). This micro-costing was conducted from a public sector, multi-agency perspective as a component of a pragmatic randomized controlled trial (RCT) evaluating the IY Toddler Parenting Programme in Wales. The IY Toddler Parenting Programme is an evidence-based 12-week programme, which teaches praise, promotes children's self-esteem, teaches coping strategies, and encourages social and emotion competences. Two group leaders delivered weekly 2–2.5 hour sessions attended by a maximum of 10 parents. In the trial, group leaders were typically health visitors and childcare practitioners.

Case study

Micro-Costing Framework for the IY Toddler Parenting Programme Example

Charles, J.M., Edwards, R.T., Bywater, T., and Hutchings, J. Micro-costing in public health economics: Steps towards a standardized framework, using the Incredible Years Toddler Parenting Program as a worked example. *Prevention Science* 2013, *14*:377–89.

Step 1—Development of cost diaries

A cost diary developed with group leader focus groups and the IY Wales Centre by Edwards and colleagues was used in the current RCT to establish the costs to set up and deliver the IY Toddler Parenting Program (Edwards et al., 2007). Activities such as the purchase of raffle prizes, felt-tip pens, paper, and photocopying were listed as examples under the heading of 'administrative costs' in the diary to guide and inform leaders. The categories were listed in a spreadsheet, with a column for each week of programme delivery.

Step 2—Cost data gathering from group leaders taking part in the RCT

Group leaders were first contacted by the first author (JMC) by phone to explain the study, and to ask if they would consent to completing a cost diary. We endeavored to obtain diaries from every group leader participating in the RCT in order to provide us with as much cost information as possible. Ten of the 18 group leaders consented to complete the diaries. Costs were gathered from two of the three groups in South Wales, two of the five groups in North Wales, and the single group run in Mid Wales. Eight leaders were unable to complete cost diaries due to time restrictions.

The consenting group leaders received the diary via email as a spreadsheet. Group leaders were requested to give as much detail as possible about length of time spent on different tasks; for example, travel to group sessions, room preparation, and running the group sessions. The leaders completed their electronic diaries weekly, and returned their completed cost diary by e-mail at the end of the 12 weeks to the first author. Leaders received a £20 book token in recognition of their time in completing the diary. During engagement and recruitment of parents, 8 of the 10 group leaders stated the same amount of time to complete these tasks; therefore, the mode values were used in the tables. In the case of group running costs such as time to prepare the room for the session, time to conduct catch-up home visits, costs of crèche facilities, rental of halls, and additional administrative costs, the group leaders provided a range of time taken and costs. Therefore, a mean was calculated to provide the average cost for these tasks across the groups and was presented in the tables. It should be noted that the ranges and standard deviations for these costs were small, and the final costs reported in the table were endorsed by the leaders who completed the diaries.

Step 3—Cost data gathering from additional sources as required

Gathering cost data from additional sources was necessary to ascertain costs not retrieved through the diaries (e.g. salaries of group leaders, group material costs, and training costs). We used national costs where available, and referred to service managers and the IY Wales Centre when these costs were unavailable. The hourly wage for health visitors was extracted from the UK Health and Social Care Unit Costs (Curtis, 2008) to provide a UK-average hourly wage for health visitors, which was checked and approved by the group leaders and service managers. The hourly wage for childcare practitioners was calculated as an average from information provided by a range of participating service managers whose services deliver the IY programme. An additional 25 per cent was added to the childcare practitioner wage for national insurance and superannuation. The hourly wage presented in the tables shows the mean wage for group leaders, which formed the basis for calculation of costs for all staff-related tasks in delivering the programme. The purchase costs of the programme materials, initial training, and trainers' wages to deliver supervision were supplied by the IY Wales Centre.

Step 4—Construction of tables

Tables 5.3, 5.4 and 5.5 present the overall cost of the programme in three 'real-world' contexts, which can be used as a guide/template to calculate a cost per person of other programmes and under different contexts, to enable comparisons between other programmes and settings.

Step 5—Conduct micro-costing analysis: An IY Parenting Programmes example

Micro-costing creates a clear picture of costs if conducted accurately and sensitively. For the year 2008/2009; the total costs to set up and deliver the programme as part of normal service delivery were £9326.73 (total costs from Table 5.3 £3305.73, plus total costs from Table 5.4 £6021.00). Thus, the total cost to set up and deliver the programme to a group of eight parents was £1165.84 per child. The cost of the programme, excluding initial training and initial set-up costs (e.g. materials), based on eight parents per group, was £752.63 per child. Within a research/development context, with the associated high levels of supervision the total costs for a group of eight parents including initial training, recruitment, and group running costs were £1509.28 per child. The costs of the programme without initial training and initial set-up costs (e.g. materials) were £1096.07 per child.

The tables present data from the weekly completed cost diaries. Table 5.3 presents the reported set-up costs, illustrating the total costs of materials, training, and one-day supervision, per programme. Table 5.4 presents the reported delivery costs of the IY Toddler Parenting Programme with initial training and supervision already undertaken, and materials purchased. Table 5.5 presents the reported set-up and delivery costs of the programme. This table differs from the previous two tables; the IY developer's fidelity guidelines recommend that weekly supervision should be undertaken when the programme is delivered within a trial setting by trained, but as yet uncertified, leaders (Webster-Stratton, 2004).

Table 5.3 Total costs to set up the Incredible Years Toddler Parenting Programme with one health visitor and one childcare practitioner running the group

Type of Cost	Units	Unit cost (£)	Total cost 2008/9 (£)
Set-Up Costs:			
Initial training costs:			
Materials (programme materials)	1 pack of IY toddler programme materials	£1027.89 for one pack of IY toddler materials (including *Value Added Tax*)	£1027.89
Training course fee	3-day training	£470.00 (including Value Added Tax) per leader	£940.00 (including Value Added Tax) for two leaders to attend training
Leader wages for two group leaders to attend training	3-day training (7 hours each day)	£493.92 per leader	£987.84 for two leaders to attend training
One-day supervision before start of programme:			
Supervision of group leaders before start of programme including travel	1 day (7.5 hours)	£350.00 (flat rate) for trainer wages to deliver supervision	£350.00
Total:			£3305.73

Step 6—Conduct-sensitivity analysis

Sensitivity analysis allows one to explore the extent to which the assumptions made are held, whilst adjusting key variables. Sensitivity analysis was applied to establish costs for 10 per group instead of 8 by calculating additional recruitment letters, telephone calls, home visits, and catch-up visits and calls. The costs per child reduced from £752.63 to £ 633.61 under normal service delivery (excluding initial set-up costs), and within a research trial from £1509.28 to £1238.94 (excluding initial set-up costs).

This micro-costing is based on a trial undertaken in predominantly rural Wales. To estimate parenting programme delivery costs in a high-cost, urban area such as London; a London-weighting calculation was applied for staff salaries only (e.g. group leader salaries to deliver the programme, trainer salaries to deliver supervision, and crèche staff salaries), following the use of the London Multiplier as detailed by Curtis (2009). When this London weighting was applied to the costs of set-up and delivery of the programme as part of normal service delivery, the total programme costs increased from £9326.73 to £10560.27, making programme delivery £1233.54 more expensive. If the programme was delivered as part of a research trial in London, costs would increase from £12074.25 to £13769.63, making the programme £1695.38 more expensive than if delivered in a more rural area.

Table 5.4 Total costs and cost per child to deliver the Incredible Years Toddler Parenting Programme over 12 weekly sessions with one health visitor and one childcare practitioner as the group leaders. Initial training and supervision has been undertaken and materials purchased (see Table 5.3)

Type of Cost	Units	Unit cost (£)	Total cost 2008/9 (£) based on 8 per group	Total cost 2008/9 (£) based on 10 per group
Delivery costs:				
Engagement and recruitment of parents:				
Time for 2 group leaders spent in home visits to recruit parents including travel time	90 minutes per family	90 minutes per family £35.28	720 minutes per group £282.24	900 minutes per group £352.80
Time for 2 group leaders to make telephone calls recruiting parents	120 minutes	120 minutes per family £47.04	960 minutes per group £376.32	1200 minutes per group £470.40
Administrative time for 2 group leaders to write and send out initial letter to parents	15 minutes for 1 letter	£5.88 in wages for 1 letter	£47.04 in wages to send letters to 8 families in first week	£58.80 in wages to send letters to 10 families in first week
Subtotal:			£705.60	£882.00
Group Costs: Mean (Standard Deviation)				
Time for 2 group leaders to prepare the room for the group	42 minutes (7.3)	42 minutes per week £16.46	504 minutes per programme (running for 12 weeks) £197.52 in direct wages to prep a room for 12 weeks	504 minutes per programme (running for 12 weeks) £197.52 in direct wages to prep a room for 12 weeks
Time for 2 group leaders to prepare for the session	120 minutes (0)	120 minutes per week £47.04	1440 minutes per programme (running for 12 weeks) £564.48 in direct wages to prepare group session for 12 weeks	1440 minutes per programme (running for 12 weeks) £564.48 in direct wages to prepare group session for 12 weeks

Table 5.4 Continued

Type of Cost	Units	Unit cost (£)	Total cost 2008/ 9 (£) based on 8 per group	Total cost 2008/ 9 (£) based on 10 per group
Group time for two leaders including travel time to and from the group	396 minutes per week (78.2) (198 minutes per week for 1 leader)	396 minutes per week (£155.23 wages for two leaders) 198 minutes per week (£77.62 wages for 1 leader)	4752 minutes per programme £1862.76 in wages to conduct group session including travel time to session	4752 minutes per programme £1862.76 in wages to conduct group session including travel time to session

Group Costs: Mean (Standard Deviation)

Time for 2 group leaders for Catch-up/home visits sessions	60 minutes (0)	60 minutes per week £23.52	720 minutes per programme £282.24 in direct wages	900 minutes per programme £352.80 in direct wages
Time for two group leaders to make telephone calls to parents	58 minutes (14.6)	58 minutes per week £22.74	696 minutes per programme £272.88 in direct wages	870 minutes per programme £341.04 in direct wages
Subtotal:			£3179.88	£3318.60
Provision of crèche facilities (salary of Crèche staff)	£105.75 per week (67.3)	£105.75 per week	£1269.00 per programme	£1269.00 per programme
Taxis	0.00	0.00	0.00	0.00
Rental of halls	£60.83 per week (58.3)	£60.83 per week	£729.96 per programme	£729.96 per programme
Food and Catering	£5.20 per week (1.8)	£5.20 per week	£62.40 per programme	£62.40 per programme
Other costs (e.g. photocopying)	£6.18 per week (2.9)	£6.18 per week	£74.16 per programme	£74.16 per programme
Subtotal:			£2135.52	£2135.52

Costs of delivering parenting group over a 12-week programme:

Total			£6021.00	£6336.12
Cost/child based on 8 parents per group			£752.63	
Cost/child based on 10 parents per group including additional recruitment letters, telephone calls, home visits, catch-up visits, and telephone call costs				£633.61

Table 5.5 Total costs and cost per child of set up and delivery of the Incredible Years Toddler Parenting Programme over 12 weekly sessions delivered within a research trial with one health visitor and one childcare practitioner as group leaders

Type of Cost	Units	Unit cost (£)	Total cost 2008/9 (£) based on 8 per group	Total cost 2008/9 (£) based on 10 per group
Set-Up Costs:				
Initial training costs:				
Materials (programme materials)	1 pack of IY toddler programme materials	£1027.89 for one pack of IY toddler materials (including Value Added Tax)	£1027.89	£1027.89
Training course fee	3-day training	£470.00 (including Value Added Tax) per leader	£940.00 (including Value Added Tax) for 2 leaders to attend training	£940.00 (including Value Added Tax) for 2 leaders to attend training
Leader wages for group leader to attend training	3-day training (7 hours each day)	£493.92 for one leader	£987.84 in wages for 2 leaders to attend training	£987.84 in wages for 2 leaders to attend training
Supervision before start of programme ('Set Up Day') costs:				
Supervision of group leaders before start of programme including travel	1 day (7.5 hours)	£350.00 (flat rate) for trainer wages to deliver supervision	£350.00	£350.00
Subtotal:			£3305.73	£3305.73
Delivery Costs:				
Engagement and recruitment of parents:				
Time for 2 group leaders conducting home visits to engage and recruit parents (including travel time)	90 minutes per family	90 minutes per family £35.28	720 minutes per group £282.24	900 minutes per group £352.80
Time for 2 group leaders to make telephone calls recruiting parents	120 minutes	120 minutes per family £47.04	960 minutes per group £376.32	1200 minutes per group £470.40

Table 5.5 Continued

Type of Cost	Units	Unit cost (£)	Total cost 2008/9 (£) based on 8 per group	Total cost 2008/9 (£) based on 10 per group
Administrative time for 2 group leaders to write and send out initial letter to parents	15 minutes for 1 letter	£5.88 in wages for 1 letter	£47.04 in wages to send letters to 8 families in first week	£58.80 in wages to send letters to 10 families in first week
Subtotal:			£705.60	£882.00
Group Costs: Mean (Standard Deviation)				
Time for 2 group leaders to prepare the room for the group	42 minutes (7.3)	42 minutes per week £16.46	504 minutes per programme (running for 12 weeks) £197.52 in direct wages to prep a room for 12 weeks	504 minutes per programme (running for 12 weeks) £197.52 in direct wages to prep a room for 12 weeks
Time for 2 group leaders to prepare for the session	120 minutes (0)	120 minutes per week £47.04	1440 minutes per programme £564.48 in direct wages to prepare group session for 12 weeks	1440 minutes per programme £564.48 in direct wages to prepare group session for 12 weeks
Group time for 2 leaders including travel time to and from the group	396 minutes per week (78.2) (198 minutes per week for one leader)	396 minutes per week (£155.23 wages for two leaders) (£77.62 wages for one leader)	4752 minutes per programme £1862.76 in direct wages to conduct group session including travel time	4752 minutes per programme £1862.76 in direct wages to conduct group session including travel time
Time for 2 group leaders for catch-up/home visits sessions	60 minutes (0)	60 minutes per week £23.52	720 minutes per programme £282.24 in direct wages	900 minute per programme £352.80 in direct wages
Time for 2 group leaders to make telephone calls to parents	58 minutes (14.6)	58 minutes per week £22.74	696 minutes per programme £272.88 in direct wages	870 minutes per programme £341.04 in direct wages
Subtotal:			£3179.88	£3318.60

(continued)

Table 5.5 Continued

Type of Cost	Units	Unit cost (£)	Total cost 2008/9 (£) based on 8 per group	Total cost 2008/9 (£) based on 10 per group
Weekly supervision time for 2 group leaders	180 minutes attending supervision	180 minutes per week £70.56	2160 minutes per programme in supervision £846.72	2160 minutes per programme in supervision £846.72
Mileage to and from weekly supervision for 2 group leaders	Varied depending upon group leader location. 66 miles mean round trip.	£26.40 for the round trip (40p per mile)	£316.80 per programme (travel to 12 supervision sessions)	£316.80 per programme (travel to 12 supervision sessions)
Trainer costs (wages for delivering Supervision)	180 minutes per session	£132.00 per session	£1584.00 per programme in Supervisor wages	£1584.00 per programme in Supervisor wages

Group Costs: Mean (Standard Deviation)

Provision of crèche facilities (salary of crèche staff)	£105.75 per week (67.3)	£105.75 per week	£1269.00 per programme	£1269.00 per programme
Taxis	0.00	0.00	0.00	0.00
Rental of halls	£60.83 per week (58.3)	£60.83 per week	£729.96 per programme	£729.96 per programme
Food and Catering	£5.20 per week (1.8)	£5.20 per week	£62.40 per programme	£62.40 per programme
Other costs (e.g. photocopying)	£6.18 per week (2.9)	£6.18 per week	£74.16 per programme	£74.16 per programme
Subtotal:			£4883.04	£4883.04

Costs of establishing and running parenting group over a 12-week programme:

Total			£12074.25	£12389.37
Cost/child based on 8 parents per group			£1509.28	
Cost/child based on 10 parents per group including additional letters, home visits, catch-up visits, and call costs				£1238.94

Table 5.5 Continued

Type of Cost	Units	Unit cost (£)	Total cost 2008/9 (£) based on 8 per group	Total cost 2008/9 (£) based on 10 per group
Costs of running parenting group excluding non-recurrent costs:				
Total			£8768.52	£9083.64
Cost/child based on 8 parents per group			£1096.07	
Cost/child based on 10 parents per group including additional recruitment letters, telephone calls, home visits, catch-up visits, and telephone call costs				£908.36

Summary of Chapter 5

This chapter:

♦ Presented an overview of the key elements of identifying, measuring, and valuing resource use to be considered before embarking on an economic evaluation of a PHI.

♦ Explained why the choice of perspective for an evaluation is important, and how the choice of perspective results in the broadening or narrowing of resource use that will be included in the evaluation.

♦ Outlined methods for identifying and measuring resource-use data; including patient recall, patient resource-use diaries, proxy reporting, and extracting data from patient records using HES or linked databanks.

♦ Signposted sources of national unit costs for resource use, including staff costs, medication, and hospital procedures.

♦ Offered guidance for handling time horizons and incorporating uncertainty for costs incurred and benefits accrued for PHIs.

♦ Presented a micro-costing case study of a parenting programme to detail the steps required for a thorough, bottom-up estimate of the costs of a preventative initiative.

References

Allen, G., 2011. *Early Intervention: The Next Steps, An Independent Report to Her Majesty's Government by Graham Allen MP*. London: The Stationery Office.

Bayoumi, A.M., 2004. The measurement of contingent valuation for health economics. *Pharmacoeconomics*, 22(11):691–700.

Briggs, A.H., Weinstein, M.C., Fenwick, E.A., Karnon, J., Sculpher, M.J., and Paltiel, A.D., 2012. Model parameter estimation and uncertainty analysis: A report of the ISPOR-SMDM Modeling Good Research Practices Task Force Working Group–6. *Medical Decision Making, 32*(5): 722–32.

Brody, B.L., Gamst, A.C., Williams, R.A., Smith, A.R., Lau, P.W., Dolnak, D., Rapaport, M.H., et al., 2001. Depression, visual acuity, comorbidity, and disability associated with age-related macular degeneration. *Ophthalmology, 108*(10): 1893–900.

Brouwer, W.B.F., 2018. The inclusion of spillover effects in economic evaluations: Not an optional extra. *Pharmacoeconomics*, (17). doi:10.1007/s40273-018-0730-6.

Byford, S. and Raftery, J., 1998. Economics notes: Perspectives in economic evaluation. *BMJ, 316*(7143): 1529.

Charles, J.M., Edwards, R.T., Bywater, T., and Hutchings, J., 2013. Micro-costing in public health economics: Steps towards a standardized framework, using the Incredible Years Toddler Parenting Program as a worked example. *Prevention Science, 14*(4): 377–89.

Clarke, P.M., Fiebig, D.G., and Gerdtham, U.G., 2008. Optimal recall length in survey design. *Journal of Health Economics, 27*(5): 1275–84.

Curtis, L., 2008. *Unit Costs of Health and Social Care 2008*. Personal Social Services Research Unit, University of Kent. Available at: <http://www.pssru.ac.uk/project-pages/unit-costs/> (Accessed 14 October 2018).

Curtis, L., 2009. *Unit Costs of Health and Social Care 2009*. Personal Social Services Research Unit, University of Kent. Available at: <http://www.pssru.ac.uk/project-pages/unit-costs/> (Accessed 14 October 2018).

Curtis, L. and Burns, A. 2017. *Unit Costs of Health and Social Care 2017*. Personal Social Services Research Unit, University of Kent. Available at: <http://www.pssru.ac.uk/project-pages/unit-costs/> (Accessed 14 October 2018).

Drummond, M.F., Sculpher, M.J., Claxton, K., Stoddart, G.L., and Torrance, G.W., 2015. *Cost analysis. Methods for the Economic Evaluation of Health Care Programmes.* Oxford: Oxford University Press.

Edwards, R.T., Céilleachair, A., Bywater, T., Hughes, D.A., and Hutchings, J., 2007. A parenting programme for parents of children at risk of developing conduct disorder: A cost-effectiveness analysis. *British Medical Journal, 334*(7595): 682.

Elliott, R. and Payne, K., 2005. *Essentials of Economic Evaluation in Health Care.* Pharmaceutical Press.

Ford, K., Butler, N., Hughes, K., Quigg, Z., Bellis, M.A., Barker, P., Conrad, D., et al., 2016. *Adverse Childhood Experiences (ACEs) in Hertfordshire, Luton and Northamptonshire.* Liverpool: Centre for Public Health, Liverpool John Moores University.

Friedli, L. and Parsonage, M., 2009. *Promoting Mental Health and Preventing Mental Illness: The Economic Case for Investment in Wales.* Cardiff: All Wales Mental Health Promotion Network.

Glick, H.A., Doshi, J.A., Sonnad, S.S., and Polsky, D., 2014. *Economic Evaluation in Clinical Trials.* Oxford: Oxford University Press.

H.M. Treasury, 2018. *The Green Book: Central Government Guidance on Appraisal and Evaluation.* London: Stationery Office.

Hunter, R. F., Murray, J. M., Gough, A., Tang, J., Patterson, C. C., French, D. P., McIntosh, E., et al., 2018. Effectiveness and cost-effectiveness of a loyalty scheme for physical activity behaviour change maintenance: results from a cluster randomised controlled trial. *International Journal of Behavioral Nutrition and Physical Activity*, *15*(1): 127.

Husereau, D., Drummond, M., Petrou, S., Carswell, C., Moher, D., Greenberg, D., Augustovski, F., et al., 2013. Consolidated health economic evaluation reporting standards (CHEERS) statement. *BMC Medicine*, *11*(1): 1.

Husereau, D., Drummond, M., Petrou, S., Greenberg, D., Mauskopf, J., Augustovski, F., Briggs, A.H., et al., 2015. Reply to Roberts et al.: CHEERS is sufficient for reporting cost–benefit analysis, but may require further elaboration. *Pharmacoeconomics*, *33*(5): 535–6.

Information Commissioner's Office. 2018. *Guide to the General Data Protection Regulation (GDPR)*. Available at <https://assets.publishing.service.gov.uk/government/uploads/system/uploads/attachment_data/file/711097/guide-to-the-general-data-protection-regulation-gdpr-1-0.pdf> (Accessed 31 October 2018).

Margrain, T.H., Nollett, C., Shearn, J., Stanford, M., Edwards, R.T., Ryan, B., Bunce, C., et al., 2012. The Depression in Visual Impairment Trial (DEPVIT): Trial design and protocol. *BMC Psychiatry*, *12*(1): 57.

McCabe, C., 2018. Expanding the scope of costs and benefits for economic evaluations in health: Some words of caution. *Pharmacoeconomics*, (17). doi:10.1007/s40273-018-0729-z.

Morris, S., Devlin, N., and Parkin, D., 2007. *Economic Analysis in Health Care*. Chichester: John Wiley & Sons Ltd.

National Institute for Health and Care Excellence, 2013. *Guide to the Methods of Technology Appraisal 2013*. London: National Institute for Health and Clinical Excellence.

National Institute for Health and Care Excellence, 2012. *Methods for the Development of NICE Public Health Guidance* (3rd edn). London: National Institute for Health and Care Excellence.

Palmer, S. and Raftery, J., 1999. Opportunity cost. *British Medical Journal*, **318**:1551–2.

Ridyard, C.H., Hughes, D.A., and DIRUM Team, 2012. Development of a database of instruments for resource-use measurement: Purpose, feasibility, and design. *Value in Health*, *15*(5): 650–5.

Russell, L., 1992. Opportunity costs in modern medicine. *Health Effects (Millwood)*, *11*:162–9.

Sanghera, S., Frew, E., and Roberts, T., 2015. Adapting the CHEERS statement for reporting cost–benefit analysis. *Pharmacoeconomics*, *33*(5): 533–4.

Squires, H., Chilcott, J., Akehurst, R., Burr, J., and Kelly, M.P., 2016. A systematic literature review of the key challenges for developing the structure of public health economic models. *International Journal of Public Health*, *61*(3): 1–10.

Thorn, J.C., Coast, J., Cohen, D., Hollingworth, W., Knapp, M., Noble, S.M., Ridyard, C., et al., 2013. Resource-use measurement based on patient recall: Issues and challenges for economic evaluation. *Applied Health Economics and Health Policy*, *11*(3): 155–61.

Weatherly, H., Drummond, M., Claxton, K., Cookson, R., Ferguson, B., Godfrey, C., Rice, N., et al., 2009. Methods for assessing the cost-effectiveness of public health interventions: Key challenges and recommendations. *Health Policy*, *93*(2): 85–92.

Webster Stratton, C., 2004. *Quality Training, Supervision, Ongoing Monitoring, and Agency Support: Key Ingredients to Implementing. The Incredible Years Programmes with Fidelity.* Available at: <http://www.incredibleyears.com/library> (Accessed 14 October 2018).

Withrow, D. and **Alter, D.A.,** 2011. The economic burden of obesity worldwide: A systematic review of the direct costs of obesity. *Obesity Reviews, 12*(2): 131–41.

Younger, J., McCue, R., and **Mackey, S.,** 2009. Pain outcomes: A brief review of instruments and techniques. *Current Pain and Headache Reports, 13*(1): 39–43.

Chapter 6

Identifying, measuring, and valuing outcomes within economic evaluations of public health interventions

Emma McIntosh

6.1 Introduction

Some of the costs and benefits of policy decisions can be readily valued because they impact directly on markets. But some cannot, and measures therefore have to be constructed or obtained from complementary markets. It will never be possible in practice to value all impacts, but we should aim to extend valuation to as many as we can. Valuation is implicit in most policy decisions, and it is preferable to make it explicit where possible to improve quality and transparency, whatever objections some may have.

Chris Riley, Chief Economist
UK Department for Transport, Local Government and the Regions
(Pearce and Ozdemiroglu, 2002)

Economists approach the measurement and valuation of outcomes as one component of an exercise in reconstructing the missing market, the other component being the measurement and valuation of resources. Market failure was introduced in Chapter 2 of this book as a key reason for government intervention in the provision of health care (for further reading on this topic see Donaldson, 1993; Mwachofi and Al-Assaf, 2011). In brief, for those readers new to the area of economic evaluation and in particular the role of 'outcomes' in this process, a useful way to think about them is as equivalent to the 'value' we would typically place on a good or service. We know how much we value the features of an apple or pear (e.g. tasty, satisfying) or a new pair of shoes (e.g. stylish, comfortable, long lasting) by how much we are willing to pay for them but we typically don't know how much we value the attributes or specific features of, say, a hernia repair. The reason for this is due to a lack of 'preference information' on such irregular events, so we are likely to be less knowledgeable about its features such as how much pain we will be in post-operatively, how long we will be in hospital for, how long the recovery will be, and what the chances are of side-effects such as infections. In public health interventions (PHIs) such as exercise referral programmes and self-management strategies implemented for reducing sedentary behaviour, the focus may be on short-term outcomes such as 'steps per day' and long-term outcomes including reduction in type 2 diabetes and cardiovascular disease. Other, broader outcomes such as increased well-being, happiness, increased social contact, reduced anxiety and depression, etc., as well as long-term outcomes, are also likely to be important, have an intrinsic value, and need to be included in the evaluation.

It is important to remember that as consumers we often do not have defined preferences for health care processes and outcomes which happen irregularly in comparison to other goods and services which we regularly consume. It is well documented and now commonly accepted that measuring and valuing outcomes (and costs for that matter; see Chapter 5 of this book) for public health economic evaluations will often require adoption of a wide societal perspective to capture the broader personal and spillover outcomes, as well as likely multi-sector impacts (sometimes referred to as health/non-health sector interfaces) such as social care, educational (e.g. improved academic attainment due to improved pro-social behaviour), judiciary (e.g. reduced crime through improvements in social and emotional well-being), housing (e.g. welfare impacts), transport (outcomes from laws, e.g. wearing seatbelts or not using mobile phones whilst driving), agricultural (e.g. pesticide impacts on human health), and employment-related effects (increased employment opportunities due to improved health and well-being). Capturing these outcomes will often require a long-term evaluative time horizon (Weatherly et al., 2009b; Lorgelly et al., 2015a) as highlighted by Sassi and colleagues (2010). Requirements for adoption of such a broad perspective add design and methodological complexity to the identification, measurement, and valuation of outcomes in population health economic evaluations. The aim of this chapter is to outline the key challenges associated with the identification, measurement, and valuation of outcomes in the evaluation of PHIs and outline methodological approaches and solutions for the generation of optimal outcome evidence for the purposes of decision-making.

Many PHIs are complex in nature, involve complex system interactions, and often involve 'behaviour change' initiatives (Craig et al., 2008), as discussed in Chapters 1 and 3 of this book. Examples discussed include interventions designed to help people stop smoking, increase exercise, reduce sedentary behaviour, increase the rate of vaccination uptake, promote the use of blue space (proximity/access to water) (Grellier et al., 2017) and green space (proximity/access to green areas including parks, woodlands, and gardens), and reduce alcohol intake. The identification and measurement of these outcomes for inclusion in a prospectively designed economic evaluation framework for the purpose of informing resource allocation decisions is complex in itself. Added to this complexity of evaluation, the need for a long-term time horizon is the issue of attribution of outcomes (Weatherly et al., 2009b) and challenges associated with robustly measuring such outcomes. In addition to this, there is clear evidence that public health decision-makers find it difficult to present a business case for investing in PHIs, due to a perceived lack of relevant data. Decision-makers ideally want to be able to cite concrete outcomes from an intervention over a period of one to five years (National Institute for Health and Care Excellence, 2011b) however this creates a challenge for the economic evaluation of PHIs whose impacts may not come to fruition til years later.

It is also the case that many PHI outcomes may be unidimensional. Proxies for long-term quality of life and quantity of life are multifaceted and not always amenable to traditional quality-adjusted life year (QALY) estimation (as discussed in Chapters 3 and 8 of this book). Indeed, research design methodologies such as natural experiments (see Chapter 3) have arisen to evaluate policies aimed at a whole population, and as such the outcomes are often not able to be designed or influenced by the researcher. Analysts therefore need to be highly flexible in their approach to such economic evaluations and consider adopting the use of such research designs within broader evaluative frameworks beyond traditional cost-effectiveness analysis (CEA) and cost–utility analysis (CUA) (Deidda et al., 2017). The uses of methods, frameworks, and decision support tools which can accommodate such multi-dimensional outcomes include cost–benefit analysis (CBA) (see Chapter 9), social cost–benefit analysis (Fujiwara and Campbell, 2011), CCA (see Chapter 10), social return on investment (SROI) (see Chapter 12), and multi-criteria decision analysis (MCDA) (see Chapter 13) (Devlin and Sussex, 2011). These frameworks and decision support tools are now being recommended more frequently by economists working in the evaluation of PHIs. For example, the UK's NICE public health economic evaluation guidance recommends the use of the CCA framework (National Institute for Health and Care Excellence, 2012b) and the CCA framework is also recommended in published public health economic evaluations (National Institute for Health and Care Excellence, 2011b; Edwards et al., 2013). However, there is still much work required to develop robust methodology and frameworks which produce cost and outcome data amenable to resource allocation decision-making. A key methodological challenge in broadening the evaluative outcomes space related to how these outcomes are subsequently 'valued' (as is the case with QALYs) for use in economic evaluation and assisting resource allocation decision-making. New approaches are being recommended such as using a life satisfaction approach to measuring subjective well-being (Dolan et al., 2008, 2011). Further, the meaningfulness of cost-effectiveness thresholds (see Chapter 2) for outcomes and the extent to which they are relevant for the multifaceted public health outcomes comes into play.

The use of decision analytic modelling methodology is also an important vehicle for conducting economic evaluations of PHIs which require long-term extrapolation of costs and outcomes (Squires et al., 2016; Marsh et al., 2012). Chapter 11 of this book outlines modelling methods as they have been applied to PHI economic evaluation. The challenge of attributing long-term outcome impacts to PHIs, along with differing outcomes impacting different government sectors (such as health, housing, education, employment, and the environment), is a key issue. Economists tend to approach such challenges by a full consideration of uncertainty in the analysis and the extent to which this uncertainty affects the likely conclusion about relative cost-effectiveness. Additional methodological consideration around this relates to the construction of models for extrapolating beyond economic evaluations alongside natural experiments (see Chapter 15).

This chapter aims to explore the many challenges associated with the identification, measurement, valuation, reporting, and presentation of outcomes within economic evaluations of population health interventions and policies. Drawing on the vast literature in this area, existing guidelines, government recommendations, and methodological advances, this chapter will outline the current challenges, solutions, and suggestions for appropriate inclusion of outcome information for the specific purpose of economic evaluation of PHIs with a view to informing decision-making. Chapter 8 of this book expands on this chapter by outlining health-adjusted life years (HALYs). HALYs are summary measures of population health that allow the combined impact of death and morbidity to be considered simultaneously (Gold et al., 2002). Health-adjusted life expectancy (HALE) is the life expectancy that someone can expect to live at a given age in the equivalent of full health. HALE statistics provide an overarching view of the morbidity and mortality burden of a population. Chapter 8 also provides a comparison of HALYs, QALYs, and disability-adjusted life years (DALYs), as well as providing greater detail on the use of QALYs in children and adolescents.

6.2 Outcome evaluation within complex interventions and complex systems

In PHI economic evaluation, the methodology for the evaluation of complex interventions is likely to be highly relevant (see Chapter 3). It is important to note, as reported by economists, is that whilst complex interventions of the sort discussed by the Medical Research Council (MRC) (Craig et al., 2006) are more challenging to evaluate, there is essentially nothing substantively different about how economists approach and undertake the economic evaluation of such complex interventions. In many instances no new economic methods will be required, and the problems can all be solved with time, effort, and resources (Byford and Sefton, 2003; Shiell et al., 2008), along with refinements such as a broader perspective, methods to allow for longer time horizon evaluation and the inclusion of multi-sectoral outcomes. This observation benefits from the development of a number of outcome research developments and new instruments suited to PHI evaluation (Coast et al., 2008c; Dolan et al., 2011; Al Janabi et al., 2012; Lorgelly et al., 2015a). These developments, including the growing acceptance and relevance of broader measures of outcomes, greater use of 'capability well-being' as an outcome, the development of the ICECAP-A (Al Janabi et al., 2012) and ICECAP-O (Coast et al., 2008a) instruments, combined with increased acceptance and use of alternative reporting and presenting frameworks such as CCA (National Institute for Health and Care Excellence, 2012a), MCDA (Devlin and Sussex, 2011), and social CBA (Fujiwara and Campbell, 2011) to give some examples.

Craig and colleagues state:

> Complex interventions are usually described as interventions that contain several interacting components. There are, however, several dimensions of complexity: it may be to do with the range of possible outcomes, or their variability in the target population, rather than with the number of elements in the intervention package itself. It follows that there is no sharp boundary between simple and complex interventions. Few interventions are truly simple, but there is a wide range of complexity. (Craig et al., 2008, p. 7)

The consequences of interventions in a complex system will typically not be the small-scale marginal changes usually examined by economists. Since everything is interconnected, changes in one part of the system feed through to other parts of the system and feed back on themselves (Shiell et al., 2008). As outlined by Shiell and colleagues, the economist's usual approach assumes that the effects of the intervention can be examined in *isolation* of changes in the wider context (Shiell et al., 2008). This point is explored in relation to economic modelling of PHIs through the inclusion of feedback loops in model specification, discussed in Chapter 11 of this book. Two consequences follow from this. First, spin-off effects are to be expected. The consequences of system-level change are both multiple and multiplied, with induced costs (increased or decreased) (for more on these, see Chapter 5 on costing in public health evaluations) and outcomes beyond those originally envisaged in the research protocol. The practical challenge of identifying and capturing these effects within an evaluation is therefore substantial (Hawe et al., 2004).

Second, as noted by Shiell and co-workers economists often assume that the value people assign to interventions is unchanging (Shiell et al., 2008). However, this assumption is unlikely to hold true with system-level change. This has been observed most notably in tobacco control, where the concerted action of public health advocates to reduce the harm associated with tobacco use has changed behaviours and social norms. Support for banning smoking in public places often increases after the policy is implemented (Siahpush and Scollo, 2001). The relevance of this phenomenon for outcomes assessment is that the value of an intervention that changes the dynamic of a complex system is likely to be a *function of the intervention*, that is, where people may value the intervention more after implementation than before it. Preferences are no longer stable, and this may undermine the validity of the methods economists use to ascertain value. It has been argued that as a consequence of this, more collective, deliberative methods of eliciting social value are needed (Shiell et al., 2008).

Byford and Sefton highlight that for some health care interventions, outcomes are relatively easy to quantify. Many interventions are judged by their success in reducing mortality or disease-specific morbidity easily amenable to quantitative measurement, such as blood pressure or symptom reduction (Byford and Sefton, 2003). They note that this is particularly true for conditions that are localized, physical, and readily treatable such as broken bones. Other health care interventions seek to make a more 'holistic' impact on conditions that influence many aspects of a person's life such as mental health problems. Such impacts are much harder to measure and compare with accuracy since they are less amenable to objective measurement and can be multiple in nature, affecting psychological, social, family, and physical functioning. The researchers add that the social care field is similar: the aims and outcomes are often multiple and subjective in nature and an accurate representation of changes in outcomes can thus be difficult (Byford and Sefton, 2003). The outcomes of many PHIs will fall into this category of being 'multiple and subjective in nature' and as such, economic evaluation of PHIs will benefit from evidence in the field of social care economic evaluation. In their systematic review of social care interventions, Faria and colleagues note that 'more methodological research and guidance is needed on standardised outcome measures on general wellbeing, on informal carer's burden and on how to trade-off the costs and benefits in different sectors' (Faria et al., 2015).

6.3 Outcomes used within 'traditional' health care economic evaluations

> Public health is overwhelmingly concerned with health as the primary (if not sole) objective. However, numerous studies demonstrate that, for the public, life is very much not all about health, but the balance of a number of aspects of life that yield welfare, or more recently 'happiness'. Wider interventions ... therefore need an approach which emphasizes—and, crucially, reconciles—the range of outcomes, or consequences, relevant to that intervention, which will likely be quite context dependent.
>
> Smith and Petticrew, 2010, p. 4

The aim of the following section is briefly to summarize and classify the main outcomes as they have traditionally been defined and described within their relevant economic evaluation framework, as has typically been the case in classic economic evaluation texts (e.g. Drummond et al., 2015). The purpose of this next section is to give the reader an insight into the types of outcomes typically used in health care economic evaluations before concentrating on developments in the outcomes research field with a particular focus on those outcomes suited to the economic evaluation of PHIs which will be discussed in later sections of this chapter.

6.3.1 Cost-effectiveness analysis (CEA) outcomes

Cost-effectiveness analysis (CEA) measure outcomes in natural units such as life years gained, disability days avoided, asthma-free days, surgical infections avoided, or cases detected (see Chapter 7 of this book). When combined with costs and compared to at least one comparator, the results of CEA are often presented as a ratio of incremental cost over incremental effect or incremental cost-effectiveness ratio (ICER). This idea was introduced in Chapter 2 of this book. An example of a CEA of a PHI is reported by McIntosh and colleagues in their economic evaluation of an intensive home visiting programme for vulnerable families (McIntosh et al., 2009). The outcomes reported in this economic evaluation were the maternal sensitivity and infant cooperativeness components of the CARE Index instrument (Crittenden, 2001). The point estimates for the ICERs for these outcomes were £2,723 and £2,033, respectively; that is, an extra unit of maternal sensitivity costs an extra £2,723 in home visiting resources, and an extra unit of improvement in infant cooperativeness costs an additional £2,033 to achieve. Notwithstanding the limitations of such narrow outcome measures for this broad context, the authors reported mean 'societal costs' for the battery of outcomes in the control and intervention arms, and reported that these incremental benefits were delivered at an incremental societal cost of £3,246 per woman. Further, the authors explored an additional outcome variable created from the data, namely 'infants identified and removed from a maltreating environment'. By way of a sensitivity analysis and by constructing a new variable entitled 'time exposed to abuse and neglect', the authors were able show the cost-effectiveness acceptability curve (CEAC) for reducing exposure to abuse and neglect. The results suggested that if decision-makers were willing to pay £1400 to reduce exposure to abuse and neglect by one month, the home-visiting intervention would have a 75 per cent probability of being cost-effective. A decision-maker's willingness to pay of £2700 to reduce exposure to abuse and neglect by one month gives it a 90 per cent probability, and a willingness to pay of £3100 returns a 95 per cent probability that the intervention would be cost-effective. The authors note that the extent to which these potential outcomes are worth the costs, however, is a matter of judgement. Given the specific context of this study as well as the relatively narrow outcome measures used, the generalizability of these results must always be a consideration. The authors highlight that it is important to interpret these results within the context of the study performed and to be cautionary about interpreting the results beyond such a context. Similarly, in their cost-effectiveness analysis of the Incredible Years (IY) parenting programme to reduce conduct disorder, Edwards and colleagues reported their economic evaluation using the primary outcome of the trial, the Strengths and Difficulties Questionnaire (SDQ), which is a measure of child behaviour (Edwards et al., 2016). The authors reported that the IY programme has a high probability of being cost-effective as judged by the investment of between £1,612 and £3,418 per child in the study required to shift an additional 23 per cent of children from above the clinical concern to below the cut-off on the SDQ, compared to the control group. The lack of a generic outcome such as a QALY in this example, akin to the home visiting example (McIntosh et al., 2009), highlights the need for an extra valuation step to decide whether these outcomes are *worth* the investment. The findings of the IY study have led to ongoing implementation of the IY programme; it is therefore an example of judgements about investment spend being made within a preventive setting without using generic preference-based outcomes. These examples show the options available when using 'effectiveness' outcomes for decision-making within public health economic evaluations but it also highlights the additional 'valuation' which needs to be carried out when using such outcomes (either explicitly or implicitly, as evidenced by the implied valuation in the IY study). In the United Kingdom, NICE Public health economic evaluation guidance states explicitly: 'If there are not enough data to estimate QALYs gained, an alternative measure of cost effectiveness may be considered (such as life years gained, cases averted or a more disease-specific outcome)' (National Institute for Health and Care Excellence, 2011a).

6.3.2 Cost–utility analysis (CUA) outcomes

In health economics, CUA has become synonymous with the QALY framework (see also Chapter 8 of this book). The main difference between CUA and CEA is that CUA typically uses generic preference-weighted health-related quality of life attributes as its outcome measure and therefore outcomes are represented in terms of QALYs instead of the natural units within CEA. CUA can, therefore, be seen as an improvement on CEA as it attempts to combine more than one outcome measure, takes account of both quality and quantity of life, and facilitates comparability across programmes. Indeed, the original development of the generic QALY framework was so that comparisons could be made across different health care interventions in different clinical areas (McIntosh and Luengo-Fernandez, 2006). In the United Kingdom, QALYs are the recommended measure of health outcomes for economic evaluations submitted to the UK's regulatory body, NICE. A QALY combines data on length of life with data on health-related quality of life (HRQoL) (Bala et al., 1998), and more recently the QALY is being increasingly used in public health economic evaluations (National Institute for Health and Care Excellence, 2012b). The HRQoL component of the QALY represents the value placed on different levels of health. This component is anchored at 0, which represents a state as poor as being dead, and 1, which represents full health. Scores of less than 0 are theoretically possible and sometimes observed; these represent levels of health that are considered to be worse than being dead. Thus, one QALY represents one year in full health. For the purposes of health care economic evaluation, QALYs are typically summed over time or across individuals. There are a variety of approaches and techniques for valuing states of HRQoL. In the United Kingdom, the NICE reference case prefers the generic EQ-5D in adults as reported by the patient or their close carer when they are unable to report themselves (see <http://www.euroqol.org>). The EQ-5D comes with a pre-existing value set obtained from a representative sample of the UK general population using the time trade-off (TTO) technique (Dolan et al., 1995). Indeed, the EQ-5D-3L (EQ-5D 3 level) is available in more than 160 translated versions and the EQ-5D-3L (EQ-5D 5 level) is available in more than 125 translated versions (for updates, please see the EQ-5D website: <http://www.euroqol.org>). Other generic preference-based measures are available such as the HUI3 (Horsman et al., 2003) and the SF-6D (Brazier and Roberts, 2004). For a comprehensive summary of preference-based outcomes, see Brazier et al., 2016. See also Chapter 8 of this book, citing Owen and colleagues show that many PHIs evaluated by the UK's NICE have a cost per QALY estimate well below the NICE threshold of between £20,000 and £30,000 per QALY (Owen et al., 2012).

Lorgelly and colleagues note that one of the limitations of QALYs is that they focus on health outcomes and many PHIs seek to impact on broader aspects of quality of life, not just health but also non-health outcomes such as empowerment, participation, and crime (Lorgelly et al., 2010). These researchers conclude that QALYs and their associated quality of life measures like the EQ-5D or SF-6D are likely to underestimate the relative benefits of PHIs when compared to health care interventions (Lorgelly et al., 2010).

6.3.3 Cost–benefit analysis outcomes: Willingness to pay (WTP)

The contingent valuation (CV) method is a stated preference approach designed to estimate monetary welfare gains/losses directly. These welfare gains/losses are typically referred to as individuals' willingness to pay (WTP)/willingness to accept (WTA). WTP values are typically used to as outcomes within CBA studies although there are other methods including the human capital approach (Brouwer et al., 1997; Pritchard and Sculpher, 2000; Lensberg et al., 2013). With CBA, economists often refer to the 're-construction of the missing market' (Smith, 2003). Frew's coverage of the CV methods in Chapter 6 in McIntosh et al. (2010) provides a summary of the outcomes side of CBA. Incorporating the well-known methodological challenges associated with valuing outcomes in monetary terms, the CBA framework has been less frequently used in health economic evaluations compared to evaluations in areas such as environmental economics (Boxall et al., 1996; Adamovicz, 2000). Chapter 9 provides detailed coverage of the economic evaluation framework of CBA.

In a typical WTP outcomes exercise, individuals are asked to consider a hypothetical scenario where they are asked to *imagine* that a market exists for the benefits or losses of a public programme. The exercise then proceeds on the hypothetical contingency that such a market exists. A number of design instruments can then be applied to ask individuals to state their WTP to ensure that a welfare gain occurs or WTA to tolerate the welfare loss from the programme. The WTP or the WTA amount is then taken as a measure of the individual's perceived value of the programme (i.e. the demand) which is then aggregated across all individuals. With its ability to place a value any attribute or feature (subject to good design and description of these feature), CV has the potential to offer substantial advantages over other outcomes such as effectiveness measures and QALYs (Ryan and Shackley, 1995; Donaldson and Shackley, 1997; Jan et al., 2000; Shackley and Donaldson, 2002;). With an increasing recognition of the need for the measurement and valuation of broad-ranging multi-sector outcomes for PHIs, there is a move towards the use of a CBA framework. Researchers are more frequently referring to the monetary valuation of these outcomes to facilitate decision-making, hence the need for economic evaluation of PHIs is likely to benefit from a renewed focus on WTP methods. There exists a vast literature on the design of CV studies considering each of the methodological topics including the use of the arguably more flexible discrete choice experiment (DCE) approach to estimating WTP (McIntosh et al., 1999; Ryan et al., 2004; Lancsar and Savage, 2004a, 2004b; Kleinman et al., 2002; Santos Silva, 2004). In particular, there is substantial evidence of potential biases within CV studies. Useful discussions of how these can be overcome with good study design are available (Desvousges et al., 1983; Smith, 1985; Johannesson, 1996; Ryan et al., 1998; Smith, 2000; Olsen and Smith, 20010; Shackley and Donaldson, 2002; Frew, 2010; Donaldson and Shackley, 1997; Donaldson et al., 1997; Blackorby and Donaldson, 1990). There are some examples of using WTP to value outcomes in public health including WTP for sport activities and WTP for text-messaging services in relation to type II diabetes (Herens et al., 2015; Islam et al., 2015). Chapter 9 provides more detail on WTP design formats and associated biases.

6.3.4 Cost–consequence analysis (CCA) outcomes

The role of CCA for decision-making in health economics and health technology assessment (HTA) has recently been recommended by UK's NICE as a possible option for the economic evaluation of PHIs (National Institute for Health and Care Excellence, 2011a). CCA is a form of economic evaluation where disaggregated costs and a range of outcomes are presented to allow readers to form their own opinion on relevance and relative importance to their decision making context (Drummond et al., 2015). Chapter 10 covers the CCA framework in more detail.

CCAs have often been recommended for complex interventions that have multiple effects, for example lifestyle education in the prevention of diabetes (Drummond et al., 2015). Increasingly, this disaggregated framework is being seen as suited to PHIs which have an array of health, non-health, and multi-sector outcomes such as educational attainment, employment, judiciary, housing, and so on, that are difficult to measure in a common unit such as a QALY (National Institute for Health and Care Excellence, 2012b). The recent recommendation of CCA in the economic evaluation of PHIs and policies in the United Kingdom most likely stems from the challenges associated with valuing the multi-sectoral outcomes in one common unit such as the QALY. Consider an example of an intervention to increase pro-social behaviour delivered in a school setting which may have long-term impacts on many sectors including education, employment, housing, and the judiciary. Capturing these outcomes within a health-related QALY may not be realistic or feasible, hence disaggregated, 'sector-relevant' outcomes may be more relevant. In addition, different government sectors may not have thresholds (or operate different thresholds) for the valuation of outcomes, and unlike the UK's health sector, which typically uses a threshold of between £20,000 and £30,000 per QALY gained (Devlin and Parkin, 2004), there is little evidence of the education, judicial, and other sectors making use of such a threshold for resource allocation. That said, recent attempts at using co-financing across sectors is promising (Remme et al., 2017), along with attempts to strengthen CEA for use in public health policy (Russell and Sinha, 2016) and expanding HTA to include the effects of other sectors such as the environment (Marsh et al., 2016). In health economics, there has also been a push for analytical methods to reflect the opportunity cost of funding de-cisions more formally (Sculpher et al., 2017).

It is also important to note the challenges and critique associated with the use of CCA in decision-making with particular attention to interpretation of CCA outcomes for resource allocation decisions. CCA has been criticized for lacking generalizability, not providing guidance on thresholds for valuations. and decisions based on CCA lacking transparency. As outlined by Brazier and colleagues in their response to Coast and colleagues, not only do decision-makers have complex decisions to make, they may not be using the values of the general population or patients but instead using their own subjective opinions (Coast, 2004; Brazier 2016). Brazier and team note that any CCAs are likely to be less transparent because, given the complexity of the tasks faced, decision-makers are unlikely to be able to explain their reasoning clearly. Transparency is not the only issue, however, as forcing decision-makers to place arbi-trary values on a large number of disaggregated outcomes may encourage inaccurate, inconsistent, and biased decision-making. The implications of this within public health economic evaluations are important to weigh up when adopting a CCA framework. It may be that the identification of a suite of outcomes within a CCA may be particularly useful in feasibility or pilot studies prior to the societal valuation of those outcomes as a 'collective' using a method such as WTP (see Chapter 9).

6.4 DALYs as an outcome measure in population health economic evaluations

A number of economic evaluations of PHIs in global health use the disability-adjusted life year (DALY) as an outcome measure. This is most likely due to the DALY's focus being on averting ill health which fits with the 'preventive' nature of many population health inter-ventions (Haby et al., 2006). As described in Chapter 8, the World Health Organization

(WHO) (<https://www.who.int/healthinfo/global_burden_disease/metrics_daly/en/>) has adopted the DALY as its measure of disease burden. One DALY can be thought of as one lost year of 'healthy' life. The sum of these DALYs across the population, or the burden of disease, represents the gap between current health status and an ideal health situation where the entire population lives to an advanced age, free of disease and disability (<http://www.who.int/healthinfo/global_burden_disease/daly_disability_weight/en/>). DALYs have traditionally been used as a measure of the *burden* of disease (Murray and Lopez, 2013). As such, unlike QALYs which are typically reported in terms of QALY gain, DALYs are typically reported as DALYs averted to represent burden. The DALY is often termed a 'societal measure' of the disease or disability burden in populations. They are calculated by combining measures of life expectancy and quality of life. DALYs are related to the QALYs, however QALYs only measure the benefit with and without medical intervention and as such are not used for measuring the burden of disease. Further, QALYs tend to be an individual and not a societal measure. DALYs are calculated by taking the sum of two components, years of life lost (YLL) due to dying early and years lost due to disability (YLD): DALY = YLL + YLD (Fox-Rushby, 2002). In contrast to the QALY outcome measure which is reported as a health gain, one DALY is equivalent to one year of healthy life lost. In relation to public health economic evaluations, Cobiac and co-workers report an increasing number of published economic evaluations of nutrition interventions using DALY measures (Cobiac et al., 2013).

DALYS were the main outcome in the adverse childhood experience- (ACE) prevention cost-effectiveness models (Haby et al., 2006). Haby and team reported on a new modelling approach developed for the assessing cost-effectiveness in obesity (ACE-Obesity) project and the likely population health benefit and strength of evidence for 13 potential obesity-prevention interventions in children and adolescents in Australia. The best available evidence, including evidence from non-traditional epidemiological study designs, was used to determine the health benefits as body mass index (BMI) units saved and DALYs averted. Haby and colleagues developed new methods to model the impact of behaviours on BMI post-intervention where this was not measured and the impacts on DALYs over the child's lifetime (on the assumption that changes in BMI were maintained into adulthood). A working group of stakeholders provided input into decisions on the selection of interventions, the assumptions for modelling, and the strength of the evidence. The results of the research revealed that the likely health benefit varied considerably, as did the strength of the evidence from which that health benefit was calculated. Haby and colleagues concluded that the use of consistent methods and *common health outcome measures* enables valid comparison of the potential impact of interventions, but comparisons must take into account the strength of the evidence used (Haby et al., 2006). Of note, this work was carried out alongside non-experimental studies and provides another example of such designs being commonly used in population health evaluation.

In a narrative on differences between QALYs and DALYs, Sassi provides a comprehensive formulation of QALY and DALY calculation methods, offering practical instruments for assessing the impact of health interventions (Sassi, 2006). Systematic differences between QALYs and DALYs are explained by reference to two examples: the prevention of tuberculosis and the treatment of bipolar depression. When a health intervention is aimed at preventing or treating a non-fatal disease, the relationship between QALYs gained and DALYs saved depends on age of onset and duration of the disease, as well as the quality of life and disability weightings. Sassi and team note that understanding similarities and differences between QALYs and DALYs is important to researchers and policy-makers for a sound interpretation of the evidence on the outcomes of health interventions. See Chapter 8 for further discussion of DALYs in CUA.

6.5 Alternative outcomes suited to the evaluation of public health economic interventions

It is now commonly accepted that focusing solely on health as an outcome measure is likely to underestimate the impact of many PHIs (Coast et al., 2008c; Lorgelly and Lawson, 2010). This section therefore introduces a number of other outcomes likely to be suited to the economic evaluation of PHIs. Public health focuses in part on behavioural risk factors like consuming unhealthy foods, drinking excessive alcohol, and smoking, as well as population-level problems of inequality and poverty. As noted earlier in this chapter, this has resulted in the interventions seeking to improve population health becoming more complex, with this complexity evident not only in the design and delivery of the intervention but in the resources, outcomes, the context, and the evaluation itself. This has given rise to an increased attention to outcomes which relate to behaviours, capabilities, and well-being, and as such there has seen an increased role for measuring outcomes beyond physical health. Some of these recent developments have stemmed from the work of Nussbaum, who identified what she regards as central human capabilities (Nussbaum, 2003): life; bodily health; bodily integrity; senses, imagination and thought; emotions; practical reason; affiliation; other species; play; and control over one's environment. This has provided the focus for the development of instruments based on these 'capability well-being' attributes.

6.5.1 Capability well-being

The capability approach was introduced by Amartya Sen in *Choice, Welfare and Measurement* (Sen, 1982). Sen proposed the capability approach as an alternative to standard utilitarian welfare economics and argues that outcomes, in the form of 'functional utilities', should not be the sole object of welfare assessments, and that capabilities (things that people are free to do or be) should also be included in the overall assessment of a person's well-being. The central concepts of Sen's capability approach include multidimensionality, the intrinsic value of freedom of choice, equity, and the objective valuation of welfare for use in interpersonal comparisons and social policies.

In recent years there has been an increase in the attention paid to the role of capabilities within health economics, stemming from Sen's research (Sen, 1987, 1993) and Nussbaum's development of this work (Nussbaum, 2003). Sen's capability approach suggests that well-being should be measured not according to what individuals actually do (functionings) but what they can do (capabilities). To this end he reports that 'functionings' represent parts of the state of a person—in particular, the various things that he or she manages to do or be in leading a life—and the 'capability' of a person reflects the alternative combinations of 'functionings' the person can achieve, and from which he or she can choose one vector of functionings (Lorgelly and Lawson, 2010). The capability approach is therefore based on a view of living as a combination of various 'doings and beings', with quality of life to be assessed in terms of the capability to achieve valuable functionings (Sen, 1993). Lorgelly and colleagues advocate the use of Sen's capabilities approach within PHIs due to the need to undertake economic evaluations across a wider range of interventions encompassing both health and non-health outcomes. There are numerous benefits of using the capability approach. It offers a much richer set of dimensions for evaluation which, given the nature of public health and social interventions and their many and complex outcomes, makes the approach ideal for capturing all these outcomes, rather than focusing solely on health status. The equitable underpinnings of the approach are also appropriate for use with PHIs which often involve reducing inequalities across groups (namely, improving deprivation) as an overriding aim (Lorgelly and Lawson, 2010).

Attempts have been made to operationalize the capabilities approach for use in health economics with the development of the preference-based capability well-being instruments including the OCAP_18, the OXCAP_MH, ICECAP-A, and the ICECAP-O (Coast et al., 2008a, 2008b; Flynn et al., 2013; Lorgelly et al., 2015a, Greco et al., 2016). Each of these will be introduced in the following.

6.5.2 **OCAP_18**

Using Nussbaum's original list of capabilities, Lorgelly and her team reduced it and developed a summary measure of well-being and capability for the purposes of using it within public health economic evaluation (Lorgelly et al., 2015b). Nussbaum's original capabilities questionnaire was reduced from 60 to 24 questions (including demographic questions). Each of Nussbaum's 1- central human capabilities are measured using one (or more) of the 18 specific capability items which are included in the questionnaire (referred to as the OCAP_18). The resulting index of capability was found to be highly correlated with a measure of health (EQ-5D) and well-being (global quality of life (QoL)), although some differences were apparent. This project operationalized the capability approach to produce an instrument to measure the effectiveness (and cost-effectiveness) of PHIs; the resulting OCAP_18 is reported to be responsive and measure something supplementary to health and well-being, hence adding to the current suite of outcome measures that available for economic evaluations of PHIs.

6.5.3 **OXCAP_MH**

Despite the limitations of the QALY approach in capturing non-health benefits and broader welfare inequalities, there have been very limited applications of the capability approach in a mental health context where these issues are imperative (Simon et al., 2013). Simon and co-workers developed the OxCAP_MH instrument which aims to operationalize the capability approach for outcome measurement in mental health research. The research focused on the identification of capabilities domains most affected by mental illness and their association with socio-demographic and clinical factors and other measures of well-being such as the EQ-5D and global assessment of functioning (GAF) scales. The OxCAP_MH item revealed significant correlations between service users' overall capability scores and the GAF scales (Goldman et al., 1992), EQ-5D VAS and EQ-5D-3L utilities (Group, 2011). The most affected capability domains were: 'daily activities', 'influencing local decisions', 'enjoying recreation', 'planning one's life', and 'discrimination'. Simon and colleagues' results support the feasibility and validity of directly measuring human capabilities for the mentally ill and the potential for applying the approach to outcome measurement (Simon et al., 2013).

6.5.4 **ICECAP-A**

The ICECAP-A (ICEpop CAPability measure for Adults) is a measure of capability for the general adult (18+) population for use in economic evaluation (Al-Janabi et al., 2012). The ICECAP-A focuses on well-being defined in a broader sense rather than health. The measure covers attributes of well-being that were found to be important to adults in the United Kingdom. The ICECAP-A comprises five attributes (lay terms in parentheses):

♦ Attachment (an ability to have love, friendship and support)

♦ Stability (an ability to feel settled and secure)

♦ Achievement (an ability to achieve and progress in life)

♦ Enjoyment (an ability to experience enjoyment and pleasure)

♦ Autonomy (an ability to be independent)

In addition to the ICECAP-A descriptive system just described, a set of UK index values for ICECAP-A were estimated using the best to worst scaling method (Flynn et al., 2013). A number of qualitative and quantitative studies of the validity of the ICECAP-A has been conducted with general population and patient samples (Al-Janabi et al., 2013; Mitchell and Iezzi, 2015; Mitchell et al., 2015)

6.5.5 **ICECAP-O**

Developed by the same group who developed the ICECAP-A instrument, the ICECAP-O (ICEpop CAPability measure for Older people) is a measure of capability in older people for use in economic evaluation (Grewal et al., 2006). As with the ICECAP-A instrument, the ICECAP-O focuses on well-being defined in a broader sense, rather than health. The measure covers five attributes of well-being that were found to be important to older people in the United Kingdom (lay terms in parentheses):

♦ Attachment (love and friendship)

♦ Security (thinking about the future without concern)

♦ Role (doing things that make you feel valued)

♦ Enjoyment (enjoyment and pleasure)

♦ Control (independence)

The ICECAP-O descriptive system was developed using qualitative methods. A set of index values for the ICECAP-O has been estimated using a best to worst scaling study of older people in England. Finally, on this topic of capabilities, although measures have been developed to assess capability in economic evaluation, there has been much less attention paid to the decision rules that might be applied alongside. Sen's capability approach has been discussed by Mitchell and co-workers with regards to 'sufficient capability' (Mitchell et al., 2015). They argue that focusing on the objective of achieving 'sufficient capability' more closely reflects the concern with equity that pervades the capability approach, and the method has the advantage of retaining the longitudinal aspect of estimating outcome that is associated with QALYs, whilst also drawing on notions of shortfall associated with assessments of poverty (Mitchell et al., 2015).

6.5.6 Experienced utility

The notion of 'experienced utility', closely related to 'happiness', was re-introduced to modern day thinking by Kahneman and colleagues (Kahneman et al., 1997), latterly explored by Carter and McBride (2013), and more recently referred to in the context of measuring outcomes in public health economic evaluations (Lorgelly and Lawson, 2010). The modern economist's notion of utility differs substantially from that of utilitarian theory where utility was the sum of experienced pleasures minus pains. This hedonic view of utility fell out of favour in the early twentieth century when critics argued that pleasures and pains could not be measured (Fleurbaey and Hammond, 2004). Economists instead redefined utility to be a representation of preferences revealed through observed behaviour and commenced the reconstruction of economic theories—the familiar preference-based territory of today's approaches to outcome development in health and environmental economics (Bateman et al., 2002). Although this 'behaviourist' view of utility still dominates economics, Kahneman and others have recently instigated this renewed interest in a notion of utility corresponding to experienced utility which, they argue, is not only measurable but also of fundamental importance for both understanding behaviour and selecting public policies because, as shown in various studies, experienced utility (enjoying) differs from decision utility (wanting or desiring) in significant ways (Kahneman et al., 1997). As such, these observations have given rise to researchers often alluding to experienced utility within the often, 'behavioural' context of population health economic evaluations.

6.5.7 Happiness/life satisfaction/well-being

Arguably, if all else is equal, more income—or gross domestic product (GDP)—allows us to satisfy more of our preferences, hence GDP is often used as a proxy for well-being. According to standard economic theory, more choice allows us to satisfy more of our preferences, and this idea has informed the design of policies in health and education (Dolan et al., 2011). A traditional 'preference satisfaction' approach is closely associated with the economists' account of well-being (Dolan et al., 2008). Preference satisfaction has also been used widely in policy appraisal, as outlined in Chapter 8. Related to the fundamental doubts with the preference satisfaction approach, Wilson and Gilbert note that we are often unable to predict the impact of future states of the world (Wilson and Gilbert, 2003), we frequently act against our 'better judgment' (Strack and Deutsch, 2004), and we are influenced by irrelevant factors of choice (Kahneman, 1999), as well as by a host of other behavioural phenomena (DellaVigna, 2009). More recently, there has been a renewed interest by the Organisation for Economic Co-operation and Development (OECD) and the UK government to measure population 'happiness' using subjective well-being measures (Di Tella and MacCulloch, 2006; Dolan et al., 2008, 2011). Put simply, using the words of Rafael Di Tella and Robert MacCulloch:

> Economists are trained to infer preferences from observed choices; that is, economists typically watch what people do, rather than listening to what people say. Happiness research departs from this tradition. Instead, happiness researchers have been particularly interested in self-reports of well-being, which may be as simple as an answer to a question with the general form 'Are you very happy, pretty happy, or not too happy?' (Di Tella and MacCulloch, 2006, p. 25).

In 1974, Richard Easterlin introduced happiness data into economics and observed that happiness is based on relative rather than absolute income and that it adapts to changes in the level of income (Easterlin, 1974). In relation to this, work by Stiglitz (2009) was highly influential in UK government's Budget 2010 Report :

> the Government is committed to developing broader indicators of well-being and sustainability, with work currently underway to review how the Stiglitz (Commission) ... should affect the sustainability and well-being indicators collected by DEFRA, and with the ONS and the Cabinet Office leading work on taking forward the report's agenda across the UK. (HM Treasury, Budget 2010)

Dolan and colleagues argue that the measurement of well-being is central to public policy and recommend three uses for any well-being measure: (i) monitoring progress;(ii) informing policy design; and (iii) policy appraisal (Dolan et al., 2011; see this reference also for a summary of recommended measures of subjective well-being).

6.5.8 Human development index (HDI)

Sen's capabilities framework, referred to in section 6.5.1, was also highly influential in development economics and led to the introduction of the human development index (HDI) by the United Nations (UN) development programme in 1990. The HDI measures levels of national development using a composite statistic comprising national income, education, and life expectancy. According to the UN, the HDI was created to emphasize that people and their capabilities should be the ultimate criteria for assessing the development of a country, not economic growth alone. The HDI can also be used to question national policy choices, asking how two countries with the same level of gross national income (GNI) per capita can end up with different human development outcomes. The UN argues that such contrasts can stimulate debate about government policy priorities. HDI is essentially a summary measure of average achievement in key dimensions of human development: a long and healthy life, being knowledgeable, and having a good standard of living. The health dimension is assessed by life expectancy at birth, the education dimension is measured by mean years of schooling for adults aged 25 years and more and expected years of schooling for children of school-entering age. The standard of living dimension is measured by GNI per capita. The HDI is the geometric mean of normalized indices for each of the three dimensions. Figure 6.1 below represents the features of the HDI.

Components of the Human Development Index

The HDI—three dimensions and four indicators

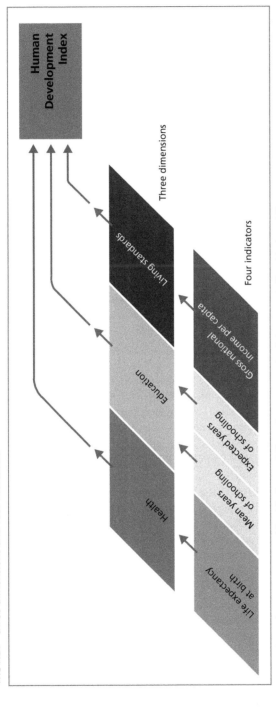

Note: The indicators presented in this figure follow the new methodology, as defined in box 1.2.
Source: HDRO.

Figure 6.1 Components of the Human Development Index.
Source: United Nations. (2010) Human Development Report 2010. Copyright © 2010 United Nations Development Programme.

There is a further version of the HDI, the inequality-adjusted human development index (IHDI) adjusts the HDI for inequality in the distribution of each dimension across the population. It is based on a distribution-sensitive class of composite inequality indices proposed by Foster, Lopez-Calva, and Szekely (Foster et al., 2005). Such an inequalities index fits with measuring the success of population health interventions whose goal is to reduce inequalities.

6.6 The relevance of perspective in outcome measurement in public health economic evaluation

The role of perspective is of particular importance for the measurement and valuation of outcomes in public health economic evaluations, due to the aforementioned challenges faced in compiling, valuing, and comparing the differing outcome units that outcomes manifest themselves across sectors (educational attainment, employment, mental health, weight, child development, dental health, etc.). The perspective from which an economic evaluation is designed reflects the costs and outcomes that will be included within the evaluation. In theory, costs can be readily identified at source and cost savings arising due to PHIs can also be readily identified and measured. With all cost investments and savings/impacts arising being in the same unit (i.e. money), the issue of perspective is arguably less challenging when it comes to cost. This book has repeatedly reiterated the fact that public health economic evaluations will most likely be broad ranging, but this is often likely to refer to reach in terms of outcome impacts. With costs being incurred by the health- and social care sector for an intervention to improve the mental health and well-being of children entering the foster care system, these costs are readily identifiable and measurable to the direct health- and social care service. However, the related outcomes associated with such an intervention are likely to be much broader; as children's mental health improves, they are likely to have better quality of life (health sector), improved educational outcomes (educational sector), and are more likely to enter employment later in life (employment sector). As such, the perspective adopted within a public health economic evaluation will essentially determine those outcomes which should be identified, measured, and valued. In the United Kingdom, NICE economic evaluation methods guidance advocates a health and personal social services (PSS) perspective for clinical economic evaluations. However, the methods guidance for public health economic evaluations states that a public sector perspective should be adopted. The guidance states: 'The broadening of the perspective set for public health guidance reflects the wider remit of public health and the changes in the way that it will be delivered after March 2013' (National Institute for Health and Care Excellence, 2012a).

In their review of economic evaluations in public health, Weatherly and colleagues reported the perspectives taken by each published study (Weatherly et al., 2009a). Fifty (32 per cent of the total) studies took a health service/healthcare payer/third-party payer perspective. Forty-eight (31 per cent) studies were reportedly undertaken from the societal perspective. However, this may be an overestimate. Twenty-three (48 per cent) of the studies undertaken from the societal perspective were QALY-based, and of these 19 (83 per cent) were undertaken by a first author located in the United States.

Only 5 out of the 19 (26 per cent) US-based QALY studies that were undertaken from the societal perspective included productivity changes as a cost. The perspective of the study was not stated in 37 (24 per cent) of the NHS Economic Evaluation Database (EED) abstracts. The perspective was that of the provider (e.g. hospital, local health department) for 12 (8 per cent) studies, the government in 2 (1 per cent) studies and the patient in a single study (1 per cent%). Four studies (3 per cent) included the analysis from multiple perspectives.

In addition to perspective, Drummond and team recommend that the intersectoral impacts of PHIs should be quantified (or at the very least described qualitatively) in a CCA in the way that makes the most sense for each sector. On the topic of outcomes for such broad-ranging perspectives they note that:

> Ideally each sector would use a well understood generic measure of outcome, in reference to which the shadow price of the budget constraint in the sector could be expressed. Although public sector decision makers are mostly concerned with the impacts of interventions on public sector budgets, there should be more consideration of impacts on the voluntary sector and private individuals, since taking this broader view may be required to assess more fully the effectiveness of programmes and to identify the equity implications arising from implementation. In evaluating PHIs, an analysis should be conducted of the costs and consequences by beneficiary group. These groups could be defined in terms of health status, socio-economic status or other characteristics, depending on policy relevance. (Drummond et al., 2006 p. 10)

As noted by Drummond and colleagues, the main argument for adopting a restrictive perspective in the United Kingdom is that the budget for the UK's NHS is meant to be for improving health (Drummond et al., 2006). Therefore, the relevant consideration in evaluating interventions is the opportunity cost (in other treatments forgone) on the health care budget. Alternatively, they argue, shouldn't the full social benefits of health care interventions be considered? If health care interventions have benefits outside the health care sector—for example, in the criminal justice system, transport, or education sector—shouldn't these be tracked and any budgetary adjustments sorted out separately? In addition, shouldn't health care aim to provide benefits to families and carers as well as the patient (Drummond et al., 2008)?

6.7 Incorporating outcomes from routine and linked data into economic evaluations

Chapter 3 discussed the increased use of natural experiment methodology for the evaluation and economic evaluation of policies and interventions aimed at improving population health. The use of natural experiments to evaluate population health interventions, outlined by Craig and colleagues (Craig et al., 2012), such as that reported by Dundas and co-workers, have begun to include economic evaluations (Dundas et al., 2014). Natural experiments, by virtue of their definition, are typically out of the design control of the researcher in terms of resource use and outcome data of the type usually collected for a prospective economic evaluation, and hence the use of routine and/or linked data are often relied upon for evaluative purposes. Often the identification and measurement of resource-use data such as hospital admissions are readily available; however, the equivalent identification and measurement of suitable outcome data for use in economic evaluations within such datasets are less clear. Traditionally, the types of outcomes required for decision-making purposes are preference-based utilities which, combined with health-state duration, can be used to calculate QALYs. Within routinely collected data, the type of outcomes is more likely to be 'resources' such as hospital admissions. Previous papers have discussed 'effectiveness' type outcomes such as average treatment effects (ATE's) (Duleep and Liu, 2013; Krief et al., 2013). Many published economic evaluations focus on only one intermediate outcome (e.g. ATE) which is then modelled to QALYs using utility values from the literature. As discussed frequently in relation to PHI evaluation, a focus on only one unidimensional outcome is likely to be too narrow an approach in population health economic evaluations where a battery of multi-sector outcomes may be more relevant for inclusion in an economic evaluation. Outcomes may be influenced by many factors. In their health in pregnancy natural experiment, Dundas and team outline relevant outcomes, not all of which are routinely captured, such as maternal diet, maternal work, psychological stress, abuse, exposure to toxic substance, and primary outcomes such as birth weight among singleton births (Dundas et al., 2014). Other secondary outcomes include gestation at booking, booking before 25 weeks, measures of size and stage, gestational age at delivery, weight for dates, term at birth, birth outcomes, and maternal smoking. Many 'outcomes' within such routine data collection are intermediate outcomes. Such outcomes should be treated as resources (hospitalizations) for the purposes of inclusion in economic evaluation and would need to be reconfigured into categories such as productivity, costs, consequences, and, where possible, researchers should source and attach utility values to outcomes. By the reclassifying such outcomes into 'resources' and subsequently costs, they are then treated correctly on the cost side of a CEA/CUA equation (see Gold et al., 1996, for additional discussion about handling outcomes in the CEA equation).

A key component of 'outcome methodology' using routine data (such as those data from natural experiment evaluations) will most likely be the modelling of short-term 'routine' data to long-term QALYs using additional evidence from systematic reviews to identify suitable utility values. It is likely that there will be numerous other 'outcomes' which could be collated within a CCA framework (see Chapter 10). The development of a longer-term economic model will most likely be standard to conduct a comprehensive economic evaluation allowing for the appropriate longer time horizon (see Chapter 11). Alternatives to utility values are attaching 'WTP' values to such outcomes and producing annual welfare values for use within a CBA, see Chapter 9.

6.8 The role of social capital in predicting outcomes of PHI interventions

Social capital has become a popular subject in the literature on determinants of health. The concept of social capital has been used in the sociological, political science, and economic development literatures, as well as in the health inequalities literature (Macinko and Starfield, 2001). The term 'social capital' has been used to describe a number of phenomena pertaining to social relations at the individual and societal levels. In a recent review, Ferguson and co-authors find that 'families with high social capital are more likely to produce children who fare positively in areas of general wellbeing, including mental and physical health, educational attainment and formal labour-market participation', concluding that 'social capital—after poverty—is found to be the best predictor of children's welfare' (Ferguson, 2006). Murayama and colleagues cite evidence from community and workplace PHIs in their argument that social capital can significantly affect health and well-being outcomes (Murayama et al., 2013). Social capital is a concept that has been used in recent years to explain health disparities (Baum, 2003), and it provides one possible theoretical basis for assessing the impact that community-based health promotion programmes have on the broader health and life of a community (Murayama et al., 2013). In addition to mortality, a number of research projects both in community and workplace settings have examined the relationship between individual social capital and health outcomes including self-rated health (Kouvonen et al., 2008; Väänänen et al., 2009; Giordano and Lindstrom, 2010). It is clear that there is a role for the measurement and valuation of social capital where relevant for economic evaluation purposes.

6.9 Reporting and presenting PHI economic evaluation outcomes

Earlier sections of this chapter have outlined the main types of economic evaluation frameworks commonly used by health economists. Specific forms of economic evaluation typically differ only as a function of the outcome measure (Drummond et al., 2015). Outcomes may be estimated from a single analytical (experimental or non-experimental) study, a synthesis of studies (see Chapter 4), mathematical modelling, or a combination of modelling and study information (Husereau et al., 2013). The Consolidated Health Economic Evaluation Reporting Standards (CHEERS) statement is an attempt to consolidate and update previous health economic evaluation guidelines efforts into one current, useful reporting guidance. The primary audiences for the CHEERS statement are researchers reporting economic evaluations and the editors and peer reviewers assessing them for publication (Husereau et al., 2013). For 'Choice of outcomes', the CHEERS statement advises that authors '[d]escribe what outcomes were used as the measure(s) of benefit in the evaluation and their relevance for the type of analysis performed', and for 'Measurement and valuation of preference based outcomes' the statement advises that '[i]f applicable, describe the population and methods used to elicit preferences for outcomes'. This guidance carries over to reporting and presenting the results of economic evaluations of PHIs, however with broader perspectives being used such as societal or public sector, there are likely to be a greater range of outcomes across sectors and to facilitate this, the use of frameworks such as CCA, CBA, and MCDA used. Hence, under 'Choice of outcomes' such outcomes would be described and their *relevance* to the type of analysis (i.e. CCA, CBA, and MCDA) outlined.

6.10 **Discussion**

Health economists have typically used standard economic evaluation methodology and reporting guidance as the ideal starting reference for designing and conducting economic evaluations of PHIs alongside RCTs and other study designs such as natural experiments. To this end, the use of QALYs and a plethora of effectiveness-type outcomes have been prevalent (Weatherly et al., 2009b; Owen et al., 2012; Cobiac et al., 2013; Edwards et al., 2013; Edwards et al., 2016). However, there have been attempts to broaden the evaluative space and embrace alternative methodologies in a bid to capture the wider spectrum of costs and outcomes associated with PHIs as driven by the greater use of a societal perspective for such economic evaluations (Drummond et al., 2006; Weatherly et al., 2009b). Economic evaluations of PHIs such as foster care interventions provide an excellent example of the multiplicity of potential outcomes within such a societal perspective including education, employment, financial status, marriage, children, social networks, and physical and mental disorders (Zerbe et al., 2009; Minnis et al., 2016). Such outcomes need somehow to be valued or weighted for use in decision making (see Zerbe et al., 2009, for their monetization of all outcomes, placed within a CBA framework).

Summary of Chapter 6

- ◆ Outcomes for use in PHI economic evaluations are likely to be multifaceted and arise in multiple sectors.
- ◆ Reporting and presenting these multifaceted, multi-sectoral outcomes will be facilitated by use of frameworks such as CCA and CBA
- ◆ Links between unidimensional, short-, and medium-term proxy outcomes to long-term outcomes will need to be evidenced to populate long-term economic models.
- ◆ Outcomes beyond health and quality of life such as capability well-being, subjective well-being, happiness and other multi-sectoral 'consequences' are likely to be relevant in economic evaluations of PHIs.
- ◆ Research is required into methods for valuing outcomes obtained from routinely collected data.
- ◆ Behaviour change intervention economic evaluations will benefit from the development of conceptual health economic logic models in order to map the 'outcome' pathway which may be complex, multifaceted, and multi-sectoral.
- ◆ Population health outcomes, typically used within developing country economic evaluations such as DALYs, may have an increased role to play in PHI economic evaluations in developed countries.
- ◆ Research should be conducted into the practicalities of applying the intersectoral compensation test approach.
- ◆ Monetary valuation of a generic measure of well-being is recommended.
- ◆ Frameworks for combining outcomes with costs in public health economic evaluations will most likely need to extend beyond CEA, CUA, and CBA to CCA, MCDA, and SROI.

References

2016. Metrics: Disability-Adjusted Life Year (DALY) Available: http://www.who.int/ healthinfo/global_burden_disease/metrics_daly/en/ [Accessed 19/01/2017 2017].

Adamovicz, W.L., 2000. Environmental valuation case studies. In: J. Louviere, D. Hensher and J. Swait (eds), *Stated Choice Methods: Analysis and Application.* Cambridge: Cambridge University Press, pp. 329–52.

Al-Janabi, H., Peters, T. J., Brazier, J., Bryan, S., Flynn, T. N., Clemens, S., Moody, A., et al., 2013. An investigation of the construct validity of the ICECAP-A capability measure. *Quality of Life Research, 22*: 1831–40.

Al-Janabi, H., Flynn, T., and Coast, J. 2012. Development of a self-report measure of capability wellbeing for adults: The ICECAP-A. *Quality of Life Research, 21*: 167–76.

Bala, M.V., Wood, L.L., Zarkin, G.A., Norton, E.C., Gafni, A., and O'Brien, B., 1998. Valuing outcomes in health care: a comparison of willingness to pay and quality-adjusted life-years. *Journal of Clinical Epidemiology, 51*: 667–76.

Bateman, I.J., Carson, R.T., Day, B., Hanemann, M., Hanley, N., Hett, T., Jones-Lee, M., et al. (eds), 2002. *Economic Valuation with Stated Preference: A Manual.* Cheltenham: Edward Elgar.

Baum, F.E., 2003. The effectiveness of community-based health promotion in healthy cities programmes. In: T. Takano (ed.), *Healthy Cities and Urban Policy Research.* London: Spon Press, pp. 104–30.

Blackorby, C. and Donaldson, D. 1990. The case against the use of the sum of compensating variations in cost–benefit analysis. *The Canadian Journal of Economics / Revue canadienne d'Economique, 23*: 471–94.

Boxall, P.C., Adamoviczb, W. L., Swait, J., Williams, M., and Louviere, J. 1996. A comparison of stated preference methods for environmental valuation. *Ecological Economics, 18*: 243–53.

Brazier, J., Ratcliffe, J., Salomon, J., and Tsuchiya, A., 2016. *Measuring and Valuing Health Benefits for Economic Evaluation.* Oxford: Oxford University Press.

Brazier, J. and Roberts, J., 2004. The estimation of a preference-based index from the SF-12. *Medical Care, 42*: 851–9.

Brouwer, W.B.F., Koopmanschap, M.A., and Rutten, F., 1997. Productivity costs measurement through quality of life? A response to the recommendation of the Washington Panel. *Health Economics, 6*: 253–9.

Byford, S. and Sefton, T., 2003. Economic evaluation of complex health and social interventions. *National Institute Economic Review, 186*: 98–108.

Carter, S. and Mcbride, M. 2013. Experienced utility versus decision utility: Putting the 'S' in satisfaction. *Journal of Socio-Economics, 42*: 13–23.

Coast, J., 2004. Is economic evaluation in touch with society's health values? *British Medical Journal, 329*: 1233–6.

Coast, J., Flynn, T., Natarajan, L., Sproston, K., Lewis, J., and Louvere, J.J.E.A., 2008a. Valuing the ICECAP capability index for older people. *Social Science and Medicine, 67*: 874–82.

Coast, J., Peters, T., Natarajan, L., Sproston, K., and Flynn, T., 2008b. An assessment of the construct validity of the descriptive system for the ICECAP capability measure for older people. *Quality of Life Research, 17*: 967–76.

Coast, J., Smith, R., and Lorgelly, P. 2008c. Should the capability approach be applied in health economics? *Health Economics, 17*: 667–70.

Cobiac, L.J., Veerman, L., and Vos, T., 2013. The role of cost-effectiveness analysis in developing nutrition policy. *Annual Review of Nutrition*, 33:373–93.

Craig, P., Cooper, C., Gunnell, D., Haw, S., Lawson, K., Macintyre, S., Ogilvie, D., et al., 2012. Using natural experiments to evaluate population health interventions: new Medical Research Council guidance. *Journal of Epidemiology and Community Health*, 66:1182–6.

Craig, P., Dieppe, P., MacIntyre, S., Michie, S., Narzqareth, I., Petticrew, M., et al., 2008. Developing and evaluating complex interventions: the new Medical Research Council guidance. *British Medical Journal*, 337: a1655.

Crittenden, P.M, 2001. *CARE-Index Infant and Toddlers. Coding Manual.* Miami, FL: Family Relations Institute.

Deidda, M., Geue, C., Kreif, N., Dundas, R., and McIntosh, E., 2017. *Conducting Economic Evaluations Alongside Natural Experiments: A Practical Guide.* Health Economists Study Group meeting, Birmingham, January 4–6 2017. Birmingham University.

Dellavigna, S., 2009. Psychology and economics: Evidence from the field. *Journal of Economic Literature*, 47: 315–72.

Desvousges, W.H., Smith, V.K., and McGivney, M.P., 1983. *A Comparison of Alternative Approaches for Estimating Recreation and Related Benefits of Water Quality Improvements.* Washington, DC: Office of Policy Analysis, US Environmental Protection Agency.

Devlin, N. and Parkin, D., 2004. Does NICE have a cost-effectiveness threshold and what other factors influence its decisions? A binary choice analysis. *Health Economics*, 13: 437–52.

Devlin, N. and Sussex, J., 2011. *Incorporating Multiple Criteria in HTA: Methods and Processes.* London: Office of Health Economics (OHE).

Di Tella, R. and Macculloch, R., 2006. Some uses of happiness data in economics. *Journal of Economic Perspectives*, 20:25–46.

Dolan, P., Gudex, C., Kind, P., and Williams, A., 1995. A social tariff for EuroQol: results from a UK general population survey. Discussion Paper no.138 ed. York: University of York.

Dolan, P., Layard, R., and Metcalfe, R., 2011. Measuring subjective well-being for public policy. In: O. O. N., (ed.), *Statistics.* Surrey.

Dolan, P., Peasgood, T., and White, M., 2008. Do we really know what makes us happy? A review of the economic literature on the factors associated with subjective well-being. *Journal of Economic Psychology*, 29: 94–122.

Donaldson, C., Gerard, K., Jan, S., Mitton, C., Wiseman, V., 1993. *Economics of Health Care Financing: The Visible Hand.* London: Macmillan.

Donaldson, C. and Shackley, P., 1997. Does 'process utility' exist? A case study of willingness to pay for laparoscopic cholecystectomy. *Social Science and Medicine*, 44: 699–707.

Donaldson, C., Shackley, P., and Abdalla, M., 1997. Using willingness to pay to value close substitutes: carrier screening for cystic fibrosis revisited. *Health Economics*, 6: 145–59.

Drummond, M.F., Sculpher, M.J., Torrance, G.W., O'Brien, B., and Stoddart, G.L., 2015. *Methods for the Economic Evaluation of Health Care Programmes.* Oxford: Oxford University Press.

Drummond, M.F., Weatherly, H., Claxton, K., Cookson, R., Ferguson, B., Godfrey, C., Rice, N., et al., 2006. *Assessing the Challenges of Applying Standard Methods of Economic Evaluation to Public Health Interventions.* York: University of York. <http://phrc.lshtm.ac.uk/papers/PHRC_D1-05_Final_Report.pdf> (Accessed 14 October 2018).

Drummond, M., Weatherly, H., and Ferguson, B., 2008. Economic evaluation of health interventions. *British Medical Journal, 337*: a1204.

Duleep, H. and Liu, X., (2016). *Estimating More Precise Treatment Effects in Natural and Actual Experiments*. Edmonton: University of Alberta.

Dundas, R., Ouédraogo, S., Bond, L., Briggs, A.H., Chalmers, J., Gray, R., Wood, R., & Leyland, A.H., 2014. Evaluation of health in pregnancy grants in Scotland: A protocol for a natural experiment. *British Medical Journal Open*, 4: e006547.

Easterlin, R. 1974. Does economic growth improve the human lot? Some empirical evidence. In: P. David and M. Reder (eds). *Nations and Households in Economic Growth: Essays in Honour of Moses Abramovitz*. London: London Academic Press.

Edwards, R.T., Charles, J.M., and Lloyd-Williams, H., 2013. Public health economics: A systematic review of guidance for the economic evaluation of public health interventions and discussion of key methodological issues. *BMC Public Health, 13*: 1001.

Edwards, R.T., Jones, C., Berry, V., Charles, J., Linck, P., Bywater, T., and Hutchings, J., 2016. Incredible Years parenting programme: cost-effectiveness and implementation. *Journal of Children's Services, 11*: 54–72.

Faria, R., Kiss, N., Aspinal, F., Harden, M., and Weatherly, H., 2015. Economic evaluation of social care interventions: Lessons drawn from a systematic review of the methods used to evaluate reablement. *Health Econ Outcome Res Open Access, 1*.

Ferguson, K.M., 2006. Social capital and children's wellbeing: A critical synthesis of the international social capital literature. *International Journal of Social Welfare, 15*: 2–18.

Fleurbaey, M.P. and Hammond, C., 2004. Interpersonally comparable utility. In: S. Barbera, P. Hammond, and C. Seidl (eds). *Handbook of Utility Theory*. Dordrecht: Springer, pp. 1179–285.

Flynn, T.N., Huynh, E., Peters, T.J., Al Janabi, H., Clemens, S., Moody, A., and Coast, J., 2013. Scoring the ICECAP—A Capability instrument: Estimation of a UK general population tariff. *Health Economics, 24*(3): 258–69.

Foster, J., Lopez-Calva, L., and Szekely, M., 2005. Measuring the distribution of human development: Methodology and an application in Mexico. *Journal of Human Development and Capabilities, 6*: 5–25.

Fox-Rushby, J. 2002. *Disability Adjusted Life Years (DALYs) for Decision Making? An Overview of the Literature*. London: Office of Health Economics.

Frew, E., 2010. Benefit assessment for CBA studies in health care using CV methods. In: E. McIntosh (ed.), *Applied Methods of Cost–Benefit Analysis in Health Care*. Oxford: Oxford University Press, pp. 119–38.

Fujiwara, D. and Campbell, R., 2011. Valuation techniques for social cost–benefit analysis: Stated preference, revealed preference and subjective well-being approaches a discussion of the current issues. In: *Pensions*. London: HM Treasury.

Giordano, G.N. and Lindstrom, M., 2010. The impact of changes in different aspects of social capital and material conditions on self-rated health over time: A longitudinal cohort study. *Social Science and Medicine, 70*: 700–10.

Gold, M.R., Siegel, J.E., Russell, L.B., and Weinstein, M.C., 1996. *Cost-effectiveness in Health and Medicine*. New York, NY: Oxford University Press.

Gold, M.R., Stevenson, D., and Fryback, D.G., 2002. HALYS and QALYS and DALYS, Oh My: similarities and differences in summary measures of population health. *Annual Review of Public Health, 23*: 115–34.

Goldman, H., Skodol, A.E., and Lave, T.R., 1992. Revising axis V for DSM-IV: a review of measures of social functioning. *American Journal of Psychiatry*, *149*: 1148–56.

Greco, G., Lorgelly, P., and Yamabhai, I., 2016. Outcomes in economic evaluations of public health interventions in low- and middle-income countries: health, capabilities and subjective wellbeing. *Health Economics*, *25*: 83–94.

Grellier, J., White, M.P., Albin, M., Bell, S., Elliott, L.R., Gascón, M., Guald, S., et al., 2017. BlueHealth: A study programme protocol for mapping and quantifying the potential benefits to public health and well-being from Europe's blue spaces. *British Medical Journal Open*, *7*: e016188. doi:10.1136/bmjopen-2017-016188.

Grewal, I., Lewis, J., Flynn, T., Brown, J., Bond, J., and Coast, J., 2006. Developing attributes for a generic quality of life measure for older people: preferences or capabilities? *Social Science and Medicine*, *62*: 1891–901.

Haby, M.M., Vos, T., Carter, R., Moodie, M., Markwick, A., Magnus, A., Tay-Teo, K.S., et al., 2006. A new approach to assessing the health benefit from obesity interventions in children and adolescents: The assessing cost-effectiveness in obesity project. *International Journal of Obesity*, *30*: 1463–75.

Hawe, P., Shiell, A. Riley, T., and Gold, L., 2004. Methods for exploring implementation variation and local context within a cluster randomised community intervention trial. *Journal of Epidemiology and Community Health*, *58*: 788–93.

Herens M.C., Van Ophem J.A.C., Wagemakers A.M.A.E., and Koelen M.A., 2015. Predictors of willingness to pay for physical activity of socially vulnerable groups in community-based programs. *SpringerPlus*, *4*: 527.

HM Treasury, 2010. Budget 2010. London: The Stationery Office.

Horsman, J., Furlong, W., Feeny, D., and Torrance, G.W., 2003. The Health Utilities Index (HUI®): Concepts, measurement properties and applications. *Health and Quality of Life Outcomes*, *1*: 54.

Husereau, D., Drummond, M., Petrou, S., Carswell, C., Moher, D., Greenberg, D., Augustovski, F., et al., 2013. Consolidated health economic evaluation reporting standards (CHEERS) statement. *International Journal of Technology Assessment in Health Care. 2000 Winter*, *29*: 117–22.

Islam, M.S., Lechner, A., Ferrari, U., Seissler, J., Holle, J., and Niessen, L.W. 2015. Mobile phone use and willingness to pay for SMS for diabetes in Bangladesh. *Journal of Public Health*, *38*: 163–9.

Jan, S., Mooney, G., Ryan, M., Bruggemann, K., and Alexander, K.,2000. The use of conjoint analysis to elicit community preferences in public health research: A case study of hospital services in Australia. *Australian and New Zealand Journal of Public Health*, *24*: 64–70.

Johannesson, M. 1996. A note on the relationship between ex ante and expected willingness to pay for health care. *Social Science and Medicine*, *42*: 305–11.

Kahneman, D., Diener, E., and Schwarz, N. (eds), 1999. *Well-being: The Foundations of Hedonic Psychology*. New York, NY: Russell-Sage.

Kahneman, D., Wakker, P.P., and Sarin, R., 1997. Back to Bentham? Explorations of experienced utility. *Quarterly Journal of Economics*, *112*: 375–405.

Kleinman, L., McIntosh, E., Ryan, M., Schmier, J., Crawley, J., Locke G.R., and De Lissovoy, G., 2002. Willingness to pay for complete symptom relief of gastroesophogeal reflux disease. *Archives of Internal Medicine*, *162*: 1361–6.

Kouvonen, A., Oksanen, T., Vahtera, J., Väänänen, A., De Vogli, R., Elovainio, M., Pentti, J., et al., 2008. Work-place social capital and smoking cessation: The Finnish Public Sector Study. *Addiction, 103*: 1857–65.

Krief, N., Grieve, R., Radice, R., and Sekhon, J.S., 2013. Regression-adjusted matching and double-robust methods for estimating average treatment effects in health economic evaluation. *Health Services and Outcomes Research Methodology, 13*: 174–202.

Lancsar, E. and Savage, E., 2004a. Deriving welfare measures from discrete choice experiments: A response to Ryan and Santos Silva. *Health Economics Letters, 13*: 919–24.

Lancsar, E. and Savage, E., 2004b. Deriving welfare measures from discrete choice experiments: Inconsistency between current methods and random utility and welfare theory. *Health Economics Letters, 13*: 901–7.

Lensberg, B.R., Drummond, M.F., Danchenko, N., Despiégel, N., and François, C., 2013. Challenges in measuring and valuing productivity costs, and their relevance in mood disorders. *ClinicoEconomics and Outcomes Research, 5*: 65–73.

Lorgelly, P.K., Lawson, K.D., Fenwick, E.A.L., and Briggs, A.H., 2010. Outcome measurement in economic evaluations of public health interventions: A role for the capability approach? *International Journal of Environmental Research and Public Health, 7*: 2274–89.

Lorgelly, P., Lorimer, K., Fenwick, E., Briggs A.H., and Anand, P., 2015a. Operationalising the capability approach as an outcome measure in public health: The development of the OCAP-18. *Social Science & Medicine, 142*: 68–81.

Lorgelly, P.K., Lorimer, K., Fenwick, E.A.L., Briggs, A.H., and Anand, P., 2015b. Operationalising the capability approach as an outcome measure in public health: The development of the OCAP-18. *Social Science & Medicine, 142*: 68–81.

Macinko, J. and Starfield, B., 2001. The utility of social capital in research on health determinants. *Milbank Quarterly, 79*: 387–427.

Marsh, K., Ganz, M.L., Hsu, J., Strandberg-Larsen, M., Gonzalez, R.P., and Lund, N., 2016. Expanding health technology assessments to include effects on the environment. *Value in Health, 19*: 249–54.

Marsh, K., Phillips, C.J., Fordham, R., Bertranou, E., and Hale, J., 2012. Estimating cost-effectiveness in public health: A summary of modelling and valuation methods. *Health Economics Review, 2*: 17.

McIntosh, E., Barlow, J., and Stewart-Brown, S., 2009. Economic evaluation of an intensive home visiting programme: A cost-effectiveness analysis from a societal perspective. *Journal of Public Health Medicine, 31*: 423–33.

McIntosh, E., Donaldson, C., and Ryan, M., 1999. Recent advances in the methods of cost–benefit analysis in health care: Matching the art to the science. *Pharmacoeconomics, 15*: 357–67.

McIntosh, E. and Luengo-Fernandez, R., 2006. Economic evaluation. Part 1: Introduction to the concepts of economic evaluation in health care. *Journal of Family Planning and Reproductive Health Care, 32*: 107–12.

Minnis, H., Boyd, K., Fitzpatrick, B., Forde, M., Gillberg, C., Henderson, M., McMahon, L., et al., 2016. Protocol 15PRT/6090: The Best Services Trial (BeST?): effectiveness and cost-effectiveness of the New Orleans Intervention Model for Infant Mental Health— NCT02653716. *Lancet*. Available at: <https://www.thelancet.com/protocol-reviews/15PRT-6090> (Accessed 7 November 2018).

Mitchell, P.M., A.-J.H., Richardson. J., and Iezzi, A.C.J., 2015. The relative impacts of disease on health status and capability wellbeing: A multi-country study. *PLoS ONE*, **10** (12): e0143590.

Mitchell, P.M., Roberts, T.E., Barton, P.M., and Coast, J., 2015. Assessing sufficient capability: A new approach to economic evaluation. *Social Science & Medicine*, (139): 71–9.

Murayama, H., Kondo, K., and Fujiwara, Y., 2013. Social capital interventions to promote healthy aging. In: I. Kawachi, S. Takao, and S. Subramanian (eds), *Global Perspectives on Social Capital and Health*. New York, NY: Springer, pp. 205–38.

Murray, C.J.L. and Lopez, A.D., 2013. Measuring the Global Burden of Disease. *New England Journal of Medicine, 369*: 448–57.

Mwachofi, A. and Al-Assaf, A.F., 2011. Health care market deviations from the ideal market. *Sultan Qaboos University Medical Journal, 11*: 328–37.

National Institute for Health and Care Excellence, N.I.F.H.A.C.E., 2011a. <http:// publications.nice.org.uk/methods-for-the-development-of-nice-public-health-guidance-third-edition-pmg4/incorporating-health-economics>

National Institute for Health and Care Excellence, N.I.F.H.A.C.E., 2011b. Supporting investment in public health: Review of methods for assessing cost-effectiveness, cost impact and return on investment. Proof of Concept Report. London: National Institute for Health and Clinical Excellence.

National Institute for Health and Care Excellence, N.I.F.H.A.C.E., 2012a. Methods for the development of NICE public health guidance (third edition).

National Institute for Health and Care Excellence, N.I.F.H.A.C.E., 2012b. *Methods for the Development of NICE Public Health Guidance: Incorporating Health Economics*. Available at: <https://www.nice.org.uk/process/pmg4/chapter/incorporating-health-economics>.

Nussbaum, M., 2003. Capabilities as fundamental entitlements: Sen and social justice. *Feminist Economics, 9*: 33–59.

Olsen, J.A. and Smith, R.D., 2001, *Theory* versus *practice*: A review of 'willingness-to-pay' in health and health care. *Health Economics*, 10:39–52.

Olsen, J.A., Donaldson, C., and Pereira, J., 2004. The insensitivity of 'willingness-to-pay' to the size of the good: New evidence for health care. Journal of Economic Psychology, 25(4):445–60.

Owen, L., Morgan, A., Fischer, A., Ellis, S., Hoy, A., and Kelly, M., 2012. The cost-effectiveness of public health interventions. *Journal of Public Health, 1*(1March): 37–45.

Pearce, D. and Ozdemiroglu, E.E.A., 2002. Economic valuation with stated preference techniques summary guide. In: Department of Transport. London: HMSO.

Pritchard, C. And Sculpher, M., 2000. *Productivity Costs: Principles and Practice in Economic Evaluation*. London, Office of Health Economics.

Remme, M., Martinez-Alvarez, M., and Vassall, A., 2017. Cost-effectiveness thresholds in global health: Taking a multisectoral perspective. *Value in Health*, 20: 699–704.

Russell, L.B. and Sinha, A., 2016. Strengthening cost-effectiveness analysis for public health policy. *American Journal of Preventive Medicine, 50*: S6–S12.

Ryan, M., Scott, D.A., and Donaldson, C., 1998. Econometric issues raised in the analysis of payment scale and closed-ended contingent valuation data sets in health care. *Health Technology Assessment, 5*(5): 1–186.

Ryan, M., Scott, D.A., and **Donaldson, C.**, 2004. Valuing health care using willingness to pay: A comparison of the payment card and dichotomous choice methods. *Journal of Health Economics*, *23*(2): 237–58.

Ryan, M. and **Shackley, P.**, 1995. Assessing the benefits of health care: How far should we go? *Quality in Health Care*, *4*: 207–13.

Santos Silva, J.M.C., 2004. Deriving welfare measures in discrete choice experiments: A comment to Lancsar and Savage (2). *Health Economics Letters*, *13*: 913–18.

Sassi, F., 2006. Calculating QALYs, comparing QALY and DALY calculations. *Health Policy and Planning*, *21*: 402–8.

Sassi, F., 2010. *Obesity and the Economics of Prevention*. Cheltenham: Edward Elgar Publishing.

Sculpher, M., Claxton, K., and **Pearson, S.D.**, 2017. Developing a value framework: The need to reflect the opportunity costs of funding decisions. *Value in Health*, *20*: 234–9.

Sen, A., 1982. *Choice, Welfare and Measurement*. Cambridge, MA: Harvard University Press.

Sen, A., 1987. *Commodities and Capabilities*. Oxford, Oxford University Press.

Sen, A., 1993. Capability and well-being. In: M.C. Nussbaum and A.K. Sen (eds), *The Quality of Life*. Oxford: Clarendon Press.

Shackley, P. and **Donaldson, C.**, 2002. Should we use willingness to pay to elicit community preferences for health care? New evidence from using a 'marginal' approach. *Journal of Health Economics*, *21*: 971–91.

Shiell, A., Hawe, P., and **Gold, L.**, 2008. Complex interventions or complex systems? Implications for health economic evaluation. *British Medical Journal*, *336*: 1281–3.

Siahpush, M. and **Scollo, M.**, 2001. Trends in public support for smoking bans in public places in Australia. *Australian and New Zealand Journal of Public Health*, *25*: 473.

Simon, J., Anand, P., Gray, A., Rugkåsa, J., Yeeles, K., and **Burns, T.**, 2013. Operationalising the capability approach for outcome measurement in mental health research. *Social Science & Medicine*, *98*:187–96.

Smith, R.D., 2003. Construction of the contingent valuation market in health care: A critical assessment. *Health Economics*, *12*:609–28.

Smith, R.D., 2000. The discrete willingness-to-pay question format in health economics: Should we adopt environmental guidelines? *Medical Decision Making*, *20*: 194–206.

Smith, R.D. and **Petticrew, M.**, 2010. Public health evaluation in the twenty-first century: Time to see the wood as well as the trees. *Journal of Public Health*, *32*: 2–7.

Smith, V.K., 1985. Some issues in discrete response contingent valuation studies. *Northeastern Journal of Agricultural and Resource Economics*, *1*: 156–75.

Squires, H., Chilcott, J., Akehurst, R., Burr, J., and **Kelly, M.P.**, 2016. A framework for developing the structure of public health economic models. *Value in Health*, *19*: 588–601.

Stiglitz, J.E., Sen, A., and **Fitoussi, J.P.**, 2009. Report by the Commission on the Measurement of Economic Performance and Social Progress. Paris: OECD.

Strack, F. and **Deutsch, R.**, 2004. Reflective and impulsive determinants of social behavior. *Personality and Social Psychology Review*, *8*: 220–47.

Väänänen, A., Kouvonen, A., Kivimäki, M., Oksanen, T., Elovainio, M., Virtanen, M., Pentti, J., et al., 2009. Workplace social capital and co-occurrence of lifestyle risk factors: The Finnish Public Sector Study. *Occupational and Environmental Medicine*, *66*: 432–7.

Weatherly, H., Drummond, M., Claxton, K., Cookson, R., Ferguson, B., Godfrey, C., Rice, N., et al., 2009a. Methods for assessing the cost-effectiveness of public health interventions: key challenges and recommendations. *Health Policy*, **93** (2–3): 85–92.

Weatherly, H., Drummond, M.F, Claxton, K., Cookson, R., Ferguson, B., Godfrey, C., Rice, N., et al., 2009b. Methods for assessing the cost-effectiveness of public health interventions: Key challenges and recommendations. *Health Policy*, *93*: 85–92.

Wilson, T.D. and Gilbert, D., 2003. Affective forecasting. *Advances in Experimental Social Psychology*, *35*: 345–411.

Zerbe, R.O., Plotnick, R.D., Kessler, R.C., Pecora, P.J., Hiripi, E.V.A., O'Brien, K., Williams, J., et al., 2009. Benefits and costs of intensive foster care services: The Casey family programs compared to state services. *Contemporary Economic Policy*, *27*: 308–20.

Chapter 7

Cost-effectiveness analysis of public health interventions

Rhiannon T. Edwards

7.1 Introduction

With the increasing influence of cost-effectiveness evidence in UK health care, the application of such methods to PHIs and programs has gathered momentum. The Wanless Reports (2002; 2004) challenged health economists to apply our methods of economic evaluation to interventions to improve public health.

Chapter 2 of this book introduced the reader to the purpose, principles, and statistical methods of cost-effectiveness analysis. This chapter provides an example of a cost-effectiveness analysis undertaken alongside a pragmatic randomized controlled trial (RCT) of a public health intervention. In the United Kingdom, the CHARISMA trial was one of the first collaborations between a local authority, Wrexham County Borough Council (who paid for the housing modifications), National Health Service (NHS) primary care, and Bangor University working with Public Health Wales who undertook the evaluation. In retrospect, a wider range of outcomes could have been collected to inform decision-making but this study is still one of the few published economic evaluations of housing interventions to improve health. The following chapters of this book illustrate a range of other methods applicable to the evaluation of such public health interventions.

7.2 Case study: Improving heating and ventilation in homes of children with asthma

The following case study is reproduced in full from Edwards, R.T., Neal, R.D., Linck, P., Bruce, N., Mullock, L., Nelhans, N., Pasterfield, D., Russell, D., Russell, I., and Woodfine, L., 2011. Enhancing ventilation in homes of children with asthma: cost-effectiveness study alongside randomised controlled trial. *British Journal of General Practice, 61*(592), pp. e733–e741.

7.2.1 Introduction

A recent update of a previous systematic review of the health effects of housing improvements (Thomson et al., 2001; Thomson et al., 2009) identified 39 controlled prospective studies, covering a variety of environmental modifications, most of which were ineffective. Nevertheless, there is some evidence that improving home ventilation and heating may be beneficial in managing childhood asthma (Warner et al., 2000; Wright et al., 2009). In the only comprehensive published study of the economics of housing modification to improve health, Chapman and colleagues used cost–benefit analysis alongside a randomized trial to show that retrofitting houses in New Zealand with insulation yielded benefits worth up to twice the cost of refurbishment (Chapman et al., 2009).

More than one in 10 children between the ages of 5 and 14 years in the United Kingdom has asthma, and it is the most common long-term medical condition in children (Asthma UK, 2011). Asthma is estimated to cost the NHS £1000 million a year (Cohen et al., 2007).

This paper describes an incremental cost-effectiveness analysis (Drummond et al., 2015; Ramsey et al., 2005; Glick et al., 2007) conducted alongside the CHARISMA trial (Children's Health in Asthma: Research to Improve Status through Modifying Accommodation), a pragmatic RCT of housing modification to improve ventilation, and central heating if necessary, in homes of children with moderate to severe asthma, in comparison with a delayed intervention (Woodfine et al., 2011).

7.2.1.1 Method

Study population The trial took place from 2004 to 2006 in Wrexham, North Wales. Children were recruited through their GPs; 20 out of the 23 practices within Wrexham Local Health Board participated. Households were randomly allocated to the intervention group or to a delayed-intervention control group who received housing modification after the end of the trial.

Intervention Each child's household was visited by a local authority housing officer who assessed the improvements needed. Ventilation systems were installed in the roof spaces of houses. Improvements were made to bring central heating systems to a defined standard; new systems were installed if none existed. There was no cost to the families for these improvements. The companion paper by Woodfine and colleagues gives more detail about the study population, inclusion and exclusion criteria, and intervention (Woodfine et al., 2011).

How this fits in The association between poor housing and ill-health has long been recognized. This study is the first cost-effectiveness analysis alongside a pragmatic RCT of improving ventilation in the homes of children with asthma. It reports that tailored ventilation and heating modifications led to a 17 per cent shift of children in the intervention group from 'severe' to 'moderate' asthma, as compared with a 3 per cent shift for the control group, at an average cost to the council of £1718 per child; but the package had no apparent effect on health-service costs. Improving ventilation in homes of children with moderate to severe asthma is likely to be a cost-effective use of public resources.

Measurement of effectiveness The main outcome measure in this cost-effectiveness study was the parent-reported asthma module of PedsQL™, a validated quality-of-life measure for children with asthma (Varni et al., 2004). The study used the total score for asthma-related quality of life on a 100-point scale, measured at the final follow-up

12 months after randomization. This asthma-specific measure was chosen, as there is no generally accepted technique for measuring utility in young children (Brazier et al., 2007) (Please see section 8.6 discussion of CHU-9D, which is now available to measure utility in young children). Data were also collected on the frequency of primary and secondary health care use and asthma-related prescribing.

Measurement of costs Cost-effectiveness analysis was undertaken from a multi-agency, public sector perspective. This combined the perspectives of Wrexham County Borough Council, which bore the cost of housing improvements in this trial, and the NHS, which bears the health care costs associated with childhood asthma. Wrexham County Borough Council provided information on the housing modification received by each household in the intervention group, and associated costs. As this study takes a public-sector perspective, it has not included the running costs of ventilation systems, estimated at £15 a year, or costs to families of running central heating.

Parents were asked to use the validated Client Service Receipt Inventory (Patel et al., 2005) adapted to recall their child's contacts with health services over the study period. A researcher later visited each participating practice to abstract from children's notes a structured record of the type and frequency of consultations, visits to emergency departments or outpatient clinics, inpatient stays, and prescribed drugs. It was found that parents' and practices' reports of health care use were not entirely consistent. However, both approaches led to similar conclusions about differences between groups, and thus about cost-effectiveness. After consideration, it was decided to report estimates of resource use from general practice records, because these records included prescribing information.

National costs were obtained from the report by Curtis and Netten for units of health and social care (Curtis and Netten, 2007), the Department of Health for NHS reference costs (Department of Health, 2006), and the Health and Social Care Information Centre for prescribing costs (NHS Information Centre, 2006). All costs are in pounds sterling for 2006. As participants were followed for only 12 months, discounting was not necessary (Eichler et al., 2004).

Analysis of effects Like the primary effectiveness analysis in the companion paper, the economic analysis focused on 177 of the 192 children randomized in the trial. Fifteen children who had no follow-up questionnaire were excluded. For 8 children who did not complete a 12-month PedsQL questionnaire, scores at 12 months were imputed by regression on scores at baseline and 4 months. Baseline PedsQL and complete cost data were available for all 177 children. Analysis of covariance was used to adjust effects for baseline scores.

Analysis of costs Health-service use and prescribing of asthma drugs were compared between the intervention and control groups. As distributions of both frequencies and costs were skewed, frequencies were compared by non-parametric tests, and costs by bootstrapping.

Costs in the 12 months before randomization did not differ significantly between groups. The possibility of adjusting costs for the corresponding costs before randomization, as for effects, was investigated. Although primary care costs before and after randomization were related, secondary care costs were highly skewed, and extreme values before randomization hardly related to extreme values after randomization. Hence, adjusting for past history did not improve the precision of estimates. For consistency, therefore, the analysis did not adjust any costs.

Cost-effectiveness analysis As the trial used a condition-specific outcome rather than a utility measure, cost-effectiveness analysis, rather than cost–utility analysis, was used (Drummond et al., 2015). This analysis compared children's adjusted change over 12 months in asthma-related PedsQL score with their health care costs, augmented by the household cost of housing modifications in the intervention group.

Incremental cost-effectiveness ratios (ICERs) were estimated, and bootstrapping was used with 1000 replications to generate confidence intervals (CIs). A cost-effectiveness plane was generated, showing the joint distribution of bootstrapped costs and effects, and a cost-effectiveness acceptability curve was also generated, covering a range of cost-effectiveness thresholds. Where possible, a bootstrapped 95 per cent CI for the ICER was derived from the cost-effectiveness acceptability curve.

Choice of threshold ICER Cost-effectiveness acceptability curves were used to show the probability that the intervention is cost-effective over the range £0 to £600 per PedsQL point. There is no guidance from the National Institute for Health and Clinical Excellence (NICE) or the literature as to what society should be prepared to pay for improvements in disease-specific quality-of-life measures like the PedsQL (Eichler et al., 2004; Raftery, 2001). The results of this study therefore show how this intervention has shifted distributions of PedsQL scores in the intervention and control groups, and relate this to the average cost per child of the intervention to Wrexham County Borough Council.

Sensitivity analyses Economic evaluation uses sensitivity analysis to investigate how sensitive findings are to basic assumptions, by varying those assumptions. Building costs vary across the United Kingdom, so the ICER was recalculated to test whether the study findings depend on building costs in North Wales, which are lower than those in London but higher than those in Northern Ireland (Johnson, 2007).

Following recent guidance that economic analysis of public health interventions should give more weight to equity (Weatherly et al., 2009, the study tested whether its findings would change if the criterion for housing improvements (asthma severity) were more stringent. The sample of children was subdivided at the median of baseline asthma scores (median = 67), and each half of the sample was analysed separately. As PedsQL does not distinguish between moderate and severe asthma, this equal division maximizes the power of the comparison and offers a working definition of 'severe' asthma.

7.2.1.2 Results

Effectiveness At baseline, the 177 children analysed in this and the companion paper were similar in all respects to the 15 children excluded for lack of follow-up data. The distributions of PedsQL scores at baseline were similar in the intervention and control groups, as was the distribution of costs. After 12 months, the PedsQL showed a mean (adjusted) improvement of 8.65 in the intervention group and 1.58 in the control group. The resulting difference of 7.07 (95% CI = 2.79–11.36) between groups is equivalent to a standardized effect size of 0.42.

Costs of housing modification The housing officers assessed 38 children (19 intervention, 19 control) as needing both ventilation and heating improvements, and the remaining 139 (69 intervention, 70 control) as needing only ventilation. However, six of the intervention group assessed as needing only ventilation subsequently received both ventilation systems and central heating improvement.

In contrast, two intervention households received neither ventilation systems nor central heating improvement, for family reasons. These were analysed by 'intention to treat'. Table 7.1 includes the costs of housing modification to improve ventilation, and heating if necessary, as estimated by Wrexham County Borough Council. These programme-specific building costs include a standard 12 per cent managerial overhead including surveying costs. The mean total cost of housing modification was £1718. The mean cost of improving ventilation and heating (excluding six houses described above) was £3675; the mean cost of improving ventilation alone was £1179 (including these six).

Health service use by children Table 7.2 summarizes the costs of health service use by children in the intervention and control groups over 12 months. There was no consistent difference between the two groups. Primary care costs were similar in the two groups, while the costs relating to secondary care over 12 months were lower, but not significantly lower, in the intervention group, mainly through fewer outpatient consultations. The total NHS costs were £61 lower for the intervention group than the control group, but this difference was also not significant. However, the total costs, including the costs of housing improvements, are inevitably much lower in the control group: £560 compared with £2217. The mean difference is £1657 with bootstrapped 95% CI = £1282–£2036.

Prescribing In the year before randomization, mean prescribing costs in primary care were £106 for the intervention group and £111 for the control group. Over the next year these costs rose to £122 in the intervention group and £136 in the control group; this difference was not significant. Table 7.2 shows the costs of prescribing over 12 months by category within the *British National Formulary*. Most costs arise from prescribing bronchodilators and corticosteroids. Although bronchodilators cost more in the intervention group, corticosteroids cost more in the control group; neither difference was statistically significant.

Total NHS costs at baseline and follow-up In the year before randomization (baseline), mean NHS costs in the intervention and control groups were £476 and £663, respectively. Although in the year after randomization (follow-up) these costs rose to

Table 7.1 Unit costs of health care and housing modifications in UK pounds (£)

Type of cost	Unit	Unit cost[a]	Details
Healthcare resources			
GP surgery consultation	Consultation	25	Per consultation lasting 10 min[15]
GP phone consultation	Consultation	31	Per consultation lasting 10.8 min[15]
GP home visit	Consultation	69	Per consultation lasting 13.2 min plus 12 min travel time[15]
Practice nurse consultation	Consultation	10	Per consultation lasting 15.5 min[15]
Paediatric thoracic out-patient clinic	Consultation	226	Mean of first and follow-up thoracic consultation (£240 and £213)[16]
Paediatric outpatient clinic	Consultation	188	Mean of first and follow-up appointment general paediatric (£228 and £149)[16]
Accident and emergency visit	Consultation	80	Department of Health (2006)[16]
Inpatient stay (asthma-related cost)	Day	453	Mean cost per bed day[16]
Prescribing	Item	Various	Department of Health (2006)[17]
Local authority housing modifications[b]			
Costs by intention to treat	**Ventilation only (n = 69)**	**Ventilation plus heating (n = 19)**	**Whole sample (n = 88)**
Mean [SD]	1179 (1100)	3675 (1999)	1718 (1685)
Range (minimum to maximum)	0 to 6924	0 to 7430	0 to 7430
Total intervention cost	81 325	69 827	151 152
Costs by treatment received	Ventilation only (n = 63)	Ventilation plus heating (n = 69)	Housing improvement (n = 88)
Mean [SD]	913 (279)	3746 (2027)	1718 (1685)
Range (minimum to maximum)	0 to 1734	0 to 7430	0 to 7430
Total intervention cost	57 507	93 645	151 152

[a]NHS costs include salary, on-costs, qualifications, overheads, and capital costs all rounded to the nearest £.
[b]Local authority costs depend on system required for each house. Costs include 12 per cent administration cost. One house from each subgroup had no modification.

Table 7.2 Mean NHS and local authority costs (£) over 12 months by group

Type of cost	Intervention (n = 88)[a] mean (SD)	Control (n = 89)[a] mean (SD)	Mean difference (bootsrapped 95% CI)
NHS primary care sector			
GP consultations			
Surgery	77(62)	78(81)	-0.83
Telephone	7 (17)	10(24)	-3.06
Home visits	2 (10)	1 (7)	0.79
Out-of-hours GP consultations			
Surgery	3 (14)	2 (10)	1.16
Telephone	4 (13)	2(19)	1.79
Home visits	0(0)	3 (14)	-3.10
Practice nurse consultations	16(12)	13(14)	3.33
Total primary care consultations	**109 (72)**	**109 (99)**	**0 (–26 to 25)**
Primary care prescribing[b]			
3.1. Bronchodilators short-term	20(26)	14(19)	6.41
3.1. Bronchcdilators long-term	28(81)	25(83)	2.30
3.1 All bronchodilators	**48(94)**	**39(86)**	**9 (–16 to 36)**
3.2 Single drug corticosteroids	23(29)	17(24)	6.39
3.2 Combination corticosteroids	23(58)	36 (104)	−13.05
3.2 All corticosteroids	**46 (58)**	**53(106)**	**−7 (−30 to 21)**
3.3–3.10	**21(51)**	**27(74)**	**−6 (−26 to 12)**
All *BNF* 3 Respiratory	**114 (135)**	**120 (173)**	**−6(−52 to 38)**
5.1 Antibacterial	3(9)	2(4)	1.26
6.3 Gluocosteroids	< 1(1)	< 1 (1)	−0.10
12.2. Drugs acting on the nose	1 (6)	< 1 (3)	0.68
13.2–5 Emollient, barriers, top-ical corticosieroids and eczema preparations	5(18)	10(33)	−5.23
Peak flow meters and other devices	1(3)	2(4)	−0.38
Total primary care prescribing	**122(143)**	**136(185)**	**−15(−83 to 14)**
Total primary care	**231(164)**	**245 (239)**	**−14(−92 to 23)**
NHS secondary sector			
Outpatients			

(continued)

Table 7.2 Continued

Type of cost	Intervention ($n = 88$)[a] mean (SD)	Control ($n = 89$)[a] mean (SD)	Mean difference (bootsrapped 95% CI)
Consultation	157(269)	219(376)	−62(−158 to 39)
Inpatients			
Inpatient hospital days (all causes)	93(308)	71 (312)	21(−68 to 114)
Prescribing	< 1(< 1)	1(6)	−0.94
Accident and emergency			
Attendances	19(38)	24(46)	−5 (−18 to 7)
Total secondary care	**269(490)**	**315(559)**	**−46(−272 to 101)**
Total NHS cost	**499 (538)**	**560(669)**	**−61(−272 to 91)**
Local authority intervention cost	1718(1695)	0(0)	1718
Housing adaptation package			
Total NHS and	**2217(1766)**	**560(669)**	**1657(1282 to 2036)**
Local authority cost			

[a]Costs rounded to nearest £. [b]British National. Formulary.

£499 in the intervention group and fell to £560 in the control group, there was again no statistically significant difference at baseline, at follow-up, or in the change from baseline to follow-up.

Cost-effectiveness Using the cost-and-effect data gathered over 12 months for 88 intervention households and 89 control households, an ICER was estimated. The difference between groups in mean total cost (£1657) was divided by the difference between groups in mean effect (7.07 PedsQL points), to yield an estimated ICER of £234 per unit change in the PedsQL asthma-specific quality of life.

Analysis of uncertainty Figure 7.1A shows the resulting cost-effectiveness plane. All 1000 bootstrapped points fall within the north-east quadrant of this plane, where the intervention is both more costly and more effective than usual treatment (Briggs and Gray, 1999). Figure 7.1B shows the corresponding cost-effectiveness acceptability curve, plotting the probability that housing modification is cost-effective against the range of thresholds below which decision-makers are willing to pay for such modifications (Fenwick et al., 2004; Koerhamp et al., 2007). As all points are in the north-east quadrant, the curve intercepts the y axis at 0.0 and approaches 1.0 as the threshold increases. The probability of the intervention being cost-effective is 2.5 per cent at a threshold of £140, and 97.5 per cent at £590. In other words, the bootstrapped 95 per cent CI for the ICER of £234 per unit change in the PedsQL asthma-specific quality of life score, runs from £140 to £590.

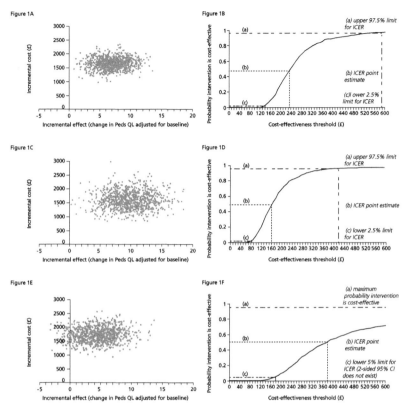

Figure 7.1 Cost-effectiveness planes (1A, 1C, 1E) and cost-effectiveness acceptability curves (1B, 1D, 1F) for all children (1A, 1B), children with severe asthma (1C, 1D) and children with moderate asthma (1E, 1F). Figures 1A, 1B: 88 in intervention group and 89 in control group. Figures 1C, 1D: 42 in intervention group and 44 in control group. Figures 1E, 1F: 46 in intervention group and 45 in control group.

Sensitivity analyses The ICER and estimated probability that housing modifications are effective depends on local building costs (Curtis and Netten, 2007). The authors estimate that in Wales, where the study took place, the intervention has an ICER of £234 (95% CI = £140–£590); with the same effectiveness. This intervention in London would have an ICER of £294 (95% CI = £174– £770), and in Northern Ireland, the ICER would be £166 (95% CI = £98– £430).

For the 44 children in the control group and 42 children in the intervention group with more severe asthma (i.e. baseline PedsQL score below the median of 67), the mean difference in costs was £1590, and the mean difference in effect was 9.67 PedsQL points, yielding an ICER of £165 (bootstrapped 95% CI = £84– £424; Figures 7.1C and 7.1D). For the 45 children in the control group and 46 children in the intervention group with more moderate asthma (i.e. baseline PedsQL score at or above the median of 67), the mean difference in costs was £1730, and the mean difference in effect was

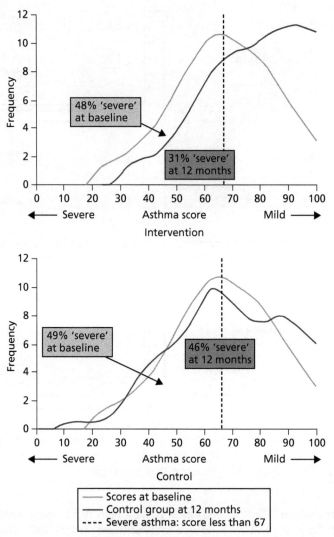

Figure 7.2 Changes in the distribution of asthma scores from baseline to 12 months. All distribution curves are smoothed. Baseline distributions are very similar in the two groups, and the baseline median of both intervention and control groups is 67 (although the proportions are marginally different, as a few score exactly 67), so the same baseline curve is used in both graphs.

4.56 PedsQL points, yielding a higher ICER of £379 (Figures 7.1E and 7.1F). Because 5 per cent of bootstrapped points fell in the north-west quadrant of the cost-effectiveness plane, where the intervention is more costly and less effective than usual treatment, it was not possible to derive a two-sided 95% CI for the subsample with more moderate asthma. Instead, a one-sided 95% CI was derived: if society were willing to pay only up to £180 (the 'threshold') per point improvement on the PedsQL scale, housing modification would be less cost-effective than no action. At a threshold of £300 per unit improvement on the PedsQL score, housing modification has a 93 per cent probability of being cost-effective for children with more severe asthma, compared with 35 per cent for children with more moderate asthma (and 76 per cent for all children). This difference is due mainly to a larger (although not significantly larger) effect in the subsample of children with more severe asthma.

Costs of shifting the distribution of asthma scores in children Figure 7.2 shows that tailored heating and ventilation housing modifications led to a 17 per cent shift of children in the intervention group from 'severe' to 'moderate' asthma, compared with a 3 per cent shift for the control group. The cost to Wrexham County Borough Council was £1718 per child in the intervention group or £12,300 per child shifted from 'severe' to 'moderate'.

7.2.1.3 Discussion

Summary This economic evaluation extends the findings of the CHARISMA trial (Woodfine et al., 2011). The analysis estimates the cost of a single-point improvement in the PedsQL asthma-specific quality of life score at £234. At baseline, the median reported asthma-related quality of life score was 67, with a lower quartile of 56 and an upper quartile of 79; 12 months later, parents of children in the intervention group reported a median score of 76, with a lower quartile of 64 and an upper quartile of 87. In summary, tailored ventilation and heating modifications moved 17 per cent of children in the intervention group from below the original median ('severe asthma') to above that median ('moderate asthma'), while only 3 per cent of controls moved from 'severe' to 'moderate'. Thus, a net 14 per cent of children (or 29 per cent of children with 'severe' asthma) became 'moderate'. The cost to Wrexham County Borough Council was £1718 per child in the intervention group, or £12,300 per child shifted from 'severe' to 'moderate'. Thus, the installation of a ventilation system, and central heating where necessary, in the homes of children with moderate to severe asthma improves their respiratory health and quality of life. These housing modifications are likely to be cost-effective.

Strengths and limitations The CHARISMA trial shows that there is scope to apply a rigorous economic approach alongside a pragmatic trial to evaluate community-based public health interventions (Edwards et al., 2008). As resources were limited, however, participating children were only followed for one year, and the study did not assess benefits to siblings or parents, measure children's respiratory function, or analyse mould spores in their houses. The measurement of respiratory function is difficult and expensive, and was too variable to contribute to a recent trial of heating alone (Howden-Chapman et al., 2008).

Comparison with existing literature A recent Cochrane Review of chemical and physical methods to control asthma concluded that they were ineffective, and recommended that further studies should be more rigorous (Gøtzsche and Johansen, 2008). By using an RCT to show that ventilation systems improve respiratory quality of life, CHARISMA has responded to this challenge. Furthermore, it has added the first rigorous cost-effectiveness analysis of housing modifications to address child-hood asthma.

Implications for practice and research Wanless, in his report, previously challenged health economists to produce rigorous evidence of the cost-effectiveness of public health interventions (Wanless, 2004). In response, CHARISMA provides evidence that improving ventilation, and heating where necessary, in homes of children with moderate to severe asthma is an effective use of public resources.

Nevertheless, the findings of this study almost certainly underestimate the full value of the effects of housing modification. Given the net benefit of 7 PedsQL points to children in the intervention group after 12 months, it is inconceivable that they gain no benefit after that. Furthermore, several parents with asthma spontaneously reported that they too had benefited. Both observations illustrate the published guidance on the economic analysis of public health interventions (Weatherly et al., 2009). This re-commended that analysts should strive not only to estimate benefits in the long term but also to consider benefits to individuals not directly targeted by the intervention. Although this guidance cannot be followed directly, the indirect evidence about long-term and parental benefits allows a conclusion that housing modification is likely to be cost-effective.

Despite the clear improvement in the health of children in the intervention group, their health care costs, notably repeat prescriptions, continued at their previous level. As the beneficial effects of housing modification become more widely known, the authors hope that the potential for reducing the prescription of asthma drugs will be recognized.

Sensitivity analysis showed that the cost-effectiveness of housing modifications was dependent on local building costs. As CHARISMA almost certainly underestimated the full value of housing modification, the authors see little reason for geographical variation in the uptake of these modifications. Sensitivity analysis also showed that cost-effectiveness differed between children with more severe asthma (whose ICER was £165), and those with less severe asthma (whose ICER was £379).

Although this subgroup analysis had lower power than the main trial, the authors conclude that the case for improving the housing of children with 'severe' asthma is even more cogent than for children with 'moderate' asthma.

Although the findings of CHARISMA are encouraging, NICE needs research of two kinds before recommending that local authorities install ventilation systems in the houses of children with asthma. First, a multi-centre trial is recommended, following children for at least two years and measuring a wider range of benefits, including benefits to other members of the family. Second, NICE should commission research to measure utility in children.

7.3 **Summary of case study**

Title	**Enhancing ventilation in homes of children with asthma: cost-effectiveness study alongside randomized controlled trial (The CHARISMA Study)**
Setting	Wrexham, North Wales.
Participants	177 children (5–14 years) with severe or moderate asthma (88 intervention, 89 control).
Recruitment	GP practices.
Intervention	Heating and ventilation modification to private and public housing.
Follow-up period	12 months.
Outcome measures	PedsQL-Asthma specific health related quality of life measure completed by parents about their child (100-point scale); school attendance; prescribed medicine.
Measurement of Costs	Wrexham County Borough Council bore the cost of housing improvements and the NHS bore the health care costs associated with childhood asthma.
	Wrexham County Borough Council provided information on the housing modification received by each household in the intervention group, and associated costs. As this study takes a public sector perspective, it has not included the running costs of ventilation systems, estimated at £15 a year, or costs to families of running central heating.
	Parents were asked to use the validated Client Service Receipt Inventory, adapted to recall their child's contacts with health services over the study period.
	National unit costs were obtained from the report by Curtis and Netten for units of health and social care (Curtis and Netten, 2007); the Department of Health for NHS reference costs (Department of Health, 2006); and the Health and Social Care Information Centre for prescribing costs (NHS Information Centre, 2006). All costs are in pounds sterling for 2006. As participants were followed for only 12 months, discounting was not necessary.
Perspective	Multi-agency, public sector perspective.
Study type	An incremental cost-effectiveness analysis alongside a pragmatic randomized controlled trial.
Previous economic evidence	UK: Somerville et al., (2002); International: Howden-Chapman et al., (2008); Chapman et al., (2009).
Existing evidence of effectiveness	There have been 39 studies, 3 of which were randomized, looking at the clinical effects of improving housing on health (Thompson and Petticrew, 2007). There has been little rigorous economic analysis of the relationship between asthma and improved housing (Howden-Chapman et al., 2008).

Title	Enhancing ventilation in homes of children with asthma: cost-effectiveness study alongside randomized controlled trial (The CHARISMA Study)
Existing evidence of cost-effectiveness	Chapman and colleagues argued for a wide perspective, taking account of economic, environmental, and health impacts of improving housing stock (Chapman et al., 2009). They used cost–benefit analysis alongside a randomized trial to show that retrofitting houses in New Zealand with insulation yielded economic benefits worth up to twice the cost of refurbishment.
Objective	To evaluate the cost-effectiveness of installing ventilation systems, and central heating if necessary, in homes of children with 'moderate' or 'severe' asthma.

Summary of Chapter 7

♦ The Wanless Reports (2002; 2004) challenged health economists to apply methods of economic evaluation public health interventions.

♦ In the United Kingdom, the CHARISMA trial was one of the first pragmatic randomized control trails of a housing modification intervention. It demonstrates that it is possible to undertake pragmatic trials in the community, and that these benefit from collaboration between agencies, in this case a local health authority, a university, and the NHS.

♦ Though a range of outcomes were measured spanning parental assessment of child asthma symptoms, prescribing and school absenteeism, in retrospect the study could have measured an even wider range of outcomes including health status of siblings, number of rooms heated and any impact on fuel poverty.

♦ In retrospect, a wider range of outcomes could have been collected to inform decision-making such as school absenteeism information.

♦ Housing is recognized as an important determinant of health and inequalities in health. Housing initiatives should routinely include an evaluative component, including analysis of cost-effectiveness. This study is still one of the few published economic evaluations of housing interventions to improve health. (See Bray et al., 2017 for an example of a more recent housing study using a cohort design).

References

Asthma, U.K., 2011. *For journalists: Key facts and statistics*. Available at: <http://www.asthma.org.uk/news_media/media_resources/for_journalists_key.html> (Accessed 15 October 2018).

Bray, N., Burns, P., Jones, A., Winrow, E. and Edwards, R.T., 2017. Costs and outcomes of improving population health through better social housing: A cohort study and economic analysis. *International Journal of Public Health*, **62**(9): 1039–50.

Brazier, J., 2007. *Measuring and Valuing Health Benefits for Economic Evaluation*. Oxford: Oxford University Press.

Briggs, A.H. and Gray, A.M., 1999. Handling uncertainty in economic evaluations of health care interventions. *British Medical Journal*, *319*(7210): 635.

Chapman, R., Howden-Chapman, P., Viggers, H., O'Dea, D., and Kennedy, M., 2009. Retrofitting houses with insulation: A cost–benefit analysis of a randomised community trial. *Journal of Epidemiology & Community Health*, *63*(4): 271–7.

Cohen, S., Taitz, J., and Jaffé, A., 2007. Paediatric prescribing of asthma drugs in the UK: Are we sticking to the guideline? *Archives of Disease in Childhood*, *92*(10): 847–9.

Curtis, L. and Netten, A., 2007. Unit costs of health and social care. Personal Social Services Research Unit. Canterbury: University of Kent PSSRU. Available at: <http://www.pssru.ac.uk/pdf/uc/uc2006/uc2006.pdf> (Accessed 15 October 2018).

Department of Health, 2006. *NHS reference costs 2006-07*. DOH: London. Available at: <http://webarchive.nationalarchives.gov.uk/20070701084335/http://www.dh.gov.uk/en/Publicationsandstatistics/Publications/PublicationsPolicyAndGuidance/DH_074472> (Accessed 2 November 2018).

Drummond, M.F., Sculpher, M.J., Claxton, K., Stoddart, G.L., and Torrance, G.W., 2015. *Methods for the Economic Evaluation of Health Care Programmes*. Oxford: Oxford University Press.

Edwards, R.T., Hounsome, B., Linck, P., and Russell, I.T., 2008. Economic evaluation alongside pragmatic randomised trials: Developing a standard operating procedure for clinical trials units. *Trials*, *9*(1): 1.

Edwards, R.T., Neal, R.D., Linck, P., Bruce, N., Mullock, L., Nelhans, N., Pasterfield, D., et al., 2011. Enhancing ventilation in homes of children with asthma: Cost-effectiveness study alongside randomised controlled trial. *British Journal of General Practice*, *61*(592): e733–e741.

Eichler, H.G., Kong, S.X., Gerth, W.C., Mavros, P., and Jönsson, B., 2004. Use of cost-effectiveness analysis in health-care resource allocation decision-making: How are cost-effectiveness thresholds expected to emerge? *Value in Health*, *7*(5): 518–28.

Fenwick, E., O'Brien, B.J., and Briggs, A., 2004. Cost-effectiveness acceptability curves–facts, fallacies and frequently asked questions. *Health Economics*, *13*(5): 405–15.

Glick, H.A., Doshi, J.A., Sonnad, S.S., and Polsky, D., 2007. *Economic Evaluation in Clinical Trials*. Oxford: Oxford University Press.

Gøtzsche, P.C. and Johansen, H.K., 2008. House dust mite control measures for asthma: Systematic review. *Allergy*, *63*(6): 646–59.

Howden-Chapman, P., Pierse, N., Nicholls, S., Gillespie-Bennett, J., Viggers, H., Cunningham, M., Phipps, R., et al., 2008. Effects of improved home heating on asthma in community dwelling children: Randomised controlled trial. *BMJ*, *337*: a1411.

Johnson, V.B. and Partners, 2007. *Laxton's Building Price Book—Major & Small Works*. Oxford: Laxtons.

Koerhamp, B.G., Hunink, M.M., Stijnen, T., Hammitt, J.K., Kuntz, K.M., and Weinstein, M.C., 2007. Limitations of acceptability curves for presenting uncertainty in cost-effectiveness analysis. *Medical Decision Making*, *27*(2): 101–11.

NHS Information Centre, 2006. *Prescription cost analysis*. Available at: <https://digital.nhs.uk/data-and-information/publications/statistical/prescription-cost-analysis/prescription-cost-analysis-2006> (Accessed 2 November 2018).

Patel, A., Rendu, A., Moran, P., Leese, M., Mann, A., and Knapp, M., 2005. A comparison of two methods of collecting economic data in primary care. *Family Practice*, *22*(3): 323–7.

Raftery, J., 2001. NICE: Faster access to modern treatments? Analysis of guidance on health technologies. *British Medical Journal, 323*(7324): 1300.

Ramsey, S., Willke, R., Briggs, A., Brown, R., Buxton, M., Chawla, A., Cook, J., et al., 2005. Good research practices for cost-effectiveness analysis alongside clinical trials: The ISPOR RCT-CEA task force report. *Value in Health, 8*(5): 521–33

Thomson, H., Petticrew, M., and Morrison, D., 2001. Health effects of housing improvement: Systematic review of intervention studies. *British Medical Journal, 323*(7306): 187–90.

Thomson, H., Thomas, S., Sellstrom, E., and Petticrew, M., 2009. The health impacts of housing improvement: A systematic review of intervention studies from 1887 to 2007. *American Journal of Public Health, 99*(S3): S681–S692.

Varni, J.W., Burwinkle, T.M., Rapoff, M.A., Kamps, J.L., and Olson, N., 2004. The PedsQL™ in pediatric asthma: Reliability and validity of the Pediatric Quality of Life Inventory™ generic core scales and asthma module. *Journal of Behavioral Medicine, 27*(3): 297–318.

Wanless, D., 2002. *Securing Our Future Health: Taking a Long-Term View.* London: HM Treasury.

Wanless D., 2004. *Securing Good Health for the Whole Population. Final Report.* London: HM Treasury

Warner, J.A., Frederick, J.M., Bryant, T.N., Weich, C., Raw, G.J., Hunter, C., Stephend, F.R., et al., 2000. Mechanical ventilation and high-efficiency vacuum cleaning: A combined strategy of mite and mite allergen reduction in the control of mite-sensitive asthma. *Journal of Allergy and Clinical Immunology, 105*(1): 75–82.

Weatherly, H., Drummond, M., Claxton, K., Cookson, R., Ferguson, B., Godfrey, C., Rice, N., et al., 2009. Methods for assessing the cost-effectiveness of public health interventions: Key challenges and recommendations. *Health Policy, 93*(2): 85–92.

Woodfine, L., Neal, R.D., Bruce, N., Edwards, R.T., Linck, P., Mullock, L., Nelhans, N., et al., 2011. Enhancing ventilation in homes of children with asthma: Pragmatic randomised controlled trial. *British Journal of General Practice, 61*(592): e724–e732.

Wright, G.R., Howieson, S., McSharry, C., McMahon, A.D., Chaudhuri, R., Thompson, J., Donnelly, I., et al., 2009. Effect of improved home ventilation on asthma control and house dust mite allergen levels. *Allergy, 64*(11): 1671–80.

Chapter 8

Cost–utility analysis of public health interventions

Rhiannon T. Edwards and Eira Winrow

8.1 Introduction

This chapter builds upon Chapter 6 by introducing the reader to the origins and use of health-related quality of life, cost–utility analysis (CUA), quality-adjusted life years (QALYs), and payer thresholds. The aim of this chapter is to outline in more depth the role of applied CUA in the economic evaluation of PHIs. The chapter then reproduces an article by Owen and colleagues at the National Institute for Health and Care Excellence (NICE) in the United Kingdom. This article shows that many PHIs often have a cost per QALY considerably lower than the £20,000 payer threshold conventionally used by the National Institute for Health and Care Excellence (NICE) in the United Kingdom.

8.2 Definition of cost–utility analysis

It is accepted that decisions have to be made about how best we allocate our scarce health and public health resources. A frequently used and recommended approach by NICE in the United Kingdom is the framework of CUA. This approach facilitates the comparison of the costs of different procedures with their outcomes measured in utility-based units. One of the most commonly used units is the quality-adjusted life year (QALY) (see Chapter 6). QALYs are calculated by estimating the total life years gained from a procedure or intervention and weighting each year to reflect the quality of life in that year (Robinson, 1993; Gold et al., 2002). Putting a value on health can be controversial and health gains are often valued differently across different societies and different age groups (Schwappach, 2002).

Chapter 6 outlined the QALY as an outcome for use in CUA. The estimation of an incremental cost per QALY aids decision-making and helps policy-makers to compare the value of different interventions that may have diverse health benefits. This ability for CUA to facilitate comparisons both across and within disease areas/specialties/programmes is a result of the use of the generic QALY outcome as compared to those narrower, typically disease-specific clinical measures used in CEA. This type of analysis alone may not provide sufficient evidence on which to make resource allocation decisions, but it increases the transparency of the resource allocation procedure (World Health Organization, 2016).

CUA is the recommended economic evaluation framework for submissions to the Canadian Agency for Drugs and Technologies in Health, in Australia for submissions to the Pharmaceutical Benefits Advisory Committee (PBAC) (PBAC, 2016), in Sweden for submissions to the Swedish Council on Health Technology Assessment (SBU) (SBU, 2013), in New Zealand for submissions to the Pharmaceutical Management Agency (PHARMAC) (PHARMAC, 2012), and other countries.

8.3 Health-adjusted life years (HALYs)

'Health-adjusted life years (HALYs) are summary measures of population health that allow the combined impact of death and morbidity to be considered simultaneously' (Gold et al., 2002, p. 116).

In essence, HALYs is an umbrella term representing attempts to adjust life expectancy to reflect health-related quality of life. Conventionally, a scale is used where 0 represents the worst imaginable state of health or sometimes death, and 1 represents perfect health. Health-adjusted life expectancy (HALE) is the life expectancy that someone can expect to live at a given age in the equivalent of full health. HALE offers an overarching view of the morbidity and mortality burden of a population. What is interesting is that although quality-adjusted life years (QALYs) and disability-adjusted life years (DALYs) essentially spring from this concept of HALYs, both have developed in different ways, have historically been used for different purposes internationally, and are not directly comparable. Table 8.2 captures the key features of HALYs, QALYs, and DALYs explored in more detail in the sections that follow.

8.4 Quality-adjusted life years (QALYs)

QALYs were developed during the 1960s by economists, operations researchers, and psychologists, primarily for use in cost-effectiveness analysis (CEA). In both the United States and the United Kingdom, they represented an important paradigm in conceptualizing the health outcome (denominator) in a cost-effectiveness (CE) ratio (Gold et al., 1996).

In the United States, the idea of adjusting life expectancy to reflect health-related quality of life emerged in the 1960s. In a speech to the American Public Health Association at the Ninetieth Annual Meeting in Miami Beach, Florida on 17 October 1962, Barkev Sanders, in his presentation of findings from the Kit Carson County survey 1962, clearly shifted the emphasis from measuring health processes to measuring health outcomes.

> In my judgment, measurement of the efficiency of health care should be made in terms of its end product-namely, its contribution to increasing the productive man-years from a given cohort, and not in terms of efforts put forth by health agencies, as is often done when we judge the adequacy of care by such units as the number of nursing visits or the volume of expenditures. (Sanders, 1964, p. 1069)

Sanders focused on economically productive years as an appropriate outcome of health care, after childhood and before old age, and referred to these years as 'disability-free, productive life' (Sanders, 1964, p. 1069).

In the United Kingdom, Alan Williams published a seminal paper in the *British Medical Journal* illustrating the use of QALYs for coronary artery bypass grafting.

> Before a well informed judgment can be made of whether it is in the public interest to increase, decrease, or keep constant the number of operations for coronary artery bypass grafting reliable comparisons must be made with other potential users of resources. Such information is not readily available, and the assumptions that I have made are not entirely satisfactory. Clearly, further research is needed and should be focused much more on measurement of the quality of life and on costs (both public and private). Far too much attention has been paid to the rate of survival, which, in the case of coronary artery bypass grafting and many other therapeutic procedures in which the main benefit is improved quality of life, is potentially misleading. Resources need to be redeployed at the margin to procedures for which the benefits to patients are high in relation to the costs. (Williams, 1985, p. 329)

A CE ratio sets out the incremental cost obtaining a unit of health effect from a health intervention (preventive or curative, population-based, or clinical). When the denominator of the CE ratio is calculated using QALYs, the cost-effectiveness analysis is referred to as CUA (Gold, 2002).

CUA is appropriate when it is necessary to have a common unit of measurement to compare between types of interventions and programs in situations where quality of life is 'the' or 'an' important outcome of health care.

Economic evaluations can make a valuable contribution to informing health care decision-making and can help to assess whether an intervention is justifiable on grounds of relative cost and outcome. QALYs provide an estimate of the extra quantity and quality of life provided by an intervention. In a public health context, an intervention to provide access to green space for young people could potentially generate QALYs as shown in Figure 8.1.

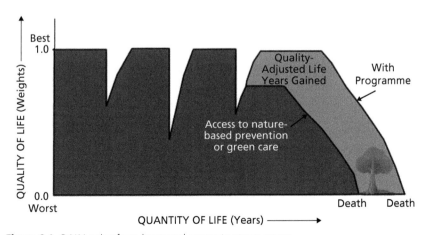

Figure 8.1 QALY gains from increased access to green space.

A QALY is an outcome measure which considers both the quantity and the quality of the extra life years provided by a health care intervention (Phillips, 2009) and can be represented by the following equation:

$$QALY = \text{length of life} \times \text{quality of life}$$

This cost–utility analysis provides a common unit (cost per QALY) and results in an estimate of the cost of provision of one year of perfect health following an intervention. It therefore helps to quantify the value for money that an intervention provides.

Due to space restrictions, in this book we do not discuss the methods of time trade-off (TTO), standard gamble (SG), and visual analogues (VA) that can be used to generate quality of life weights. Instead, we direct the reader to Chapter 10 of Morris et al. (Morris et al., 2007).

The US Panel on Cost-Effectiveness in Health and Medicine and the National Institute of Health and Care Excellence (NICE) in the United Kingdom have both adopted the QALY for their 'reference case' (National Institute for Health and Care Excellence, 2013). This provides a standardized method to promote comparability in cost-effectiveness analyses of different health care interventions.

8.5 QALY league table approach and threshold approach

An underlying and often implicit assumption associated with the use of QALYs is that the major objective of health care decision-makers is to maximize health or health improvement across the population subject to resource constraints (Weinstein et al., 2009). The fact that NICE uses a higher threshold for medicines to be used in end of life care or orphan drug medicines implies a weakening of this principle, perhaps reflecting societal values.

Two methods to assess whether an estimate of cost per QALY represents good value for money are the league table approach and the threshold approach. By using these approaches, estimates of the cost per QALY can be calculated for an intervention, such as the prescription of a drug and determining whether or not the prescription of that drug is good value for money.

Cost per QALY league tables are used to categorize interventions by their average cost per QALY estimate. In theory, such league tables can help to inform decisions as to how a limited amount of money might be efficiently spent in order to achieve the greatest health gain for the population. QALY league tables make comparisons possible between interventions in the same disease/ therapy area such as the efficiency of conventional surgery compared to keyhole surgery for uterine fibroids. Comparisons can also be made across therapy areas, for example, surgery for uterine fibroids compared to bowel cancer screening.

QALY league tables have been criticized for oversimplifying complex clinical conditions and for too simplistic resource allocation decisions (Drummond et al. (1993). Gerard and Mooney outline four QALY league table issues which require 'handling with care'. They are: (i) the relevant measure of cost in QALY league tables must be restricted to health service resource use; (ii) the relevant measure of benefit in QALY league tables is clearly restricted to QALYs, thereby restricted to the utility of health gains and indeed the maximization of the utility of health gains; (iii) in incorporating the results of CUA studies into QALY league tables there is a need for greater clarification of where we are at the margin, that is, scale of service delivery; and (iv) those who might use CUA results in QALY league tables need to ascertain whether the original context of the study will allow the results to be transferred to the local context of the decision-maker. Finally, the authors argue that the only legitimate (and clearly important) goal of QALY league tables is the maximization of the utility of health gains within a health service budget (Gerard and Mooney, 1993).

QALYs may also lack sensitivity when attempting to compare similar treatments in the same therapy area. They may not take into consideration the stage of the disease and may not reflect what is important either clinically or to the patient. Possibly the greatest area of controversy for the QALY metric has been how 'quality' values have been chosen. It is not always recognized that preferences for health states are often dependent on factors such as age and lifestyle, and that they may, therefore, be different for different people in similar health states.

The threshold approach is often used together with the league tables in assessing whether or not an intervention provides good value for money. The threshold measurement is made by calculating whether or not the cost per QALY estimate falls above or below a specific 'threshold' value. A useful guide to the threshold approach is provided by McCabe and colleagues (McCabe et al., 2008). As discussed in Chapter 2, cost-effectiveness analysis is the process of comparing the incremental cost-effectiveness ratio of a new technology (which may be more costly than existing alternatives) with an accepted or established cost-effectiveness threshold. This cost-effectiveness ratio, such as a cost per QALY, tells us whether the anticipated health gain from a new intervention exceeds the health expected to be lost elsewhere as other health care activities are displaced, that is, its opportunity cost (McIntosh, 1999). This threshold represents the added cost that has to be borne by the NHS, or wider society with respect to PHIs, to forgo one quality-adjusted life year (QALY) of health through

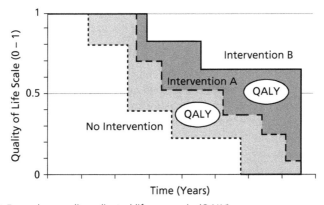

Figure 8.2 Example—quality-adjusted life year gain (QALY).

displacement. Interventions above a given threshold value would not be considered good value for money. However, since thresholds may vary by country, it is therefore likely to vary in different societies and cultures, depending on how they themselves value health care. In the United Kingdom, the National Institute for Health and Care Excellence (NICE) has been using a cost-effectiveness threshold ranging from £20,000 pound and £30,000 pound (without formal empirical justification) since around 2001 (<http://www.nice.org>). However, recently authors have argued the threshold is more like £13,000 (Claxton et al., 2015). Later in this chapter, a case study by Owen and colleagues shows that many public health interventions are highly cost-effective using this threshold approach (Owen et al., 2012).

Critics of QALYs are of the opinion that the method is too imprecise and arbitrary to be the basis of determining who will or will not receive treatment (Lorgelly et al., 2010). Supporters suggest that since health care resources are limited, difficult decisions have to be made, and that QALYs enable those decisions to be made in a way which may not be precise but at least is approximately optimal for patients and society.

8.6 Measuring health-related quality of life and utility in children and young people

Many public health prevention initiatives are aimed at young children and adolescents, often delivered in school settings. Thorrington and Eames published a systematic review of measuring health utilities in children and adolescents (Thorrington and Eames, 2015). They evaluated 90 studies from a total of 1780 selected from the databases. The EuroQol EQ-5D instrument was the most frequently used single method, selected for 41 studies. Fifteen of the methods used were generic methods and the remaining 7 were disease-specific. Forty-eight of the 90 studies (53 per cent) used some form of proxy, with 26 (29 per cent) using proxies exclusively to estimate health utilities (Thorrington and Eames, 2015). More recently, PHIs to reduce obesity in children have been using the CHU-9D instrument (Frew et al., 2015). Table 8.1 provides a summary of commonly used health-related quality of life measures that can be used to measure outcomes in children, some of which can provide preference-based utility weights for QALY calculations and subsequently for utilizing with CUAs of interventions aimed at children and young people.

8.7 Disability-adjusted life years (DALYs)

In order to measure the burden of disease, injury, and disability in a population, a metric is needed which provides a consistent and comparative description of the prevalence and severity of ill-health, disability, and premature death in a population. This assessment is an important factor in public health planning, decision-making, resource allocation, and the monitoring and evaluation of health programmes. Traditionally, a country's burden of disease was expressed using one measure, namely years of life lost (YLL), that is, from a population's average life expectancy. This measure, however, did not take into account that not only were years of life lost through premature death but that they could also be lost through disability or poor health. Chapter 6 introduced the concept of the disability-adjusted life years (DALY). DALYs were developed by researchers at Harvard University as a measure which takes account of disability by combining mortality and morbidity into one metric. In 1990, the World Health Organization's Global Burden of Disease Study was the first publication to use this method (Murray, 1994; Lopez and Murray, 1998). Since then, DALYs have become increasingly common as a measure in the spheres of public health and health impact assessments, and in providing a measure of the burden of disease of a country

Although DALYs have been used both to measure outcomes in micro-economic evaluations and to set priorities in league tables of cost-effectiveness, they have been controversial since they are dependent upon imprecise assumptions about life years. This has also made it difficult for them to be used as comparative measures or in different contexts (Anand and Hanson, 1997). They have, however, been the basis of the WHO Global Health Estimates which provide comprehensive mortality and loss of health statistics for all regions of the world. This information can be useful in assessing the comparative importance of diseases and injuries in causing premature death, loss of health, and disability in different populations, and it has particularly been applied in developing countries. Changes in data and methods have meant that WHO estimates since 2000 are not comparable with previous WHO estimates, and this consequently makes identifying long-term trends difficult. To meet the need for DALY estimates which are consistent with the Global Health Estimates for cause-specific mortality, the WHO has released estimates of DALYs by cause, age, and sex at a regional level for the years 2000 and 2011 (World Health Organization, 2013).

8.8 Summary of HALYs, QALYs, and DALYs

Table 8.2 summarizes the concepts of HALYs, DALYs and QALYs discussed in this chapter.

8.9 Case study: The cost-effectiveness of PHIs

The following case study is reproduced in full from Owen, L., Morgan, A., Fischer, A., Ellis, S., Hoy, A., and Kelly, M.P., 2012. The cost-effectiveness of PHIs. *Journal of Public Health*, 34(1), pp. 37–45.

8.9.1 Introduction

The need to make the best use of limited resources in the UK's NHS has always been a priority but this imperative is now greater than ever. The economic case for PHIs to contribute to this endeavour hitherto has lacked a systematic compilation of evidence, in both the breadth and the depth that would allow informed decisions about the allocation of resources between prevention and treatment options, and between options within prevention options.

Butterfield and colleagues argue that the current 4 per cent of the NHS budget spent on prevention needs to be at least maintained to ensure that current levels of health

Table 8.1 Standardized and validated questionnaires to calculate QALYs in adolescents and children

Questionnaire	Short description of questionnaire	Source of tariffs	Key reference	Registration and cost of questionnaire use in research
EQ-5D (3L)	This is a standardized measure of health status developed by the EuroQol Group. It is intended for use with adults (16 years and over, though it can be used with 12 years and above depending on study design). The questionnaire is two-pages long and consists of five dimensions (mobility, self-care, usual activities, pain/discomfort, and anxiety/depression) with three possible responses (no problems, some problems, extreme problems) and a visual analogue scale.	Health Utility scores from this questionnaire can be compared to UK norms collated by the EuroQol Group. A calculator is available from the EuroQol group website to calculate QALYs from the Health Utility Index Scores obtained by the answers to the five dimensions.	The EuroQol Group (1990). EuroQol: A new facility for the measurement of health-related quality of life. *Health Policy* 16(3):199–208.	Permission to use the EQ-5D (3L) must be obtained from the EuroQol Group via the online registration form on their website https://euroqol.org/>). The costs of using the questionnaire are determined by the information provided on the registration form. The cost is dependent upon the type of study, funding source, sample size, and number of requested languages.
EQ-5D (5L)	This is a standardized measure of health status developed by the EuroQol Group. It is intended for use with adults (16 years and over). Like the 3L version it consists of five dimensions (mobility, self-care, usual activities, pain/discomfort, anxiety/depression). However, there are five possible responses (no problems/slight problems/moderate problems/severe problems/extreme problems). The EQ-5D (5L) also consists of a visual analogue scale.	Value sets of the EQ-5D (5L) were published in 2016 and are taken from stated preference data of 996 members of the public in England. A calculator is also available from the EuroQol group website to download in order to calculate QALYs from the Health Utility Index Scores obtained by the answers to the five dimensions.	Janssen, M.F., Pickard, A.S., Golicki, D., Gudex, C., Niewada, M., Scalone, L., Swinburn, P., et al. Measurement properties of the EQ-5D-5L compared to the EQ-5D-3L across eight patient groups: A multi-country study. *Quality of Life Research*, 22(7):1717–27. doi:10.1007/s11136-012-0322-4.	Permission to use the EQ-5D (5L) must be obtained from the EuroQol Group via their online registration form on their website. The costs of using the questionnaire are determined by the information provided on the registration form. The cost is dependent upon the type of study, funding source, sample size, and number of requested languages.

EQ-5D-Y	This is the Youth version of the EQ-5D (3L). It is intended to be used with children aged 8–15 years old. For children above 15 years old the adult version of the EQ-5D (3L) may be used depending upon study design. For children under 8 years old a parental proxy is recommended to obtain responses to the five dimensions. The wording of the questionnaire as a whole has been simplified and made more relevant to children (e.g. naming school, hobbies, and sports as examples of usual activities). The questionnaire has three levels of severity of responses to the five dimensions (no problems/some problems or a bit/ a lot (of) problems.	At present, a value set for the EQ-5D-Y is not yet available. It is not recommended to use the 3L value set as proxy value set for the EQ-5D-Y. The EuroQol Group is currently developing valuation for the EQ-5D-Y.	Ravens-Sieberer, U., Wille, N., Badia, X., Bonsel, G., Burström, K., Cavrini, G., Devlin, N., et al., 2010. Feasibility, reliability, and validity of the EQ-5D-Y: results from a multinational study. *Quality of Life Research* 19(6): 887–97.	Permission to use the EQ-5D-Y must be obtained from the EuroQol Group via the online registration form on their website. The costs of using the questionnaire are determined by the information provided on the registration form. The cost is dependent upon the type of study, funding source, sample size, and number of requested languages.
Health Utilities Index (HUI®)	The Health Utilities Index (HUI®) is a family of generic preference-based systems for measuring comprehensive health status and health-related quality of life (HRQoL). The questionnaires are appropriate for broad range of subjects (5 years of age and older). For ages 5–8 years, HUI Inc recommends a proxy-assess, self-, or interviewer-administered version. For ages 8–12 years, the self-assess, interviewer-administered version and for individuals 13 years or older self-assess, self-, or interviewer-administered version is appropriate. There are three versions of HUI*: HUI Mark1 (HUI1); HUI Mark 2 (HUI2); and HUI Mark 3 (HUI3). Each version of the HUI* includes a health status classification system and formula for calculating utility scores. HUI2 describes 24,000 unique health states and HUI3 describes 972,000 unique health states.	Scoring information for each HUI* questionnaire is available from the HUInc website from the HUI manual. Population norms are available for the HUI2 and HUI3 on the HUInc website.	Horsman, J., Furlong, W., Feeny, D., and Torrance, G., 2003. The Health Utilities Index (HUI®): Concepts, Measurement Properties and Applications'. *Health and Quality of Life Outcomes* 1(54), October 16.	An application form to use the HUI* questionnaires must be completed by researchers before use. HUInc has a three-tier licensing fee schedule for its standard 'paper and pencil' survey instruments and instruction/ application manual. The 'tiered' fee schedule greatly reduces the total price to studies using multiple 'off-the-shelf' versions of either self-complete or interviewer-administered format HUI questionnaires. The new fee schedule (in US$), in 2018 prices, is as follows:

(continued)

Table 8.1 Continued

Questionnaire	Short description of questionnaire	Source of tariffs	Key reference	Registration and cost of questionnaire use in research
	HUI® provides descriptive evidence on multiple dimensions of health status, a score for each dimension of health, and an HRQL score for overall health. Health dimensions include vision, hearing, speech, ambulation/mobility, pain, dexterity, self-care, emotion, and cognition. Each dimension has 3– 6 levels. HUI® systems describe almost a million unique health states. HUI questionnaires are available in two major formats: generically referred to as the 15Q and 40Q. [Note that, despite the designation '15Q' or '40Q', each version of the HUI has at least one additional (optional) question. These extra questions are not HUI questions and thus do not figure into the scoring algorithms for either the HUI2 or HUI3.			**I:** $5,000.00 for the base package of manual and one version of questionnaire plus $2,500.00 for each of the next five questionnaires (2-3-4-5-6) in same format. **II:** $1,875.00 for each of the next six questionnaires (7-8-9-10-11-12) in same format. **III:** $1,250.00 for each additional questionnaire (13th and more) in same format as the original.
SF-36	This is a comprehensive short-form health survey with 36 questions yields an 8-scale health profile as well as summary measures of health-related quality of life. The eight scales are: physical functioning, role physical, bodily pain, general health, vitality, social functioning, role emotional, and mental health. The SF-36 is suitable for self-administration, computerized administration, or administration by a trained interviewer in person or by telephone, to individuals aged 14 and older.	Scoring information is available from the SF-36 manual. Population norms are available for the SF-36 from SF-36 organization's website and manual.	Brazier, J.E., Harper, R., Jones, N.M., O'Cathain, A., Thomas, K.J., Usherwood, T., and Westlake, L., 1992. Validating the SF-36 health survey questionnaire: New outcome measure for primary care. *BMJ*, *305*(6846):160–4.	A survey request form must be completed and a license fee may apply to use the SF-36 questionnaire.

Measure	Description	Reference	Scoring information	Access/License
SF-12	This is a short-form version of the SF-36. The questionnaire still has eight scales; physical functioning, role physical, bodily pain, general health, vitality, social functioning, role emotional, and mental health. However, the number of questions referring to each scale has been reduced substantially. There are standard (4-week) and acute (1-week) recall versions of the questionnaire for self-administration as well as scripts for personal interviews. Like the SF-36, it is recommended for use with individuals aged 14 years and older.	Ware, J.E., Kosinski, M., and Keller, S.D., 1996. A 12-item short-form health survey: Construction of scales and preliminary tests of reliability and validity. *Medical Care, 34*(3):220–33.	Scoring information is available from the SF-12 manual. Population norms are available for the SF-12 from SF-36 organization's website and manual.	A survey request form must be completed and a license fee may apply to use the SF-12 questionnaire.
SF-8	This questionnaire is an even more reduced version of the SF-36. It uses a single item to measure each of the eight domains of health (physical functioning, role physical, bodily pain, general health, vitality, social functioning, role emotional, and mental health). The SF-8 is recommended for use with individuals aged 14 years and older.	Ware, J., Kosinski, M., Dewey, J., and Gandek, B, 2001. *How to Score and Interpret Single-Item Health Status Measures: A Manual for Users of the SF-8 Health Survey.* Boston, MA: QualyMetric.	Scoring information is available from the SF-8 manual. Population norms are available for the SF-8 from SF-36 organization's website and manual.	A survey request form must be completed and a license fee may apply to use the SF-8 questionnaire.
Child Health Utility 9D (CHU-9D)	This is a paediatric generic preference-based measure of health-related quality of life. It consists of a descriptive system and a set of preference weights, giving utility values, allowing the calculation of QALYs. It has nine dimensions (worried, sad, pain, tired, annoyed, school-work/homework, sleep, daily routine, able to join in activities). Each of the nine dimensions has five possible responses. The questionnaire is validated for use with children aged 11–17 years.	Stevens, K., 2012. Valuation of the Child Health Utility 9D Index. *Pharmacoeconomics* 30:8:729–47.	Scoring information and population norms are available from CHU-9D's developer, Dr Katherine Stevens, University of Sheffield (<https://www.sheffield.ac.uk/scharr/sections/heds/mvh/paediatric>).	A user licence registration form must be completed in order to receive the CHU-9D, available from the CHU-9D website. For commercial users a fee may apply for use of the CHU-9D.

Table 8.2 Summary of HALYs, QALYs, and DALYs

	Definition	Method of Calculation	Source of HQoL/Utility Adjustment	Example Publication
HALYs	HALYs is an umbrella term representing attempts to adjust life expectancy to reflect health-related quality of life.	In order to develop a HALY measure, it is necessary to: describe 'health' in context with the health state or condition; develop health-related quality of life values for the health state or condition; calculate values for combinations of health states and life expectancy for this health state or condition (Gold et al., 2002).	Depends on the type of HALY being measured (QALY or DALY).	Gold et al., 2002; Sassi, 2006.
QALYs	A QALY is an outcome measure that combines the quantity and quality of extra life years gained by a health care intervention in a single index.	Length of Life × Quality of Life	e.g. EQ-5D CHU-9D SF-6D HUI	Williams, 1995; Drummond et al., 2015.
DALYs	DALYs measure the burden of disease in terms of years lost due to ill-health, disability, or early death, and is often used in international comparisons of health and health inequalities across countries.	YLD + YLL (YEARS LIVED WITH DISABILITY + YEARS OF LIFE LOST)	Epidemiological or hospital data WHO Global Burden of Disease	Devleesschauwer et al., (2014); WHO Global Burden of Disease (Mathers et al., 2008).

in England do not worsen compared with other European countries Butterfield et al., 2009). They also highlight that there is much variation in spending on prevention by primary care trusts. This may reflect the original observation by Wanless (2004) that lack of information about cost-effectiveness of interventions hinders priority setting at a local level.

8.9.2 Preventable disease: The scale of the problem

The health and economic effects of lifestyle diseases are substantial. In 2008 an estimated 170,000 deaths in England and Wales, around a third of all deaths, were premature (under the age of 75) (Office of National Statistics, 2008a). Many of these deaths could have been prevented by lifestyle changes undertaken at an earlier time of life (Office for National Statistics, 2008b; Kelly, 2009) The diseases associated with smoking, lack of physical activity, obesity, and alcohol misuse feature among the leading causes of premature death in the United Kingdom. In 2006, around 30 per cent of premature deaths among men and 21 per cent among women were from cardiovascular disease (CVD), accounting for just over 40,000 premature deaths in that year (ONS, 2008a) In addition, there are an estimated 7 million people in the United Kingdom living with CVD (British Heart Foundation, 2018).

In 2008, the total disease burden attributable to preventable deaths in England and Wales (i.e. under the age of 75 but excluding deaths below the age of 28 days) was 44 years of life lost per 1000 population or about 2.6 million life years lost each year (ONS, 2008a). If the NHS is prepared to pay £20,000 per life year gained at full health, as the lower boundary of the cost-effectiveness threshold used by NICE implies, the value of this loss, for England and Wales as a whole, is about £51 billion per year.

The current level of tobacco use is estimated to cost the NHS around £2.7 billion every year (Callum, 2008), while treating people with health problems related to being overweight or obese is estimated to cost the NHS £4.2 billion annually, a figure which is forecast to more than double by 2050 in terms of current prices (Foresight, 2007). Physical inactivity is estimated to cost the NHS £1.06 billion per year (Allender, 2007), and the costs of treating the chronic and acute effects of alcohol misuse up to £1.7 billion per year. It is estimated that up to 35 per cent of all accident and emergency attendances and ambulance costs are alcohol related (Strategy Unit Alcohol Harm Reduction Project, 2003).

Despite this, only 4 per cent of NHS funding is spent on prevention (Marmot, 2010). Some have suggested that this may be because the economic evidence in favour of prevention is largely missing or of poor quality (Wanless, 2002; Marsh et al., 2013). For example, a recent systematic review of economic evaluations of primary prevention targeting CVD or risk reduction found that the vast majority of these evaluations focused on clinical prevention (Schwappach et al., 2007). Another rapid review of PHIs found that only 27 per cent provided sufficient economic evidence for assessing cost-effectiveness (Marsh et al., 2013). There may also be more practical reasons for underinvestment which relate to decision-making processes at a local level such as the need for short-term planning and pressures to deliver. Perhaps, there is also a view that the NHS contribution to public health goals is limited compared to the impact that can be made at a population level (e.g. mass-media campaigns or other sectors). All this points to the need to improve both the evidence of cost-effectiveness of PHIs and how these data can be fed into the reality of local decision-making processes.

8.9.3 Methodological challenges and the NICE approach

The methodological challenges of assessing the cost-effectiveness of PHIs are well documented (Kelly et al., 2005; Drummond et al., 2007; Schwappach et al., 2007; Weatherly et al., 2009). In the absence of an established approach, a range of different economic methods have been employed making it difficult to compare PHIs. In a review undertaken by Drummond and colleagues, 37 per cent of the studies identified adopted a cost-effectiveness analysis, 36 per cent a cost–consequence analysis, and 27 per cent a cost–utility analysis (Drummond et al., 2007). When NICE took on responsibility for public health in 2005, it offered an opportunity to build a more systematic approach to assessing the cost-effectiveness of PHIs.

The main method used—cost–utility analysis—considers the quality of life someone will experience as well as the extra life they will gain as a result of intervening in a particular way. For PHIs, the perspective adopted is usually that of the NHS or public sector. The costs of lost production due to illness or incapacity are not routinely included.

The time horizon is chosen to ensure that all important costs and effects are captured, in most cases a lifetime horizon. An annual discount rate of 3.5 per cent is applied to the costs and benefits. Sensitivity analyses are undertaken to handle parameter uncertainty.

The comparator against which the cost-effectiveness of an intervention is assessed varies from study to study. It may be usual practice, best practice, or 'no intervention'. Comparators described as 'no intervention' typically involve the assessment of the intervention against a background rate where this is known.

In general, interventions costing less than £20,000 per QALY are considered by NICE to be cost-effective. Interventions costing between £20,000 and £30,000 per QALY may be considered cost-effective if certain conditions are satisfied. NICE does not usually recommend an intervention if it costs more than £30,000 per QALY (other than for certain end-of-life treatments) unless a strong case can be made that it is an effective use of NHS resources.

8.9.4 Methods

We examined the cost-effectiveness estimates produced for all public health guidance published until June 2010. The topics for the guidance are referred to NICE by the Department of Health and although the assessment of cost-effectiveness has focused on interventions, the published guidance reflects a broader understanding of public health which takes into account the systems and structures for improving public health as well as the interventions.

For the analysis in this chapter, we focused on the 21 (of 26) publications which included base-case cost–utility analyses (i.e. those that were based on a cost per QALY). The estimates were extracted from economic models commissioned by Centre for Public Health Excellence. Full details of the models are available on the NICE website (<https://www.nice.org.uk/media/default/about/what-we-do/into-practice/costing_manual_update_050811.pdf>).

8.9.5 Results

The 21 publications studied yielded 200 base-case cost-effectiveness estimates given in terms of QALYs gained (see Table 8.3). Of these, 30 were cost saving (i.e. the intervention was more effective and cheaper than the control). A further 141 were estimated to cost less than £20,000 per QALY, and of these 69 cost less than £1000 per QALY. Seven cost between £20,000 and £30,000. Eleven estimates were above £30,000 per QALY and a further 11 interventions were dominated (i.e. the intervention was more costly and less effective than the comparator).

The median cost per QALY was £365 for the interventions costing less than £20 000 per QALY (including interventions that were cost saving). Even including those estimated to cost more than £20,000 per QALY and interventions that were dominated, the total median cost per QALY is estimated to be £633.

Table 8.4 presents a summary of the findings by topic. Interventions targeting smoking accounted for the majority of the estimates (63.5 per cent). Physical activity accounted for 10.5 per cent, alcohol prevention 7.5 per cent, and prevention of sexually transmitted diseases 7 per cent. A minority of estimates concerned social and emotional wellbeing (5.5 per cent), substance misuse (3 per cent), long-term sickness and incapacity (1.5 per cent), behaviour change (0.5 per cent), and population strategies to prevent CVD (0.5 per cent).

Interventions that were found to be cost-effective at a £20,000 per QALY threshold ranged from those targeted at individuals using face-to-face interventions to those targeted at whole populations such as mass media campaigns and legislative measures. Interventions aimed at the general population tended to have a somewhat lower cost per QALY than those targeted at disadvantaged groups. Although the vast majority of interventions were aimed at adults, interventions aimed at children and young people were also found to be cost-effective. It is noteworthy that interventions aimed at the population as a whole are among the cheapest in terms of cost per QALY; examples

Table 8.3 Number (%) and median values of ranges of the estimated incremental cost per QALY for PHIs

	Cost saving (intervention dominates)	£0 to < £20 000	£20,000 to £30,000	> £30,000	Intervention was dominated
Number (%)	30(15)	141(70.5)	7(3.5)	11(5.5)	11(5.5)
Median	N/A	£1030	£25,150	£90,786	N/A

Table 8.4 Median and range of values of incremental cost-effectiveness estimates for PHIs assessed by NICE

Guidance topic classification	Comparator	Median cost/QALY (£)	Range (£) (minimum–maximum)	Number of estimates included in median
*PH1: Brief interventions (BA) and referral for smoking cessation				
BA only (5 mins)	Background quit rate	732	577–1677	8
BA [5 mins plus nicotine replacement therapy (NRT)]	Background quit rate	2110	1664–4833	8
BA [5 mins plus self- help)	Background quit rate	370	292–847	8
PH2: Four commonly used methods to increase physical activity (PA)				
Interview	Advice	84	NA	1
Exercise prescriptions	Advice	77	20–159	4
Interviews with exercise voucher	Advice	227	NA	1
Intensive interviews	Advice	105	NA	1
Exercise prescription and exercise information	Advice	425	NA	1
Exercise prescription with intensive general	Advice	437	NA	1
Practitioner (GP) training				
Intensive interviews with exercise voucher	Advice	430	NA	1
PH3: Prevention of sexually transmitted infections and under 18 conceptions				
Tailored skill session	Usual care, didactic messages	3200	NA	1
Accelerated partner therapy: Doxycycline	Patient referral	14,025	9350–18,700	2
Accelerated partner therapy: Azithromycin	Patient referral	19,425	12,950–25,900	2
Brief counselling	Didactic messages	12,194	12,308–25,900	2
Information and behaviour skills	Didactic information	10,286	NA	1
Information, motivation, and behaviour skills	Didactic information	14,143	10,286–18,000	2

Table 8.4 Continued

Guidance topic classification	Comparator	Median cost/QALY (£)	Range (£) (minimum–maximum)	Number of estimates included in median
Enhanced counselling	Didactic messages	45,606	39,600–51,613	2
Intensive counselling	Treatment as usual	24,000	N/A	1
Behavioural skills counselling	Standard 15 min risk reduction counselling	96000	N/A	1
PH4: Interventions to reduce substance misuse among vulnerable young people				
Life-skills training	Normal education	3492	1296–6846	3
'Say yes first'	Normal education	90,786	N/A	1
Teacher training		157,384	N/A	1
The Abecedarian Project	Normal child rearing	195,225	NA	1
PH5: Workplace interventions (WIs) to promote smoking cessation				
Brief advice plus self-help material	Background quit rate	Dominates	NA	1
Brief advice plus self-help material plus NRT	Background quit rate	Dominates	NA	1
Brief advice plus self-help material plus NRT plus	Background quit rate	Dominates	NA	1
Specialist clinic				
Less intensive counselling and bupropion	Background quit rate	Dominates	NA	1
More intensive counselling and bupropion	Background quit rate	Dominates	NA	1
BA	Background quit rate	Dominates	NA	1
PH6: Behaviour change				
Mass media to promote healthy eating	No intervention	87	NA	1
PH8: PA and the environment				
Urban trail	No intervention	10445	2640–25 150	4

(*continued*)

Table 8.4 Continued

Guidance topic classification	Comparator	Median cost/QALY (£)	Range (£) (minimum–maximum)	Number of estimates included in median
PH10: smoking cessation services				
Brief advice	Background quit rate	Dominates	NA	1
Nicotine patch, pharmacy consultation	Background quit rate	Dominates	NA	1
Nicotine patch, pharmacy consultation + behavioural programme	Background quit rate	Dominates	NA	1
Brief advice plus self-help material	Background quit rate	984	NA	1
Brief advice plus self-help material plus NRT	Background quit rate	Dominates	NA	1
Brief advice plus self-help material plus NRT plus	Background quit rate	Dominates	NA	1
Specialist clinic				
Less intensive counselling and bupropion	Background quit rate	Dominates	NA	1
More intensive counselling and bupropion	Background quit rat	Dominates	NA	1
Nicotine patch, group counselling	Background quit rate	Dominates	V	1
Nicotine patch, individual counselling	Background quit rate	Dominates	NA	1
Nicotine patch—no counselling	Background quit rate	Dominates	NA	1
PH12: Social and emotional well-being in primary education				
Universal intervention (emotional function only)	No intervention	10,594	NA	1
Universal intervention (emotion + cognition)	No intervention	5278	NA	1
Focused intervention (1 level improvement)	No intervention	988,404	NA	1
Focused intervention (two level improvement)	No intervention	177,560	NA	1
PH13: Promoting PA in the workplace				
PA counselling	No intervention	864	495–1234	2

Table 8.4 Continued

Guidance topic classification	Comparator	Median cost/QALY (£)	Range (£) (minimum–maximum)	Number of estimates included in median
PA walking programme	No intervention	686	NA	1
PH14: Preventing the uptake of smoking by children and young people				
Mass media intervention	Background quit rate	49	NA	1
Point-of-sale intervention	Background quit rate	1690	NA	1
PH15: identifying and supporting people most at risk of dying prematurely				
Smoking cessation—general population: incentive schemes workplace	WI with no incentive	2089	NA	1
Smoking cessation—general population: incentive schemes NRT	Intervention no NRT	358	45–671	2
Smoking cessation—general population: incentive schemes NRT	Intervention with free guide but no free aid offered	Dominated	NA	1
Smoking cessation—general population: client centred	Background quit rate no intervention or usual care	50	0–437	8
Smoking cessation—general population: proactive telephone counselling	Usual care or intervention but no telephone counselling	427	139–1602	9
Smoking cessation—general population: proactive telephone counselling	Intervention but no telephone counselling	Dominated	NA	4
Smoking cessation—general population: recruitment to quit and win	Background quit rate; no intervention or advice	260	77–13,500	15
Smoking cessation—general population: recruitment to quit and win	Intervention or no intervention	Dominated	NA	3
Smoking cessation—general population: identify smokers through others means	No intervention	504	78–4178	4

(continued)

Table 8.4 Continued

Guidance topic classification	Comparator	Median cost/QALY (£)	Range (£) (minimum–maximum)	Number of estimates included in median
Smoking cessation—general population: identify smokers through others means	No intervention	Dominated	NA	1
Smoking cessation—general population: drop-in/rolling community based	Background quit rate	91	NA	1
Smoking cessation—general population: pharmacist based	Usual care	546	438–655	2
Smoking cessation—general population: dentist based	Usual care	302	269–360	3
Smoking cessation—general population: dentist based	Usual care (query contamination)	Dominated	NA	1
Smoking cessation—disadvantaged groups: client-centred social marketing	No intervention	1564	420-6412	3
Smoking cessation—disadvantaged groups: workplace	No intervention	1399	NA	1
Smoking cessation—disadvantaged groups: pregnant women	Usual care	1593	NA	1
Smoking cessation—disadvantaged groups: proactive telephone support pregnant women	Intervention but no offer of telephone support	5992	NA	1
Smoking cessation—disadvantaged groups: incentive NRT prescription	No intervention	1627	NA	1
Smoking cessation—disadvantaged groups: recruitment at paediatric unit	Usual care	1837	NA	1
Smoking cessation—disadvantaged groups: NHS SSS	No intervention	2686	2535–2837	2
Smoking cessation—disadvantaged groups: pharmacist based	No intervention	3151	1030–5272	2
Statins—general populations: pharmacist based	Usual care or no intervention	4892	1648–8234	4
Statins—disadvantaged groups: culturally sensitive screening	No intervention	4260	NA	1

Table 8.4 Continued

Guidance topic classification	Comparator	Median cost/QALY (£)	Range (£) (minimum–maximum)	Number of estimates included in median
Statins—disadvantaged groups: invitation for screening by GP	Usual care or no intervention	4346	4000–4692	2
PH16: mental well-being and older people				
Tri-weekly walking programme after six months	Information and education	7400	NA	1
Advice about PA	Usual care	35,900	26,200–45,600	2
Advice about PA	Nutrition advice	Dominated	NA	1
PH17: promoting PA for children and young people				
Walking buses	No intervention	4007	NA	1
Dance-class programme	No intervention	27,570	NA	1
Free swimming	No intervention	40,462	NA	1
Community sports	No intervention	71,456	NA	1
PH19: management of long-term sickness and incapacity for work				
WI	Usual care for musculoskeletal disorders	Dominates	NA	1
PA and education	Usual care for musculoskeletal disorders	2758	NA	1
PA and education and workplace visit	Usual care for musculoskeletal disorders	Dominates	NA	1
PH20: social and emotional well-being in secondary education				
Internet-based expert system + peer initiative to reduce bullying and victimization	No intervention	9600	NA	1

* more detailed descriptions of the interventions can be found on the individual NICE webpages associated with guidance represented here: <http://guidance.nice.org.uk/PHG/Published>

include mass media campaigns to promote healthy eating and legislation to reduce young people's access to cigarettes.

8.9.6 **Discussion**

8.9.6.1 Main findings of this study

This analysis showed that the PHIs considered by NICE are generally highly cost-effective according to the NICE threshold. As such, they represent good value for money. Given that the cost per QALY for most interventions is extremely low, it seems likely that as a nation we are not investing sufficiently in PHIs.

At the time of writing, the NHS has been undergoing major reform (Department of Health, 2010; Department of Health, 2011). The changes include the transfer of public health functions from the NHS to local authorities along with their associated financial resources. Amidst these changes, the need for evidence of what works and evidence of what is cost-effectiveness is greater than ever.

The analysis in this chapter provides a single, comprehensive source of evidence on the cost-effectiveness of PHIs. It is a first step in compiling the evidence that would allow informed decisions about the allocation of resources between different PHIs. Clearly, the analysis does not cover all PHIs and we need to continue in this endeavour.

We have not sought to suggest priorities for interventions. Aside from the fact that studies show that cost-effectiveness is not the only criterion used by decision-makers for allocating resources (Graham et al., 1998; Zwart-van Rijkom et al., 2000), local demographic and public health data, national and local policies and plans, national guidance, examples of best practice, and benchmarking data with other organizations are typically used by commissioners of services. A recent survey of 300 NHS commissioning staff showed that local public health intelligence, expert advice, and examples of best practice featured among the most sought after types of evidence (Gkeredakis and Claudia, 2011).

8.9.6.2 What is already known on this topic

Only a small percentage of the current NHS budget is spent on prevention. There is a paucity of evidence on the cost-effectiveness of PHIs. As noted earlier, a recent rapid review found that 15 of 41 published studies of PHIs contained no economic data and a further 15 which contained insufficient evidence for assessing whether the interventions were cost-effective (Marsh et al., 2013). The adoption of different economic methods makes it difficult to compare interventions.

8.9.6.3 What this study adds

With pressure on budgets and fundamental changes underway in the NHS and public health structure, there is a need for evidence to support the case for investing in PHIs. This is the first study to provide a comprehensive list of the cost-effectiveness of PHIs. Using a standard set of methods, the analysis has shown that the vast majority of PHIs considered thus far by NICE are highly cost-effective.

8.9.6.4 Limitations of this study

Estimating the cost-effectiveness of PHIs poses a number of challenges. Often there is a lack of data, or the data relate to intermediate or short-term outcomes (e.g. knowledge, attitudes, behaviour change within one year of the intervention) rather than long-term outcomes that are more relevant. Interventions are rarely well described and often differ in crucial details from those that have been modelled. Study quality varies considerably and interventions carried out elsewhere, or at a different point in time, do not necessarily apply to the United Kingdom today. Another important caveat is that there can be rapidly diminishing marginal returns to an intervention.

For some pieces of guidance, the cost-effectiveness of an intervention was determined with respect to 'usual care'. However, not all instances of 'usual care' mean the same thing. In some instances, the cost-effectiveness of an intervention may have been assessed against best practice; in others it may have been assessed against another intervention or 'nothing'. This is crucial because if, for example, one intervention is cheaper and gains more QALYs than any other, then all other interventions will be dominated by them. However, compared to doing nothing, the other interventions might be very cost-effective. In the current analysis, in most of the examples where the intervention was dominated it had been compared with another intervention. In some instances, the only difference between the intervention and the comparator was the *offer* of an additional component.

The efficacy studies underpinning the economic models rarely provide data on the relative effectiveness of individual elements within a multi-component intervention. Similarly, to the authors of this chapter's knowledge, there have been no head-to-head studies to assess any synergy between different combinations (or packages) of PHIs.

8.10 Conclusion

This synthesis of available economic evidence has shown that the vast majority of PHIs considered thus far by NICE are a highly cost-effective use of public funds. A next challenge would be to provide commissioners with a framework which combines information gained from economic analyses with other decision-making criteria so that transparent rationales for investment in particular PHIs can be made.

8.11 Summary of case study

Title	The cost-effectiveness of PHIs
Setting	Considering the cost-effectiveness data which aid and support decision-making in the National Institute for Health and Care Excellence (NICE).
Perspective	NICE, policy- and decision-makers, Public Health England.
Study type	Cost-effectiveness estimates from England which support public health guidance were collated and scrutinized.
Previous economic evidence	Before this article there was no list of cost-effectiveness estimates for PHIs in England.
Objective	To assess the cost-effectiveness of PHIs based on the existing literature which underpins public health guidance.

Summary of Chapter 8

◆ Many PHIs have a cost per QALY considerably lower than the UK's £20,000 payer threshold conventionally used by NICE.

◆ HALYs is an umbrella term representing attempts to adjust life expectancy to reflect health-related quality of life.

◆ When the denominator of the CE ratio is calculated using QALYs, the cost-effectiveness analysis is referred to as cost–utility analyses (CUA).

◆ Relative to a payer threshold, a cost per QALY tells us whether the anticipated health gain from a new intervention exceeds the health expected to be lost elsewhere as other health care activities are displaced (i.e. its opportunity cost).

◆ If the cost per QALY threshold used by NICE was reduced from £20,000 to £13,000 as has been proposed, many PHIs would still be good value for money to society.

◆ The EQ-5D is the most commonly used instrument to generate utility values for generating QALYs, in both adults and young people. With many public health prevention initiatives aimed at young children and adolescents, the newly developed preference based Child Health Utility instrument (CHU9D) is a welcome addition to the PHI economic evaluation toolkit.

◆ DALYs are used to estimate population disease burden. Total DALYs across a population can be thought of as a measurement of the gap between current health status and an ideal health situation where the entire population lives to an advanced age, free of disease and disability.

References

Allender, S., Foster, C., Scarborough, P., and Rayner, M., 2007. The burden of physical activity-related ill health in the UK. *Journal of Epidemiology and Community Health*, 61(4): 344–8.

Anand, S. and Hanson, K., 1997. Disability-adjusted life years: a critical review. *Journal of health economics*, 16(6): 685–702.

British Heart Foundation. 2018. *CVD Statistics*. Available at: <https://www.bhf.org.uk/-/media/files/research/heart-statistics/bhf-cvd-statistics—uk-factsheet.pdf> (Accessed 2 November 2018).

Butterfield, R., Henderson, J., and Scott, R., 2009. i *Public Health and Prevention Expenditure in England*. Available at: <http://citeseerx.ist.psu.edu/viewdoc/download?doi=10.1.1.372.1840&rep=rep1&type=pdf> (Accessed 2 November 2018).

Cabinet Office, 2003. *Strategy Unit Alcohol Harm Reduction Project—Interim Analytical Report*. <https://www.lemosandcrane.co.uk/dev/resources/Cabinet%20Office%20-%20Alcohol%20Misuse%20Report.pdf> (Accessed 2 November 2018).

Callum C., 2008. *The cost of smoking to the NHS. Action on Smoking and Health* Available at: <http://www.ash.org.uk> (Accessed 15 October 2018).

Claxton, K., Martin, S., Soares, M., Rice, N., Spackman, E., Hinde, S., Devlin, N., et al., 2015. Methods for the estimation of the National Institute for Health and Care Excellence cost-effectiveness threshold. *Health Technology Assessment*, 19: 14

Cornes, P., 2012. The economic pressures for biosimilar drug use in cancer medicine. *Targeted Oncology*, 7(1): 57–67.

Department of Health. 2010. *Equity and Excellence: Liberating the NHS*. Available at: <http://www.dh.gov.uk/prod_consum_dh/groups/dh_digitalassets/@dh/@en/@ps/documents/digitalasset/dh_117794.pdf> (Accessed 15 October 2018).

Department of Health. 2011. *Healthy Lives, Healthy People: Our Strategy for Public Health in England*. Available at: <http://www.dh.gov.uk/en/Publicationsandstatistics/Publications/PublicationsPolicyAndGuidance/DH_121941> (Accessed 15 October 2018).

Devleesschauwer, B., Havelaar, A.H., De Noordhout, C.M., Haagsma, J.A., Praet, N., Dorny, P., Duchateau, L., et al., 2014. DALY calculation in practice: A stepwise approach. *International Journal of Public Health*, 59(3): 571.

Drummond, M., Torrance, G., and Mason, J., 1993. Cost-effectiveness league tables: more harm than good? *Social Science & Medicine*, 37(1): 33–40.

Drummond M.F, Weatherly H.L.A, Claxton K.P et al. 2007. *Assessing the challenges of applying the standard methods of economic evaluation to public health programmes*. Public Health Research Consortium. Available at: <http://phrc.lshtm.ac.uk/papers/PHRC_D1-05_Final_Report.pdf> (Accessed 2 November 2018).

Drummond, M.F., Sculpher, M.J., Claxton, K., Stoddart, G.L., and Torrance, G.W., 2015. *Methods for the Economic Evaluation of Health Care Programmes*. Oxford: Oxford University Press.

Drummond, M., Weatherly, H., and Ferguson, B., 2008. Economic evaluation of health interventions. *British Medical Journal*, 337: a1204.

Foresight. 2007. *Tackling obesities—future choices project report*. Available at: <http://www.foresight.gov.uk/Obesity/Obesity_final_part1.pdf> (Accessed 15 October 2018).

Frew, E. J., Pallan, M., Lancashire, E., Hemming, K., and Adab, P., 2015. Is utility-based quality of life associated with overweight in children? Evidence from the UK WAVES randomised controlled study. *BMC Pediatrics*, 15: 211.

Gerard, K. and Mooney, G., 1993. QALY league tables: Handle with care. *Health Economics*, 2: 59–64.

Gkeredakis, E. and Claudia, R., 2011. Using evidence is not an open and shut case. *Health Service Journal*, 26 May, 23–25.

Gold, M.R., Stevenson, D., and Fryback, D.G., 2002. HALYS and QALYS and DALYS, Oh My: similarities and differences in summary measures of population Health. *Annual Review of Public Health*, 23(1): 115–34.

Gold, M.R., Siegel, J.E., Russell, L.B., and Weinstein, M.C., 1996. *Cost-Effectiveness in Health and Medicine*. New York, NY, Oxford University Press.

Graham, J.D., Corso, P.S., Morris, J.M., Segui-Gomez, M., and Weinstein, M.C., 1998. Evaluating the cost-effectiveness of clinical and public health measures. *Annual Review of Public Health*, 19(1): 125–52.

Kelly, M.P. and Abraham, C., 2009. *Behaviour change: The NICE perspective on the NICE guidance*. Available at: <http://dx.doi. org/10.1080/08870440802643013> (Accessed 15 October 2018).

Kelly, M.P., McDaid, D., Ludbrook, A., and Powell, J., 2005. *Economic Appraisal of PHIs*. London: Health Development Agency.

Lopez, A.D. and Murray, C.C., 1998. *The Global Burden of Disease 1990–2020*. Geneva: WHO.

Lorgelly, P.K., Lawson, K.D., Fenwick, E.A., and Briggs, A.H., 2010. Outcome measurement in economic evaluations of PHIs: a role for the capability approach? *International Journal of Environmental Research and Public Health*, 7(5): 2274–89

Marmot, M., 2010. *Fair society healthy lives.* Available at: <http://www.instituteofhealthequity. org/resources-reports/fair-society-healthy-lives-the-marmot-review/fair-society-healthy-lives-full-report-pdf> (Accessed 15 October 2018).

Marsh, K., Dolan, P., Kempster, J., and Lugon, M., 2013. Prioritizing investments in public health: A multi-criteria decision analysis, *Journal of Public Health,* **35**(3):460–6.

Mason, J.M., 1994. Cost-per-QALY League Tables. *Pharmacoeconomics,* 5(6): 472–81.

Mathers, C., Fat, D.M., and Boerma, J.T., 2008. *The Global Burden of Disease: 2004 Update.* Geneva: WHO.

McCabe, C., Claxton, K., and Culyer, A., 2008. The NICE cost-effectiveness threshold: what it is and what that means. *Pharmacoeconomics,* **26**: 733–44.

McIntosh, E., Donaldson, C., and Ryan, M., 1999. Recent advances in the methods of cost-benefit analysis in health care. *Pharmacoeconomics,* *15*(4): 357–67.

Morris, S., Devlin, N. and Parkin, D., 2007. *Economic analysis in health care.* John Wiley & Sons.

Murray, C.J.L., 1994. Quantifying the burden of disease: The technical basis for disability-adjusted life years. *Bulletin of the World Health Organization, 72*(3): 429–45. Available at: <http://apps.who.int/iris/bitstream/10665/52181/1/bulletin_1994_72%283%29_429-445. pdf?ua=1> (Accessed 15 October 2018).

National Institute for Health and Care Excellence, 2009. *Methods for the Development of NICE Public Health Guidance* (2nd edn) Available at: <http://www.wphna.org/htdocs/ downloadsmay2012/2009%20NICE%20public%20health%20guidance%20pdf.pdf> (Accessed 2 November 2018).

National Institute for Health and Care Excellence, 2010. Measuring effectiveness and cost effectiveness: the QALY. Available at: https://www.nice.org.uk/proxy/?sourceurl=http:// www.nice.org.uk/newsroom/features/measuringeffectivenessandcosteffectivenesstheqaly. jsp

National Institute for Health and Care Excellence, 2013. Guides to the methods of technology appraisal. Available at: <https://www.nice.org.uk/process/pmg9/chapter/the-reference-case> (Accessed 2 November 2018).

Office for National Statistics, 2008a. *Statistical Bulletin: Births and deaths in England and Wales.* Available at: <https://www.rcog.org.uk/globalassets/documents/news/ statsbulletin2008birthsanddeathsfina_tcm77-228125.pdf> (Accessed 2 November 2018).

Office for National Statistics, 2008b. *Mortality statistics. Deaths registered in 2008.* Available at: <https://www.ons.gov.uk/ons/rel/vsob1/mortality-statistics--deaths-registered-in-england-and-wales--series-dr-/2008/mortality-statistics--deaths-registered--series-dr-.pdf> (Accessed 2 November 2018).

Owen, L., Morgan, A., Fischer, A., Ellis, S., Hoy, A., and Kelly, M., 2012. The cost-effectiveness of public health interventions. *Journal of Public Health,* 34(1): 37–45.

Pharmaceutical Benefits Advisory Committee, 2016. *Guidelines for Preparing Submissions to the Pharmaceutical Benefits Advisory Committee (PBAC).* Available at: <https://pbac.pbs. gov.au/> (Accessed 15 October 2018).

Pharmac, 2012. *Prescription for Pharmacoeconomic Analysis: Methods for Cost-Utility Analysis.* Available at: <https://www.pharmac.govt.nz/2012/06/26/PFPAFinal.pdf> (Accessed 2 November 2018).

Phillips, C., 2009. *What is a QALY?* Available at: <http://www.bandolier.org.uk/painres/ download/whatis/QALY.pdf> (Accessed 2 November 2018).

Robinson, R. 1993. Cost–utility analysis. *British Medical Journal,* 307: 859–62.

Sanders, B.S., 1964. Measuring community health levels. *American Journal of Public Health and the Nation's Health, 54*: 1063–70.

Sassi, F., 2006. Calculating QALYs, comparing QALY and DALY calculations. *Health Policy and Planning, 21*(5): 402–8.

Schlander, M., 2010. Measures of efficiency in health care: QALMs about QALYs? *Zeitschrift für Evidenz, Fortbildung und Qualität im Gesundheitswesen, 104*(3): 214–26.

Schwappach, D.L.B., 2002. Resource allocation, social values and the QALY: A review of the debate and empirical evidence. *Health Expectations, 5*: 210–22.

Schwappach, D.L., Boluarte, T.A., and Suhrcke, M., 2007. The economics of primary prevention of cardiovascular disease–a systematic review of economic evaluations. *Cost Effectiveness and Resource Allocation, 5*(1): 1.

Thorrington, D., and Eames, K. 2015. Measuring health utilities in children and adolescents: A systematic review of the literature. *PLoS ONE, 10*: e0135672.

Wanless D., 2002. *Securing our Future Health: Taking a Long Term View. Final Report.* London: HM Treasury.

Wanless, D., 2004. *Securing Good Health for the Whole Population.* London: HM Stationery Office.

Weatherly, H., Drummond, M., Claxton, K., Cookson, R., Ferguson, B., Godfrey, C., Rice, N., Sculpher, M., et al., 2009. Methods for assessing the cost-effectiveness of PHIs: Key challenges and recommendations. *Health Policy, 93*(2): 85–92.

Weinstein, M.C., Torrance, G., and McGuire, A., 2009. QALYs: The basics. *Value in Health, 12*(s1): S5–S9.

World Health Organization, 2013. *WHO Methods and Data Sources for Global Burden of Disease Estimates 2000–2011.* Available at: <http://www.who.int/healthinfo/statistics/GlobalDALYmethods_2000_2011.pdf?ua=1> (Accessed 15 October 2018).

World Health Organization, 2016. *Introduction to Drug Utilization Research.* Available at: <http://apps.who.int/medicinedocs/en/d/Js4876e/5.4.html> (Accessed 15 October 2018).

World Health Organization, 2015. *Health Statistics and Information Systems.* Available at: <http://www.who.int/healthinfo/en/> (Accessed 15 October 2018).

Williams, A., 1985. Economics of coronary artery bypass grafting. *BMJ (Clinical research edn), 291*(6491): 326–9.

Zwart-van Rijkom, J.E., Leufkens, H.G., Busschbach, J.J., Broekmans, A.W., and Rutten, F.F., 2000. Differences in attitudes, knowledge and use of economic evaluations in decision-making in The Netherlands. *Pharmacoeconomics, 18*(2): 149–60.

Chapter 9

Cost–benefit analysis for applied public health economic evaluation

Emma McIntosh, Camilla Baba, and
Willings Botha

9.1 Introduction

This chapter introduces the reader to the stages of cost–benefit analysis (CBA) as specifically applied to public health interventions (PHI) economic evaluation. The focus of this chapter follows on from the messages of Chapter 6 on the relevance of, and methods for, quantifying the 'outcomes' of PHIs in monetary form for CBA. Two novel case studies focus on the use of stated preference discrete choice experiment (SPDCE) methodology for valuation of multi-attribute benefits comprising health, non-health, and process outcomes of the type likely to occur in PHIs. With little consensus on suitable evaluation methods in public health (Mathes et al., 2017), CBA arguably provides a useful framework for valuation of the broad-ranging costs and outcomes pertinent to the economic evaluation of PHIs. In addition to this, this chapter explores the merit in the more recent approach of social CBA (Fujiwara and Campbell, 2011). This latter approach draws heavily on the use of the subjective well-being outcomes (Dolan et al., 2008, Dolan et al., 2011) referred to in Chapter 6 of this book. This chapter does not detail costing approaches for CBA; these methods are well documented in Chapter 5 and elsewhere (Brouwer et al., 2001; McIntosh et al., 2010; Drummond et al., 2015).

The earlier handbook in this series entitled *Applied Methods of Cost–Benefit Analysis in Health Care* outlines CBA methods as applied to health (McIntosh et al., 2010). This chapter puts forward a case for the suitability of the CBA framework (in its widest and most practical sense) for use in PHI economic evaluation. As this book has outlined thus far that, contrary to standard health care interventions, PHIs are typically delivered *outwith* a health service setting hence by definition are likely to involve resources (and potential cost savings) beyond the health service. As discussed in Chapter 3, PHIs can have broad-ranging outcomes linked not only to health but education, employment, housing, and other government sectors (Kelly et al., 2005, Weatherly et al., 2009). Given these special features and as recognized in National Institute for Health and Care Excellence's (NICE) public health technical guidance for incorporating health economics into PHI evaluation (NICE, 2012; see also Appendix 9.1), the holistic CBA framework arguably provides an ideal framework for economic evaluation of PHIs, particularly in the absence of consensus of an appropriate evaluative methodology (Mathes et al., 2017). This book outlines variations on the CBA framework including the more pragmatic, yet less theoretically appealing, social return on investment (SROI) approaches, which are becoming increasingly used in public health economic evaluations (Masters et al., 2017). CBA conventionally takes a societal perspective allowing comparison of cost-benefit ratios across projects, based on a firm theoretical framework. By contrast, SROI can involve a range of stakeholder perspectives and as such is more stakeholder driven hence this makes comparison of SROI ratios across studies which have used different methods challenging (Fujiwara, 2015). The aim of this chapter is to provide guidance on up-to-date methodology and practical suggestions for carrying out applied CBA within the context of PHIs.

This chapter will:

- briefly introduce the basic welfare economic theories including Pareto optimality
- outline the key assumptions of normative economics and the basic theory of preferences
- outline the main choices of benefit measure for use in CBA, focusing on willingness to pay (WTP) methodology
- outline and describe the merits of the emerging social CBA method
- introduce Stated Preference Discrete Choice Experiments (SPDCEs) as an alternative method for valuing outcomes
- describe case studies of SPDCE in a public health evaluative context

9.2 **Why CBA for PHI economic evaluation?**

In Chapter 2 of this book we explored the notion that the market system in health care fails to allocate resources optimally, with markets for public health prevention goods particularly vulnerable to market failure. With the recent public health function in England moving from the National Health Service (NHS) to local government, joint working between the NHS and local authorities in Wales, Scotland, and Northern Ireland and increased joint working through devolution within England, there is increased demand for economic evidence to support cross-sectoral investment decisions aimed at having an impact on public health. CBA typically measures all costs and outcomes in monetary terms. These sectors all understand the language of money, making CBA and alternatives including Return On Investment (ROI) and Social ROI (SROI) ideal methods of evaluation appropriate to a wide audience of stakeholders. In the last 20 years there has been a rapid rise in the number of methodological and applied contributions to the economics of health care, mainly in the area of cost-effectiveness and cost–utility analyses (Drummond et al., 2015). Despite a fewer number of CBAs during this same period there has been a huge increase in the number of methodological applications in the area of contingent valuation (CV) and the measurement and valuation of monetary benefits necessary for the process of CBA (McIntosh et al., 2010). CV is the main technique for valuing outcomes in welfare values, or 'outcomes' which sit on the 'benefits' side of the equation in CBA. There has been a notable increase in the CV methods of both WTP (Ryan and Shackley, 1995; Ryan et al., 1997, 2004; Diener et al., 1998) and SPDCEs for estimating welfare values in health care

(Hall et al., 2002; Ryan, 2004; de Bekker-Grob et al., 2012) with some of this a response to the desire to broaden the evaluative space (Ryan and Shackley, 1995; Donaldson and Shackley, 1997). Associated methodological challenges, in a bid to reduce the inherent bias challenges arising when generating monetary values, have restricted the widespread adoption of CBA in health care research in comparison to cost–utility analysis (CUA) and cost-effectiveness analysis (CEA). More flexible and practical forms of CBA as presented in this chapter will hopefully provide some optimism for those analysts who see the merit and applicability of CBA's broad-ranging, holistic approach ideally suited to PHI economic evaluation.

The distinguishing feature of this series of handbooks from Oxford University Press is its much stronger practical flavour in comparison to existing texts, with plenty of illustrative material and worked examples provided. Given the important theoretical basis of CBA, this chapter begins by briefly introducing the basic theorems of welfare economics before progressing to outlining the particular relevance of the CBA framework for economic evaluation of PHIs. For a more detailed introduction to the basic theories of 'normative' welfare economics including Pareto-improving criteria, discussed in this book in Chapter 2, theories underlying preferences and utility maximization, as well as the theory underlying the alternative types of welfare measure (compensating variation, equivalent variation, and consumer surplus), readers are referred to Boadway and Bruce (1984), Layard and Walters (1978), Layard and Glaister (1994), and Mishan (Mishan, 1971).

While CBA is a common form of economic evaluation across other sections of the economy such as the environment and transport, other than methodological contributions in the area of benefit assessment for use in CBAs (Hanley et al., 2003; McIntosh et al., 2010), the application of the CBA methodology in the health care sector has been notably limited with a widespread reluctance to use CBA for health care evaluations because of the necessity of valuing all outcomes in monetary terms (Klose, 1999; Brent, 2003). As pointed out by Borghi, 'few WTP studies in the health sector have used their results within a CBA, an essential step to informing resource allocation decisions' (Borghi, 2008). However, with the recent increase in the interest in PHI evaluation and the call by governing bodies such as UK's NICE to widen the evaluative space there has been a shift towards an increase in the use of frameworks such as MCDA (Devlin and Sussex, 2011), and methods such as SROI (Banke-Thomas et al., 2015), both discussed later in this book. While not CBA in themselves these methods offer a practical alternative to CBA and can provide a stepping stone to the monetary valuation of outcomes.

9.3 What is cost–benefit analysis?

CBA is a theoretical framework in which both the costs and outcomes of a project, service, good, or, in the PHI context, an intervention, are quantified in monetary terms to identify the option with the greatest social ranking as judged by net monetary benefit. Where the outcomes are greater than the costs, then the decision to allocate resources is justified (Boadway and Bruce, 1984). To decide on the worth of a project involving public expenditure it is necessary to weigh up the advantages and disadvantages. As Dasgupta and Pearce state, 'cost–benefit analysis purports to be a way of deciding what society prefers' (Dasgupta and Pearce, 1978, p. 19). Where only one option or service or PHI can be chosen from a series of options, CBA should inform the decision-maker which option is socially most preferred, from a societal perspective. An important stage in this process is the unbiased and accurate identification, measurement, and valuation of gains and losses (benefits and costs) arising from the intervention or service (Dasgupta and Pearce, 1978).

9.4 **Welfare economics**

As discussed in Chapter 2, the theory of welfare economics lies at the root of applied CBA methods. Economic evaluation aims to assess the costs and consequences of a particular 'change in circumstances', for example, a new bridge, clearing of a forest for recreational purposes or in public health, the introduction of a nursery school programme of supervised tooth-brushing. It is the use of methods for measuring such *welfare change* for which applied economists have become known. Boadway and Bruce note that 'welfare economics can be viewed as an investigation of methods of obtaining a social ordering over alternative possible states of the world' (Boadway and Bruce, 1984 p. 1. Economists are interested in 'ranking different *allocations of resources*, where this is used in its broadest sense to refer to the combinations of commodities produced and consumed by each decision maker in the economy and the combinations of factors used in the production of each commodity' (Boadway and Bruce, 1984).

9.4.1 **Basic theories**

'Utility is the subjective satisfaction of the household and cannot be observed directly. It must be inferred from observable attributes of household consumption behaviour and the hypothesis of utility maximisation' (Groves, 1970). This statement is a useful starting point with which to explore the mechanisms of welfare economics. A distinction is usually made between analysing the consequences of a change (positive economics) and making judgements concerning the desirability of a particular change or policies (normative economics). It is this latter type of economics and its role in applied PHI economic evaluation, with which CBA is concerned.

9.4.2 **Welfare: What is it?**

Boadway and Bruce state that welfare economics can be 'viewed as an investigation of methods of obtaining a *social ordering* over alternative possible *states of the world*' (Boadway and Bruce, 1984, p. 1). Such a social ordering then permits the comparison of states of the world and allows the ranking of each state in terms of 'better than', 'worse than', or 'equally as good as' (Mishan, 1981; Boadway and Bruce, 1984). The term 'welfare' in economics is often referred to as the sum of individuals 'well-being', resulting from consumption of goods and services. This suggests that in order to obtain a social ranking of states, one must be able to find ways of measuring quantitatively the impact of changes in the use of resources upon human well-being. In traditional health economics terms, within a medical model, if society wishes to make the most, in terms of individuals' well-being, of its endowment of all health care resources, it must find a way of comparing the values of what society receives from any health care change (i.e. the benefits) with the values of what its members give up by taking resources from other uses (i.e. the costs) (Freeman, 1993). It should be clear to the reader of this book, with respect to public health, that finding an appropriately broad and encompassing welfare measure is a key requirement to support evidence-based policy. Standard economic theory for measuring changes in individuals' well-being was developed for the purpose of interpreting changes in the prices and quantities of goods purchased in markets. This theory became the basis for welfare measurement criteria when it was identified that the *trade-offs* people make as they choose less of one good and substitute more of some other good reveal something about the value people place on these goods. Later sections in this chapter will explain how value measures based upon such substitutability can be expressed in a number of ways, including the commonly used WTP and willingness to accept (WTA) compensation methods for changes in quantity and quality of goods. Following on from Chapters 2 and 3 we return to the concept of Pareto-improving criteria, a means by which social states can be ordered using some value judgement.

9.4.3 Welfare economics and the important role of Pareto-improving criteria

Welfare economics has historically been dominated by the notion of a social welfare function (SWF). While the SWF remains used for illustrative purposes in economics texts it plays no role in *applied* welfare economics because it is a concept difficult to define (Mitchell and Carson, 1989). An alternative, more applied approach which is also 'perhaps ethically more neutral' is the Pareto criterion (Mitchell and Carson, 1989), which states that policy changes which make at least one person better off without making anyone worse off are Pareto improving and should be undertaken. The important point to note for the purposes of applying welfare economics to PHI economic evaluation is that the criterion used by welfare economics to judge a new policy or policy change is whether that policy is 'Pareto improving'. A Pareto-improving policy change would constitute one which moves an economy or a 'society experiencing a public health intervention' to a position which is Pareto-superior (preferred) from a position which is Pareto-inferior (less preferred). Such a change is sometimes referred to as an increase in relative efficiency.

John Hicks (1939) and Nicholas Kaldor (1939) proposed a welfare criterion which has been alternatively called the potential Pareto-improvement criterion (PPIC) or the potential compensation test (Hicks, 1939; Kaldor, 1939). A potential Pareto improvement means that the gainers from the change could *hypothetically* compensate the losers from the change. The PPIC has been controversial because, without the *actual* payment of compensation, it is possible to make a very small group of people much better off while making the vast majority worse off. The PPIC has found wide acceptance and use among applied economists. Mitchell and Carson note that use of the

PPIC has been justified on several grounds. The most common of these is the argument that projects should be decided on the basis of strict economic efficiency. In addition to this is the argument that the PPIC is only one piece of information available to policy makers, who are free to reject policy changes with adverse distributional consequences if they wish (Mitchell and Carson, 1989).

The important point to note for the purposes of advocating the use of CBA for the economic evaluation of PHIs is that CBA (often referred to as the 'applied side of modern welfare economics') operationalizes a version of the Pareto criterion by placing monetary values on the gains and losses to those affected by a change in the level of provision of a good or service for which there is often no market such as public health interventions. This allows the calculation of net gain or loss from a policy change, and the determination of whether the change is potentially Pareto-improving.

9.4.4 The importance of preferences in CBA

Welfare theory starts with the premise that individuals[1] are the best judge of their own welfare, and that inferences about welfare can be drawn from each individual by observing that individual's choices among alternative bundles of goods and services. An individual chooses among available bundles on the basis of his or her preferences and budget and if an individual prefers bundle **A** over bundle **B**, then bundle **A** must provide a higher level of welfare for the individual. It is assumed that the individual can compare any two commodity bundles, or services and decide that one is at least as good as the other. Preferences are assumed to have certain properties (i.e. reflexive, transitive, complete, and continuous) such that a utility function $\mathbf{u}(\mathbf{x})$ is a suitable representation of individual preferences (McIntosh et al., 2010). As Freeman notes, the property of substitutability or 'continuity' is at the core of the economist's concept of value (Freeman, 1993). Substitutability is key as it establishes trade-off ratios between pairs of goods/attributes that matter to people. The importance of substitutability will become more evident in a later section of this chapter on the use of WTP and SPDCE methodologies to obtain measures of welfare, where substitutability is a crucial assumption for deriving welfare values for use in the CBA framework.

9.4.5 Estimating welfare change

Within the realms of economic theory, the standard context in which to measure benefits or 'outcomes' is to evaluate price changes and hence changes in individual welfare (Boadway and Bruce, 1984). The basis for determining these values stems from the underlying preference structure of the individual and the assumptions made about how preferences should 'behave'. Welfare measures are obtained by converting changes in utility to monetary values. There are three main approaches to estimating welfare changes, they are: consumer surplus (CS), equivalent variation (EV), and compensating variation (CV). It is commonly accepted that the use of Hicksian demand functions are more appropriate welfare measures in the context of policy decision-making

---

[1] The term 'individual' is used here. However, often the term 'household' is used when discussing these theories.

with CV being the preferred measure in CBA. CV is the amount of money we can take away from an individual after an economic change, while leaving her as well off as she was before it. For a welfare gain, it is the amount she would be willing to pay for a change. For a welfare loss, it is the amount she would need to accept as compensation for the change (Layard and Walters, 1978). With reference to the evaluation of PHIs, this reasoning for using CV fits in with the methods used for the economic evaluation of health care by estimating welfare gains and losses in a CBA. For readers wishing to explore theories of consumption in more depth, please refer to chapters 20 and 21 in Mishan (1981).

In the case of a good or service that is traded in a competitive market, buyers and sellers reveal their preferences directly through their actions where price and quantity signals are observed, hence allowing CV to be estimated directly. This method of eliciting welfare change is called revealed preference (RP). However, as explained in Chapter 2, in health care and in public health more broadly, market failure exists and thus extensive government intervention is required and, as a consequence, health care, preventive health care, and PHIs are often provided publicly (i.e. people are not revealing their preferences via how much they pay for health care goods and services). As a result of market failure, the measure of 'value' usually obtained by measuring individuals' responses to price and quantity changes in the competitive market is absent and preferences are not revealed in the usual manner (i.e. by how much people pay). A number of practical methods have therefore been developed to measure the individuals' willingness to pay for non-marketed goods. These include: stated preference (SP) survey techniques, the Clarke–Groves mechanism (Groves, 1970; Clarke, 1971), travel cost methods (Hotelling, 1947), and hedonic approaches (Griliches, 1971; Rosen, 1974). In environmental economics, methods of valuing amenities have traditionally been categorized as direct and indirect. Indirect methods, such as the travel cost approach, use actual choices made by consumers to develop models of choice. Direct methods ask consumers what they would be willing to pay or accept for a change in a good or service. Direct methods are examples of CV stated preference techniques in that individuals do not actually make any behavioural changes, they only *state* that they would behave in this fashion. Both methods have advantages and disadvantages. Direct methods are often criticized because of the hypothetical nature of the questions and the fact that actual behaviour is not observed (Environmental Protection Agency, 2009). However, these direct methods currently provide the main viable alternative to valuing goods and services where the consumer may have had little or no experience of the good being valued.

In health economics and public health economics, where consumers—members of the population who may be potential patients—may have had little or no experience of the health care service or good requiring valuation, and actual choices for treatments or preventative services are often heavily influenced by professional advice (asymmetry of information), the direct methods are often the best option. Direct methods allow the valuation of a quality or quantity change involving a number of attribute levels changes. The appropriate context in terms of information requirements and consumer sovereignty required for eliciting unbiased preferences can also be established within the direct methods and in doing so, a hypothetical market framework is provided for decision-making.

9.4.6 Applied welfare economics as applied to CBA

Economic evaluation is concerned with comparing costs and benefits within an evaluative framework to provide information on the 'worthwhileness' of particular allocative decisions. Chapters 7 and 8 explored the methods of cost-effectiveness and cost–utility analysis in PHI economic evaluation. Economic evaluation is commonly used to provide information for making resource allocation decisions in health care and within public health economics. As outlined in Chapter 6, the techniques vary mainly in terms of how the outcomes are identified, quantified, and valued. Chapter 6 also outlined measures of outcome of particular use in PHI economic evaluations. Essentially, if a good or service contributes positively to human well-being, it has economic value. The basic value judgement underlying economic valuation is that 'preferences count', although this does not imply that all decisions must be made on the basis of what people want. Other factors, such as what is morally appropriate, what is ethically acceptable, and what is reasonable and practical, must be taken into account, although such factors are typically less amenable to formal economic analysis.

As outlined earlier in this chapter, there are two main ways of estimating the economic values attached to non-market goods and services: revealed preferences (indirect approach) and stated preferences (direct approach). Revealed preference approaches identify the ways in which a non-marketed good influences actual markets for some other good; that is, value is revealed through a complementary (surrogate or proxy) market. An example of a revealed preference approach in health care would be the measurement of the travel costs incurred to attend a vaccination clinic. Stated preference approaches or CV methods (direct methods), on the other hand, are based on hypothetical or constructed markets; they ask people to state what economic value they attach to those goods and services. It is this latter approach which is the subject area of much of this remaining chapter. Finally, a third approach to economic valuation, more commonly used by environmental economists, relies on the build-up of case studies from revealed and stated preference studies and then seeks to 'borrow' the resulting economic values and apply them to a new context. This is termed benefits transfer (see Bateman et al., 2002 for a comprehensive summary of this method).

9.4.7 Eliciting WTP in the hypothetical health care market

In health economics, the most popular technique used to elicit monetary measures of benefit has been the use of direct survey-based stated preference (SP) CV methods to extract WTP for hypothetical goods and services designed based around new interventions or services. Typically, CV methods use surveys to elicit people's preferences for public goods by finding out what they would be willing to pay for specified improvements to services (see Chapter 6). The number of SP CV studies in health care has grown rapidly, with the majority of these being carried out for the purposes of benefit measurement to fit into a CBA framework. Diener and colleagues noted the wide variation amongst health care CV studies in terms of the types of questions being posed and the elicitation formats being used (Diener et al., 1998). Much of the research into health care CV of recent years has, in fact, concentrated on these 'methodological' issues—the ultimate aim being to obtain the most valid, reliable, consistent, and meaningful measure of maximum WTP, derived through hypothetical means. CV surveys typically aim to obtain an accurate estimate of the benefits of a change in the level of provision of a good, which can then be combined with the costs of producing the good, within a CBA. As Mitchell and Carson state: '[i[n order to do this, the survey must simultaneously meet the methodological imperatives of survey research and the requirements of economic theory' (Mitchell and Carson, 1989, p. 17). Mitchell and Carson go on to note that to meet the methodological imperatives requires that the scenario be understandable and meaningful to the respondents and free of incentives which might bias the results. Further, a survey must obtain the correct benefit measures for the good in the context of an appropriate hypothetical market setting. The following section provides a summary of the commonly used methods for eliciting WTP as a measure of benefit for CBA along with some of their key methodological challenges.

9.4.7.1 Willingness to pay

WTP as a benefit measurement tool is based on the premise that the maximum amount of money an individual is willing to pay for a commodity is an indicator of the value or utility or satisfaction to them of that good or service. Despite the theoretical merits of this approach, there has been substantial criticism of the WTP approach (Kahneman and Knetsch, 1992; Diamond and Hausman, 1994). The majority of the criticisms are associated with the possible biases which are a threat to the validity of WTP results (Svedsater, 2000). Diener and colleagues explored the main elicitation methods for WTP in health economics. They were: open-ended questions, bidding games, payment cards, closed-ended or 'take-it-or-leave-it', and closed-ended with follow-up methods (Diener et al., 1998; see also chapter 6 in McIntosh et al., 2010 for detail of these methods). The National Oceanic Administrative Association (NOAA) panel carried out an assessment of the various approaches to eliciting WTP. Their recommendations included promotion of the closed-ended format, face-to-face interviews instead of surveys, pilot surveying and pre-testing, and provision of accurate information on the good being valued (Arrow et al., 1993). The elicitation format refers to the style of questioning used to elicit the WTP value. There are a number of different formats to choose from, each with its own strengths and weaknesses and there is debate in the literature concerning which is superior (Smith, 2000). the next subsection of this chapter presents a brief summary of the most common formats used to elicit WTP values. For a more complete summary please refer to chapter 6 in McIntosh et al., 2010.

9.4.7.2 Open-ended WTP format

The open-ended question is the 'simplest' of the elicitation methods. This question asks participants to state their WTP for a health care intervention without any prompts or cues from the questionnaire or interviewer. Usually the respondents are provided with a space (a line to write on) for their final maximum WTP value. An example of an open-ended WTP question is shown in Box 9.1.

Box 9.1 Example of an open-ended WTP format

What is the maximum amount you would be willing to pay to

attend a community-based walking initiative? £_____

9.4.7.3 Iterative bidding method

This elicitation format is termed the 'bidding game' and first originated in environ-mental economics (Randall and Kriesel, 1990). The iterative bidding question is de-signed so that it resembles an auction because the respondent enters a bargaining process with the interviewer and is often likened to a 'haggle' technique that happens in real-life markets (Frew, 2010). The respondent is presented with a first bid amount and, depending on whether they accept or reject that bid, this bid is either raised or lowered till eventually the respondent's maximum WTP is reached. The amount by which the bids are raised or lowered is determined by an algorithm to ensure that each respondent participates in the same bidding process. Once the highest bid is reached in the algorithm, the question reverts to an open-ended question of the type outlined earlier.

9.4.7.4 Payment-scale method

The payment-scale question design was developed by Mitchell and Carson as an al-ternative to the bidding game approach (Mitchell and Carson, 1989, pp. 30–1). The payment-scale question presents respondents with a range of values to choose typic-ally with a series of bid amounts in a vertical list from the lowest bid to the highest bids in increments as shown in Box 9.2.

9.4.7.5 Closed-ended/dichotomous-choice/discrete question

Closed-ended questions are designed to allow a simple Yes/No response from participants. This method was developed by Bishop and Heberlein (1979). Respondents are presented with a bid value and asked if they are WTP that amount (see Box 9.3).

The bid values are varied across the sample so that it is possible to estimate the percentage of respondents who are WTP as a function of the bid (Bishop and Heberlein, 1979; Frew, 2010). The closed-ended design is recommended by Mitchell and Carson as being suitable for a mail questionnaire survey (Mitchell and Carson, 1989). It is also claimed that the question design is less stressful to the respondent.

Other direct WTP approaches include the closed-ended with follow-up and the marginal approach (for a summary of these please refer to McIntosh et al., 2010 and specifically Frew, 2010). More recently, the method of SPDCE has been used as an alternative methodology for eliciting WTP. The following section outlines SPDCE methods.

Box 9.2 Example of a payment-scale WTP format

Please place a tick (✓) next to the amounts you are sure you would be willing to pay and a cross (×) next to the amounts you would not pay. Please circle the maximum amount you would be willing to pay. If the maximum amount is not on the scale, please insert it into the space provided.

£100

£150

£200

£250

£300

£400

£500

£1000

£2000

£3000

£4000

£_____

9.4.7.6 Stated preference discrete choice experiments (SPDCEs) for eliciting WTP

SPDCEs are a quantitative technique for eliciting and valuing preferences. SPDCE allows researchers to uncover how people value individual attributes of a programme, product, or service by asking them to state their choice over different hypothetical alternatives. Analyses of these choices allows quantification of the trade-offs being made and, if cost is include as an attribute, estimation of WTP for changes in attribute levels. To date, SPDCEs have been applied to a range of health care, health policy, planning, and resource allocation decisions (Hall et al., 2002; Ryan et al., 2008), but less commonly in public health evaluation (Lowin et al., 1999). However, SPDCEs may be particular suited to economic evaluations of PHI because of their ability to incorporate

Box 9.3 Example of the closed-ended WTP format

Would you be willing to pay £10 to attend a community-based walking initiative?

☐ Yes ☐ No

broad-ranging attributes, including multi-sectoral attributes. In theory, this approach could identify, measure, and value not only attributes within different sectors but also the trade-offs *between* sectors such as health, public health, education, and judicial. SPDCE approaches allow researchers to determine not only the preferred programme characteristics of both existing as well as non-existing programs but also to quantify the importance of the measured programme characteristics relative to each other by including cost as an attributes and eliciting WTP values. Ryan and Gerard provide a useful starting point for reviewing the use of SPDCE methodology in health (Ryan and Gerard, 2003). de Bekker-Grobb and co-workers updated this review and indicated a rapid growth in SPDCEs in health, reflecting similar growth in the frequency of use of this technique in other areas (de Bekker-Grob et al., 2012).

Increasing acknowledgement, particularly pertinent in public health, that individuals derive well-being benefit (or utility) from other, non-health sources, has led to the question as to how best to measure these attributes which are beyond health outcomes (Ryan et al., 2008). Moving away from the QALY 'paradigm' to consider the multifaceted aspects of health and how best to include valuations for other elements/attributes has led health researchers in the last two decades to borrow from transport and environmental economics to adopt methodology that captures utilities with preferences (Ryan and Shackley, 1995; Reed Johnson and Adamowicz, 2011). As we showed in Chapter 8, many PHIs have a cost per QALY below the UK's NICE threshold of £20,000 to £30,000. Whilst useful in allowing the comparison of the relative cost-effectiveness of PHIs, compared with medical interventions, we acknowledge that QALYs cannot capture the wider benefits of wider public health interventions, and so methods such as SPDCEs to generate WTP values for use in CBAs may well be more appropriate in providing evidence of cost and outcomes spanning many sectors of the economy (NICE 2012; Edwards et al., 2013)

With the inclusion of a cost attribute (i.e. a payment vehicle) within an SPDCE, it is possible for these trade-offs between attributes and overall preferences for attributes to be converted into monetary units, generating WTP values, and thereby allowing for the outcome to be included in CBA and comparisons outwith one intervention area and across sectors, making this ideally suited to the public health arena with its multi-sectoral impacts. Ideally, outcomes should be valued using a generic outcome

Box 9.4 Five stages of an SPDCE

1   Identifying appropriate attributes

2   Define and assign attribute levels

3   Generate experimental design

4   Administer questionnaire (collect data)

5   Analyse data

measure which enables interventions that may have very different impacts to be compared against a common measure (McIntosh et al., 2012). The design and conduct of a SPDCE typically has five stages; see Box 9.4.

The following two novel case studies of benefit valuation for economic evaluation purposes within PHIs are empirical examples of conducting SPDCEs in population health settings.

9.5 Case study 1: Creating green spaces as a public health intervention

9.5.1 Woods In and Around Towns (WIAT)

The Woods In and Around Towns (WIAT) project in Scotland is used in this chapter as a case study to illustrate the use of SPDCE methods to value the outcomes of a PHI for use in a CBA framework. The WIAT project aims to regenerate, improve, and promote woodlands to render them safe and to increase individuals' contact with nature, potentially lowering stress levels and in turn improving the mental well-being of society (Silveirinha de Oliveira et al., 2013). The outcomes of the WIAT project are grouped into three main categories: (i) the non-health outcomes which include enhanced environment; increased woodland visits through improved behaviours and perception towards woodlands; and increased social support for environmental use; (ii) the health outcome of lowered stress levels; and (iii) the distal health outcome behaviours such as increased physical activity levels and social cohesion which could result in restoration and in turn improve mental well-being (Silveirinha de Oliveira et al., 2013). Given that these outcomes are broad, consisting of health and non-health items, the WIAT project could be considered a complex public health intervention (Craig et al., 2006). To deal with these many outcomes, a multiple economic analysis method was applied with a CUA approach adopted to value all health-related outcomes in terms of QALYs (Ward Thompson et al., 2018), alongside a CBA framework (including elicitation of WTP values of the woodland attributes from society to capture and value the broader non-health benefits in monetary unit). A cost–consequences analysis (CCA) approach was also used to present the varied results of the costs and outcomes in a balance sheet-like format (Botha, 2017). The emphasis in this case study is on the valuation of the non-health outcomes using a SPDCE approach.

9.5.2 Methods

Attributes and levels of the SPDCE were identified through a qualitative process that included literature review on predictors of woodland use; discussions with experts in landscaping, health, and environment; and pilot surveys. Five attributes each with three levels were identified as presented in Table 9.1. Respondents from the Scottish population aged 16 and older (n = 510) who were panel members of a market research company, ResearchNow were presented with 18 pairs (choice sets) of hypothetical woodlands scenarios generated from a fractional experimental design in NGene software (version 1.1.2) (Choicemetrics, 2014). The scenarios in a choice set differed systematically in their attribute levels as shown in Table 9.2, and respondents were

Table 9.1 Identified attributes and levels

Attributes	Levels
1. The woodland environmental support defined as one which allows you to do the things you want to do, either on your own or with others (such as exercise, relaxing, enjoying wildlife), and makes it easy and enjoyable to do them	No support; Some support; A lot of support
2. The time that it takes to walk from home to the woodland	◆ 5 minutes ◆ 15 minutes ◆ 50 minutes
3. The quality of the woodland environment which include cleanliness; the condition of paths and entrances; the naturalness of its appearance; the views of plants and wildlife	◆ Poor quality ◆ Average quality ◆ Good quality
4. The opportunities for social activities that the woodland offers such as meeting people, community events, guidance on how to use the woodland and about what is going on there	◆ No opportunities ◆ Some opportunities ◆ Many opportunities
5. The cost for access to the woodlands, if you imagine you lived in a country where you had to pay, in the form of an annual subscription, to go there	◆ £0 ◆ £15 ◆ £50

asked to make repeated choices between two options (woodland A and B), or to select a third, 'None of these' option. The extent to which respondents were prepared to trade off one set of attributes or levels against one another was assessed. The assumption was that respondents would choose the woodland option with attributes or levels that provided them with the overall greatest satisfaction (Hensher et al., 2015). Data were analysed in Stata (StataCorp, 2013) using a random parameter logit (RPL) model (Hauber et al., 2016).

Table 9.2 A choice set example

Characteristics	Woodland A	Woodland B
1. The **woodland environmental support** that allows you to undertake enjoyable activities easily	**Some** support	**A lot** of support
2. The **time** that it takes to walk from home to the woodland	**50**mins	**15**mins
3. The **quality of the woodland environment**	**Poor** quality	**Good** quality
4. The **opportunities for social activities**	**Some** opportunities	**Many** opportunities
5. The **cost for access** to the woodland	£50	£50

Which woodland would you prefer?   Woodland A ☐   Woodland B ☐   None of these

The inclusion of a hypothetical cost for access to the woodlands allowed the calculation of the marginal WTP for various improvements of the attributes and their associated levels through marginal rate of substitution (MRS) (Ryan et al., 2012). The inclusion of a 'time' attribute also permitted the estimation of value in terms of the amount of time in minutes that an individual was willing to 'give up' to access a woodland with a preferred attribute or level.

9.5.3 **Results**

The SPDCE results are presented in Table 9.3. A full description of this case study can be found in Botha, 2017.

Coefficients of the RPL model reveal the relative importance weights for the preferred woodland attributes and levels. All coefficients were statistically significant (p < 0.001), which implies that all the identified attributes and levels were associated with (i.e. predictors of) individuals' choices of hypothetical woodlands presented to them. The signs of the coefficients were in line with *a priori* expectations of a monotonic relationship; for example, a unit increase in walking time from home to woodlands and in cost for accessing woodlands were negatively associated with choosing a woodland.

The attribute related to quality of the woodland environment was most influential in woodland choice decisions. Respondents were 3.5 times more likely to choose a woodland with good environmental quality (odds ratio (OR) 3.50, 95% CI: 3.21–3.82) and 2.8 times more likely to choose a woodland with an average environmental quality (OR 2.83, 95% CI: 2.60–3.08) compared to a woodland with poor quality environment. This was followed by the attribute pertaining to environmental support for individual or group activities. In this case, individual were 2.8 times more likely to choose a woodland with a lot of environmental support (OR 2.80, 95% CI: 2.58–3.05); and 2.3 times for that woodland with some environmental support (OR 2.32, 95% CI: 2.14–2.53) compared to a woodland with none of the environmental support. The third preferred attribute related to the opportunities that a woodland offered for social activities. Individuals were 1.5 times more likely to choose a woodland that offered many opportunities for social activities (OR 1.53, 95% CI 1.41–1.66), and 1.4 times more likely to choose a woodland which offered some opportunities for social activities (OR 1.36, 95% CI: 1.24–1.48), compared to a woodland that had none. A unit increase in cost for accessing a woodland and in walking time from home to the woods had negative association with the woodland choice decision. Thus, OR 0.96, 95% CI: 0.96–0.97 for the cost for accessing woodlands as a yearly subscription representing a 4 per cent decrease in choosing a woodland for any unit (one British pound) increase. The same trend was shown for a minute increase in time to walk from home to the woodlands (OR 0.98, 95% CI: 0.97–0.98) which represents a 2 per cent reduction of woodland choice decisions.

Table 9.4 presents the results for WTP (in British pounds) and willingness to walk (in minutes) to access a woodland with improvements in a given attribute-level calculated as the ratio of the attribute of interest divided by the negative of the coefficient on the cost attribute and the time attribute respectively:

Table 9.3 Random parameter logit (RPL) model results

Attributes	Coefficients	Standard Errors	95% CIs	Odds ratios	Standard Errors	95%CIs	P values
The supportive woodland environment that allows you on your own or in a group to do enjoyable activities easily (Base level: No support)	-	-	-	-	-	-	-
◆ Some support	0.84	0.043	0.76–0.93	2.32	0.10	2.14–2.53	<0.001
◆ A lot of support	1.03	0.043	0.95–1.12	2.80	0.12	2.58–3.05	<0.001
The time it takes to walk from home to the woodland	−0.02	0.001	−0.03–0.02	0.98	0.00	0.97–0.98	< 0.001
The quality of the woodland environment (Base level: Poor quality)	-	-	-	-	-	-	-
◆ Average quality	1.04	0.044	0.95–1.13	2.83	0.12	2.60–3.08	< 0.001
◆ Good quality	1.25	0.044	1.17–1.34	3.50	0.15	3.21–3.82	< 0.001
The opportunities for social activities (Base level: No opportunities)	-	-	-	-	-	-	-
◆ Some opportunities	0.31	0.045	0.22–0.39	1.36	0.06	1.24–1.48	< 0.001
◆ Many opportunities	0.43	0.042	0.35–0.51	1.53	0.06	1.41–1.66	< 0.001
The cost for access to the woodland	−0.04	0.001	−0.038–0.35	0.96	0.00	0.96–0.97	< 0.001

Individuals are willing to pay, as an annual subscription, for improvements in the quality of the woodland environment: £34.45, 95% CI: £31.53–£37.57 for the change from poor environmental quality to good environmental quality, and £28.58, 95% CI: £25.83–£31.50 from poor environmental quality to an average environmental quality. The WTP for the attribute related to woodland environmental support was £28.32, 95% CI: £25.63–£31.19 for changes from a woodland with no environmental support to a lot of environmental support, and £23.18 95% CI: £20.61–£25.88 from no environmental support to some environmental support. With respect to WTP for the attribute related to opportunities that a woodland offers for social activities, individuals were willing to pay £11.76, 95% CI: £9.43–£14.14 for improvements from a woodland that offers no opportunities for social activities to that with many social opportunities; and £8.39, 95% CI: £5.94–£10.89 for a change from no social opportunities to some social opportunities. Individuals were not willing to pay anything for a unit increase in walking time (minutes) from home to access woodlands with given attributes or levels.

In terms of individuals' willingness to walk/give up time (in minutes) from home to a woodland with improvements in a given attribute, it was found that on average individuals were willing to give up 53 minutes (95% CI: 48–60 minutes) to walk from home to access a woodland with good environmental quality; and 44 minutes (95% CI: 39–50 minutes) for a woodland with an average environmental quality, compared to woodlands with poor environmental quality. Individuals were willing to give up 44 minutes in walking time (95% CI: 39–49 minutes) from home to access a woodland that offers a lot of environmental support; and 36 minutes (95% CI: 31–40 minutes) for a woodland that provides some environmental support, compared to woodlands that did not have any environmental support. It was also shown that individuals were willing to forgo 18 minutes of walking time (95% CI: 14–22 minutes) to get to a woodland with many social opportunities; and 13 minutes (95% CI: 9–17 minutes) to a woodland that provides some social opportunities, compared to woodlands without any social opportunities. Individuals were not willing to give up their time to walk to a woodland that needed paying for access.

9.5.4 **Conclusion**

The quantitative information from the SPDCE results provides insights to policy-makers such that specific areas of woodland (green space) improvements aimed at improving population health and reducing inequalities can be identified and prioritized to increase access to woodlands for the well-being of the society. The marginal WTP and total WTP values for the most preferred woodland attributes or levels could represent benefits in terms of welfare improvements and inform an economic evaluation through a CBA framework (Van Der Pol et al., 2010; Tockhorn-Heidenreich et al., 2017). For example, the marginal WTP for a preferred woodland attribute or level could be compared with the cost of its delivery or implementation and it would be possible to assess whether offering this attribute or level as part of an intervention provides a positive net benefit. Similarly, it would also be possible to aggregate the marginal WTP estimates for the configuration of the most preferred woodland attributes or levels and make comparison with the total cost of their delivery or implementation (Carlsson, 2011). The compensating

Table 9.4 WTP and willingness to walk (in minutes) to access a woodland with preferred attributes

Attributes	Coefficients	WTP (as an annual Subscription) $\left(\dfrac{\text{battribute}}{-\beta\text{cost}}\right)$	95% CIs	Willingness to walk from home to woodlands (in minutes) $\left(\dfrac{\text{battribute}}{-\beta\text{time}}\right)$	95% CIs
The supportive woodland environment that allows you to do enjoyable activities easily (Base level: No support)	-	-	-	-	-
◆ Some support	0.844	£ 23.18	£20.61–£25.88	36 minutes	31–40 minutes
◆ A lot of support	1.031	£ 28.32	£25.63–£31.19	44 minutes	39–49 minutes
The time it takes to walk from home to the woodland	–0.024	–£0.65	–£0.58–£0.71		
The quality of the woodland environment (Base level: Poor quality)	-	-	-	-	-
◆ Average quality	1.040	£ 28.58	£25.83–£31.50	44 minutes	39–50 minutes
◆ Good quality	1.254	£ 34.45	£31.53–£37.57	53 minutes	48-60 minutes
The opportunities for social activities (Base level: No opportunities)	-	-	-	-	-
◆ Some opportunities	0.305	£ 8.39	£5.94–£10.89	13 minutes	9–17 minutes
◆ Many opportunities	0.428	£ 11.76	£9.43–£14.14	18 minutes	14–22 minutes
The cost for access to the woodland	–0.036	-	-	-	-

variation approach is argued to be appropriate in deriving the total WTP estimates from SPDCEs through the log-sum formula which accounts for the probability of making a choice (Lancsar and Savage, 2004; Karlström, 2014). In health care, individuals often have one option of intervention or treatment to consume with certainty, hence the probability of making a choice is 1 (Ryan, 2004). This also holds when the SPDCE options are generic (Carlsson, 2011). These assumptions reduce the compensating variation approach to the sum of marginal WTP for the attributes or levels (Ryan, 2004; Carlsson, 2011).

9.6 Case study 2: Valuing the attributes of community empowerment in an urban regeneration context

In this next case study, a second novel SPDCE is presented which values attributes of community empowerment in an urban regeneration context. Given the broad-scale emphasis on community participation, this SPDCE focuses on the extraction of values in terms of willingness to give up time rather than money with a view to transforming these time values into monetary values for use in a CBA framework. UK-wide regeneration programmes, as a form of PHI, have sought to ameliorate resident living conditions, their health, and wider social inequalities (Williams et al., 2008; MacGregor, 2010; McCartney et al., 2017). Community empowerment, a community's ability to make choices and influence local decision-making, has become a key component of such programmes with policies striving to incorporate communities to promote a sense of involvement, control, and autonomy over events within their neighbourhood, affecting their lives; an example of a health assets-approach in public health as discussed in Chapter 1. Underpinning resource allocation to community empowerment-promoting activities is evidence suggesting that more empowered individuals report better mental well-being (Baba et al., 2016). It is theorized that incorporating community empowerment-fostering activities in urban regeneration programmes could serve as an alternative, cost-effective pathway to health gains, acting as an intermediate surrogate indicator of health (Baba et al., 2016). However, justification for the allocation of resources to community empowerment-fostering activities requires examination of the value of the outcomes associated with community empowerment activities. There is a clear need for community empowerment-promoting activities and actions to meet communities expectations and requirements, yet due to the challenging and context specific nature of urban regeneration programmes, there exists no single way to promote community empowerment. In addition, previous economic evaluations of regeneration have not captured the 'value' of community empowerment yet acknowledge the need to identify suitable methodology to do so (Tyler et al., 2010; Popay et al., 2015). Thus, adapting methodology previously used to value environmental improvements targeted through regeneration activity, a SPDCE was conducted. The aim of this SPDCE was to provide valuations of community empowerment attributes, when delivered as part of an urban regeneration programme.

9.6.1 Methods

Prior to this SPDCE, the authors first explored the hypothesis that empowerment can produce health gains in an urban regeneration context (Baba et al., 2016). The study confirmed that those householders experiencing urban regeneration in Glasgow, UK who reported a stronger sense of empowerment also had better general health and mental well-being. Therefore, concluding that investment in empowerment could lead to long-term health benefits, a systematic review with narrative synthesis was conducted to identify key components of community empowerment within an urban regeneration context (Baba, 2016). The attributes identified in this review were further validated through consultation with Greater Glasgow and Clyde Community Engagement Managers and the West and Central Voluntary Sector Network (WCVSN). These bodies are actively involved in engaging with communities throughout Glasgow. The objective of this piloting and validation was to ensure that attributes were easily comprehensible for respondents and that the levels represented a realistic range of values. The attributes and their associated levels are described in Table 9.5.

Expert guidance and existing literature highlighted that residents' time commitment' was an appropriate 'payment vehicle' as residents are seldom expected to pay for community empowerment activities. NGene software was used to create a D-efficient fractional factorial design of 18 choice-sets (Choicemetrics, 2014). A consistency and reliability check were added to test the validity of the responses. An example choice-set is shown in Table 9.6. Additionally, socio-demographic characteristics of respondents were collected.

9.6.2 Results

A UK-representative (by age and gender) sample of 302 participants was recruited by ResearchNow in May 2015. Using a mixed logit (MXL) model to account for preference heterogeneity, all attributes were considered random except the payment vehicle of residents' time commitment', which was fixed. For those attribute levels which were statistically significant ($p \leq 0.05$), it was possible to convert model output to determine respondents' willingness to give up time for community empowerment attributes, allowing the authors to produce clear guidance outlining UK population preferences. This is show in Table 9.7.

Table 9.5 illustrates that respondents were willing to give up the greatest amount of time, 19.48 hours per month, for scenarios in which they felt they know some of their neighbours and feel like a valued member in the community, and funding was the least appealing attribute (relative to the other community empowerment attributes). When broken down into weekly commitments, excluding resources/funding, it is possible to observe that overall difference in time commitment across the remaining attributes is only just over two hours (124 minutes). The results outlined the marginal increase in the preference/value exhibited by respondents between the 'worst' level and 'best' level of the community empowerment inclusion and trust in stakeholders' attributes. These results highlight that respondents place a relatively lower value for the marginal utility gain from extra resource allocation to provide the 'better' level as compared to the higher relative values for marginal gains at the low/mid level . Thus, decision-makers must consider whether the additional investment to achieve these higher levels is worthwhile. These marginal time values could be readily converted into monetary values using standard values for time such as leisure of employment (wages), and these results placed into a CBA framework.

Table 9.5 Attributes used to describe community empowerment in urban regeneration programmes

Community Empowerment features	Levels
Inclusion The extent to which you are included in community decision making processes (e.g. through local meetings, regular email/telephone contact).	◆ You never have the opportunity participate
	◆ You have the opportunity to participate sometimes
	◆ You have the opportunity to participate regularly
Trust in stakeholders The extent to which community decision making processes are explained and transparent and whether your views are included in local decisions.	◆ Decision-making processes are not explained and no consideration of your views is evident
	◆ Some decision-making is explained and some consideration of your views is evident
	◆ Decision-making processes are fully explained; you can see consideration of your views in local decisions
Sense of belonging How well you know your neighbours and how valued you feel as a member of the local community.	◆ You do not know your neighbours and do not feel a valued member of the community
	◆ You know some of your neighbours and feel a valued member in the community
	◆ You know all your neighbours well and feel a valued member of the community
Residents time commitment Amount of your own time you have to give up to ensure your views are heard.	◆ 0 hours every month
	◆ 4 hours every month
	◆ 16 hours every month
Resources/funding The level of stakeholder provided opportunities and resources for communities to develop skills/expertise and gain new community assets.	◆ None—there is no help or support of any kind
	◆ Some—limited help and support is available
	◆ Yes—help and support is available
Information/knowledge Your level of knowledge of issues and developments in the urban regeneration programme.	◆ You are not informed about the regeneration programme
	◆ You are somewhat informed about the regeneration programme
	◆ You are fully informed about the regeneration programme

The results from this second case study on valuing the attributes of community empowerment are also highly relevant to research on public health 'assets'. Historically, approaches to the promotion of population health have been based on a 'deficit' model; that is, they tend to focus on identifying the problems and needs of populations that

Table 9.6 An example choice-set from the community empowerment SPDCE

Scenario 1	Option A	Option B
Inclusion Your inclusion in the decision-making process	You have the opportunity to participate **regularly**	You **never** have the opportunity participate
Trust in stakeholders You can see your input being carried out in decision-making	**Some** decision-making is **explained** and **some consideration** of your views is evident	**Some** decision-making is **explained** and **some consideration** of your views is evident
Sense of belonging Your interaction with neighbours and feeling valued in the community	You **do not know your neighbours** and **do not feel a valued member** of the community	You know **all your neighbours well** and **feel a valued member** of the community
Residents' time commitment Time sacrificed to ensure your views are heard	**4hrs** /month	**4hrs**/month
Resources Stakeholders provision of opportunities and resources for communities	**None**—there is no help or support of any kind	**Yes**—help and support is available
Information/ knowledge Your knowledge of issues in the urban regeneration programme	**You are fully informed** about the regeneration programme	**You are not informed** about the regeneration programme
Which would you prefer?	☐	☐
Neither ☐		

require professional resources and high levels of dependence on hospital and welfare services (Morgan and Ziglio, 2007). In contrast, 'assets' models tend to accentuate positive capability to identify problems and activate solutions, focusing on promoting salutogenic resources; that is, focusing on factors that support human health and well-being rather than on factors that cause disease. These salutogenic factors are those that promote the self-esteem and coping abilities of individuals and communities, eventually leading to less dependency on professional services. An assets approach to health and development embraces a 'salutogenic' notion of health creation and in doing so encourages the full participation of local communities in the health development process. There is very little economic evaluation evidence for assets-based approaches other than a review conducted by Glasgow University (Lawson and McIntosh, 2013). The report concluded that overall, asset-based working is an increasingly used term in policy circles, partly as a response to the perceived limitations of existing services to address the persistence of inequalities in health and well-being. The good intentions of those advocating asset-based approaches are unequivocal, however there is an urgent need to test whether asset-based approaches represent value for money in terms of

Table 9.7 Willingness to give up time for community empowerment attributes

Attribute	Willingness to give up time/hrs	hrs/month	hrs/week
Inclusion	You have the opportunity to participate sometimes	12:36	3:09
	You have the opportunity to participate regularly	12:00	3:0
Trust in stakeholders	Decision-making processes are fully explained; you can see consideration of your views in local decisions	13:18	3:18
Sense of belonging	You know some of your neighbours and feel a valued member in the community	19.48	4.52
	You know all your neighbours well and feel a valued member of the community	13:24	3:21
Resources/ funding	Yes—help and support is available	6:24	1:36
Information/ knowledge	You are somewhat informed about the regeneration programme	11:12	2:48
	You are fully informed about the regeneration programme	15:36	3:54

leading to improvements in health and well-being as well as reducing health inequalities. In particular, it is imperative that economic evaluation is undertaken more routinely for both (so-called) deficit- and asset-based approaches in order to inform how scarce public resources can best be allocated.

9.6.3 Social cost–benefit analysis

Recently there has been interest in the method of social CBA. This approach essentially differs from main stream CBA approaches simply in the way in which it values and incorporates outcomes. Social CBA uses a life satisfaction approach to incorporate outcomes, as opposed to the stated and revealed preference approaches alluded to in this chapter and in Chapter 6. This life satisfaction approach estimates the value of non-market goods by looking at how they impact on people's reported well-being (life satisfaction). This new non-preference approach has been gaining popularity over the past decade (Dolan et al., 2008; Powdthavee, 2008; Greco et al., 2016). From April 2011, the UK's ONS will include four questions on subjective well-being in the Integrated Household Survey (IHS). The IHS is a composite household survey combining the answers from a number of ONS household surveys to produce a dataset of core variables. The well-being module will include a question on overall life satisfaction rated on an 11-point scale (0–10). With approximately 200,000 people interviewed each year, this will be the largest regular survey on well-being in the United Kingdom, and it provides an opportunity for analysts to use the life satisfaction method on a much larger dataset. Whilst the use of subjective well-being measurement, and its associated use in the CBA framework, is an emerging research issue, a number of valuations so far generated by the life satisfaction approach appear to be implausibly high so caution is needed when using this approach (Fujiwara and Campbell, 2011).

Summary of Chapter 9

This chapter:

◆ Introduced the reader to the basic welfare economic theories which provide the foundations for CBA.

◆ Argued the case for the suitability of the CBA framework for the economic evaluation of PHI interventions.

◆ Described the theoretical appropriateness and practical challenges with estimation of WTP for use in CBA for public health economic evaluation.

◆ Highlighted the potential role for SPDCE methods to generate outcomes for use in public health CBA using two novel case studies.

◆ Outlined the emergence of the social CBA method (as an alternative to CBA) and its use of subjective well-being outcomes.

References

Arrow, K., Solow, R., Portney, P., Leamer, E., Radner, R., and Schuman, H., 1993. Report of the NOAA Panel on Contingent Valuation. *Federal Register*, January 15, *58*(10): 4601–14.

Baba, C., Kearns, A., Mcintosh, E., Tannahill, C., and Lewsey, J., 2016. Is empowerment a route to improving mental health and wellbeing in an urban regeneration (UR) context? *Urban Studies*, *54*: 1619–37.

Baba, C.R.B., 2016. *Valuing the health and wellbeing aspects of community empowerment in an urban regeneration context using economic evalaution techniques.* PhD, University of Glasgow.

Banke-Thomas, A.O., Madaj, B., Charles, A., and Van Den Broek, N., 2015. Social Return on Investment (SROI) methodology to account for value for money of public health interventions: a systematic review. *BMC Public Health*, *15*: 582.

Bateman, I.J., Carson, R.T., Day, B., Hanemann, M., Hanleys, N., Hett, T., Jones-Lee, M., et al., 2002. *Economic Valuation with Stated Preference: A Manual*, Cheltenham, Edward Elgar.

Bishop, R. and Heberlein, T., 1979. Measuring values of extra-market goods: Are indirect measures biased? *American Journal of Agricultural Economics*, *61*: 926–30.

Boadway, R.W. and Bruce, N., 1984. *Welfare Economics*. Oxford: Oxford University Press.

Borghi, J., 2008. Aggregation rules for cost–benefit analysis: A health economics perspective. *Health Economics*, *17*: 863–75.

Botha, W.C., 2017. *A broader economic evaluative space for public health interventions: an integrated approach.* PhD, University of Glasgow

Brent, R.J., 2003. *Cost–Benefit Analysis and Health Care Evaluations.* Cheltenham: Edward Elgar.

Brouwer, W., Rutten, F., and Koopmanschap, M.A., 2001. Costing in economic evaluations. In: M.F. Drummond and A. Mcguire (eds), *Economic Evalauation in Health Care: Merging Theory with Practice.* Oxford: Oxford University Press, pp. 68–93.

Carlsson, F., 2011. *Non-Market Valuation: Stated Preference Methods.* Oxford: Oxford University Press.

Clarke, E., 1971, Multipart pricing of public goods, *Public Choice*, *11*(1):17–33.

Craig, P., Dieppe, P., Macintyre, S., Michie, S., Narzqareth, I., and Petticrew, M., 2008. Developing and evaluating complex interventions: New Medical Research Council Guidance. *British Medical Journal*, *337*: a1655. doi:10.1136/bmj.a1655.

Choicemetrics, 2014. NGene 1.1.2: User manual and reference guide. Choice Metrics Pty Ltd. Available at: <http://www.choice-metrics.com> (Accessed 30 October 2018).

Dasgupta, A., K and Pearce, D.W., 1978. *Cost–Benefit Analysis: Theory and Practice,* Basingstoke: Macmillan.

De Ayala, A., Hoyos Ramos, D., and Mariel Chladkova, P., 2012. Landscape valuation through discrete choice experiments: Current practice and future research reflections. Biltoki: Universidad del País Vasco, Departamento de Economía Aplicada III (Econometría y Estadística).

de Bekker-Grob, E.W., Ryan, M., and Gerard, K., 2012, Discrete choice experiments in health economics: A review of the literature. *Health Econ.*, *21*: 145–72. doi:10.1002/hec.1697.

Devlin, N. and Sussex, J., 2011. *Incorporating Multiple Criteria in HTA: Methods and Processes.* London: Office of Health Economics.

Diamond, P.A. and Hausman, J.A., 1994. Contingent valuation: Is some number better than no number? *Journal of Economic Perspectives*, *8*: 45–64.

Diener, A., O'Brien, B., and Gafni, A., 1998. Health care contingent valuation studies: A review and classification of the literature. *Health Economics*, *7*: 313–26.

Dolan, P., Layard, R., and Metcalfe, R., 2011. *Measuring Subjective Well-being for Public Policy.* London: Office for National Statistics.

Dolan, P., Peasgood, T., and White, M., 2008. Do we really know what makes us happy? A review of the economic literature on the factors associated with subjective well-being. *Journal of Economic Psychology*, *29*:94–122.

Donaldson, C. and Shackley, P., 1997. Does 'process utility' exist? A case study of willingness to pay for laparoscopic cholecystectomy. *Social Science and Medicine*, *44*: 699–707.

Drummond, M.F., Sculpher, M.J., Torrance, G.W., O'Brien, B. and Stoddart, G.L., 2015. *Methods for the Economic Evaluation of Health Care Programmes.* Oxford: Oxford University Press.

Edwards, R.T., Charles, J.M., and Lloyd-Williams, H., 2013. Public health economics: A systematic review of guidance for the economic evaluation of public health interventions and discussion of key methodological issues. *BMC Public Health*, *13*: 1001.

Environmental Protection Agency, 2009. Valuing Environmental Goods: A State of the Arts Assessment of the Contingent Variation Method, vol. 1. Available at: <https://yosemite. epa.gov/ee/epa/eerm.nsf/oeT/391685728EBDDC0A8525657C004B272A> (Accessed 30 October 2018).

Freeman, A.M., 1993. *The Measurement of Environmental and Resource Values: Theory and Methods,* Washington, DC: Resources for the Future.

Frew, E., 2010. Chapter 7. In: A. Gray and A. Briggs (eds), *Applied Methods of Cost Benefit Analysis in Health Care.* Oxford: Oxford University Press, pp. 119–38.

Fujiwara, D. and Campbell, R., 2011. *Valuation Techniques for Social Cost–Benefit Analysis: Stated Preference, Revealed Preference and Subjective Well-Being Approaches: A Discussion of the Current Issues.* London: HM Treasury.

Fujiwara, D., 2015. The Seven Principle Problems of SROI. SIMETRICA. <http://www. simetrica.co.uk> (Accessed 15 October 2018).

Greco, G., **Lorgelly, P.**, and **Yamabhai, I.**, 2016. Outcomes in economic evaluations of public health interventions in low- and middle-income countries: Health, capabilities and subjective wellbeing. *Health Economics, 25*: 83–94.

Griliches, Z., 1971. *Price Indexes and Quality Change.* Cambridge, MA: Harvard University Press.

Groves, T., 1970. *The allocation of resources under uncertainty: The informal and incentive roles of prices and demands in a team.* PhD, University of California, Berkeley, CA.

Hall, J., **Viney, R.**, **Haas, M.**, and **Louviere, J.**, 2002. Using stated preference discrete choice modelling to evaluate health care programs. *Journal of Business Research, 5760*: 1–7.

Hanley, N., **Ryan., M.**, and **Wright R.**, 2003. Estimating the monetary value of health care: lessons from environmental economics. *Health Economics, 12*: 3–16.

Hauber, A.B., **González, J.M.**, **Groothuis-Oudshoorn, C.G.**, **Prior, T.**, **Marshall, D.A.**, **Cunningham, C.**, **Ijzerman, M.J.**, et al., 2016. Statistical methods for the analysis of discrete choice experiments: A Report of the ISPOR Conjoint Analysis Good Research Practices Task Force. *Value in Health, 19*(4) 300–15.

Hensher, D., **Rose, J.**, and **Greene, W.**, 2015. *Applied Choice Analysis.* Cambridge: Cambridge University Press.

Hicks, J.R., 1939. *Value and Capital,* London: Oxford University Press.

Hotelling, H., 1947. *The Economics of Public Recreation. The Prewitt Report.* Washington, DC: National Parks Service.

Kahneman, D. and **Knetsch, J.L.**, 1992. Valuing public goods: The purchase of moral satisfaction. *Journal of Environmental Economics and Management, 22*: 57–70.

Kaldor, N., 1939. Welfare propositions of economics and interpersonal comparisons of utility. *Economic Journal, XLIX*: 549–52.

Karlström, A., 2014. Appraisal. In: S. Hess and A. Daly (eds), *Handbook of Choice Modelling.* London: Edward Elgar Publishing.

Kelly, M.P., **McDaid, D.**, **Ludbrook, A.**, and **Powell, J.**, 2005. *Economic Appraisal of Public Health Interventions.* London: NHS Health Development Agency.

Klose, T., 1999. The contingent valuation method in health care. *Health Policy, 47*: 97–123.

Lancsar, E. and **Savage, E.**, 2004. Deriving welfare measures from discrete choice experiments: Inconsistency between current methods and random utility and welfare theory. *Health Economics, 13*: 901–7.

Lawson, K. and **McIntosh, E.**, 2013. *A Review of the Economic Evidence for Asset-Based Approaches for Health Improvement: Findings and Recommendations.* Glasgow: Glasgow Centre for Population Health.

Layard, P. and **Walters, A.**, 1978. *Microeconomic Theory.* Singapore: McGraw-Hill.

Layard, R. and **Glaister, S.**, 1994. *Cost–Benefit Analysis.* Cambridge: Cambridge University Press.

Lowin, A., **Hall, J.**, **Viney, R.**, **Louviere, J.**, **Kenny, P.**, and **King, M.**, 1999. Discrete choice modelling: How to introduce varicella vaccination into Australia. In: J.C. Baldry (ed.), *Economics and Health 1999, Australian Studies in Health Service Administration.* Sydney: School of Health Sciences Management: University of New South Wales.

Macgregor, C., 2010. Urban regeneration as a public health intervention. *Journal of Social Intervention: Theory and Practice, 19*: 38–51.

Masters, R., **Anwar, E.**, **Collins, B.**, **Cookson, R.**, and **Capewell, S.**, 2017. Return on investment of public health interventions: A systematic review. *Journal of Epidemiology and Community Health, 71*: 827–34.

Mathes, T., Antoine, S.-L., Prengel, P., Bühn, S., Polus, S., and Pieper, D., 2017. Health technology assessment of public health interventions: A synthesis of methodological guidance. *International Journal of Technology Assessment in Health Care, 33*(2): 135–46.

McCartney, G., Hearty, W., Taulbut, M., Mitchell, R., Dryden, R., and Collins, C., 2017. Regeneration and health: A structured, rapid literature review. *Public Health, 148*: 69–87.

McIntosh, E., Clarke, P., Frew, E., and Louviere, J.J., 2010. *Applied Methods of Cost Benefit Analysis in Health Care.* Oxford: Oxford University Press.

McIntosh, E., Lawson, K., Donaldson, C., White, M., Kee, F., Deverill, M., and Bond, L., 2012. Report on a workshop on methods for the economic evaluation of population health interventions: conceptual and practical challenges. Available at: <https://www.gla.ac.uk/media/media_257001_en.pdf> (Accessed 30 October 2018).

Mishan, E.J., 1971. *Cost–Benefit Analysis.* New York, NY: Praeger.

Mishan, E.J., 1981. *Introduction to Normative Economics.* Oxford: Oxford University Press.

Mitchell, R. and Carson, R.T., 1989. *Using Surveys to Value Public Goods.* Washington, DC: Resources for the Future.

Morgan, A. and Ziglio, E., 2007. Revitalising the evidence base for public health: an assets model. *Promotion & Education, 14*: 17–22.

National Institute for Health and Care Excellence, N.I.F.H.A.C.E., 2012. *Methods for the Development of NICE Public Health Guidance: Incorporating Health Economics.* Available at: <https://www.nice.org.uk/process/pmg4/chapter/incorporating-health-economics> (Accessed 30 October 2018).

Popay, J., Whitehead, M., Carr-Hill, R., Dibben, C., Dixon, P., Halliday, E., Nazroo, J., et al. 2015. The impact on health inequalities of approaches to community engagement in the New Deal for Communities regeneration initiative: a mixed-methods evaluation. *Public Health Research, 3*(12).

Powdthavee, N., 2008. Putting a price tag on friends, relatives, and neighbours: Using surveys of life satisfaction to value social relationships. *Journal of Socio-Economics, 37*: 1459–80.

Randall, A. and Kriesel, W., 1990. Evaluating national policy proposals by contingent valuation. In: R.L. Johnson and G.V. Johnson (eds), *Economic valuation of natural resources: Issues, theory and applications.* Boulder, CO: Westview Press, pp. 153–76.

Reed Johnson, F. and Adamowicz, W.L., 2011. Valuation and cost–benefit analysis in health and environmental economics. In: E. McIntosh, P.M, Clarke, E.J. Frew, and J.J. Louviere (eds), *Applied Methods of Cost–Benefit Analysis in Health Care* (2nd edn). Oxford: Oxford University Press, pp. 79–96.

Cummings, R.C., Brookshire, D.S., Coursey, D.L., and Schulzem W.D., 1986. *Valuing Environmental Goods: A State of the Arts Assessment of the Contingent Method.* Totowa, NJ: Rowman and Allanheld.

Rosen, S., 1974. Hedonic prices and implicit markets: product differentiation in pure competition. *Journal of Political Economy, 82*: 34–55.

Ryan, M., 2004. Discrete choice experiments in health care. *British Medical Journal, 328*: 360–1.

Ryan, M., 2004. Deriving welfare measures in discrete choice experiments: A comment to Lancsar and Savage (1). *Health Economics, 13*: 909–12.

Ryan, M. and Gerard, K., 2003. Using discrete choice experiments in health economics: Current practice and future prospects. *Applied Health Economics and Policy Analysis, 2*: 55–64.

Ryan, M. and Shackley, P., 1995. Assessing the benefits of health care: How far should we go? *Qualitative Health Care, 4*: 207–13.

Ryan, M., Ratcliffe, J., and Tucker, J., 1997. Using willingness to pay to value alternative models of antenatal care. *Social Science & Medicine, 44*:371–80.

Ryan, M., Scott, D.A., and Donaldson, C., 2004. Valuing health care using willingness to pay: A comparison of the payment card and dichotomous choice methods. *Journal of Health Economics, 23*(2): 237–58.

Ryan, M., Skåtun, D., and Major, K., 2008. Using discrete choice experiments to go beyond clinical outcomes when evaluating clinical practice. In: M. Ryan, K. Gerard, and M. Amaya-Amaya (eds), *Using Discrete Choice Experiments to Value Health and Health Care*. Dordrecht: Springer, pp. 101–17.

Ryan, M., Kolstad, J., Rockers, P., and Dolea, C., 2012. How to conduct a discrete choice experiment for health workforce recruitment and retention in remote and rural areas: A user guide with case studies. *CapacityPlus. World Bank and World Health Organization.* Washington, DC: World Bank.

Silveirinha de Oliveira, E., Aspinall, P., Briggs, A., Cummins, S., Leyland, A. H., Mitchell, R., Roe, J., et al., 2013. How effective is the Forestry Commission Scotland's woodland improvement programme—'Woods In and Around Towns' (WIAT)—at improving psychological well-being in deprived urban communities? A quasi-experimental study. *British Medical Journal Open, 3*: e003648. doi:10.1136/bmjopen-2013-003648.

Smith, R.D., 2000. The discrete willingness-to-pay question format in health economics: Should we adopt environmental guidelines. *Medical Decision Making, 20*(2): 194–206.

StataCorp, 2013. Stata Statistical Software. *Release 13*. College Station, TX StataCorp LP.

Svedsater, H., 2000. Contingent valuation of global environmental resources: Test of perfect and regular embedding. *Journal of Economic Psychology*, **21**: 605–623.

Tockhorn-Heidenreich, A., Ryan, M., and Hernández, R., 2017. Discrete choice experiments. In: K.M. Facey, H. Ploug Hansen, and A.N.V. Single (eds), *Patient Involvement in Health Technology Assessment*. Singapore: Springer.

Tyler, P., Warnock, C., Provins, A., Wells, P., Brennan, A., Cole, I., Gilbertson, J., et al., 2010. *Valuing the Benefits of Regeneration*. London: Department of Communities and Local Government.

Van Der Pol, M., Shiell, A., Au, F., Johnston, D., and Tough, S., 2010. Eliciting individual preferences for health care: A case study of perinatal care. *Health Expectations, 13*: 4–12.

Vecchiato, D. and Tempesta, T., 2013. Valuing the benefits of an afforestation project in a peri-urban area with choice experiments. *Forest Policy and Economics, 26*: 111–20.

Ward Thompson, C., Silveirinha de Oliveira, E., Tilley, S., Elizalde, A., Botha, W., Briggs, A., Cummins, S., et al., 2018. Health impacts of the WIAT programme to improve local woodlands for deprived urban communities: A quasi-experimental study. *NIHR Public Health Research*, pp. 236.

Weatherly, H., Drummond, M.F., Claxton, K., Cookson, R., Ferguson, B., Godfrey, C., Rice, N., et al., 2009. Methods for assessing the cost-effectiveness of public health interventions: Key challenges and recommendations. *Health Policy, 93*: 85–92.

Williams, D.R., Costa, M.V., Odunlami, A.O., and Mohammed, S.A., 2008. Moving upstream: How interventions that address the social determinants of health can improve health and reduce disparities. *Journal of Public Health Management and Practice, 14*: S8–17.

Appendix 9.1

CBA checklist for compilers of NICE public health reviews

1. Is there a well-defined question?
2. Is there a comprehensive description of alternatives?
3. Was one of the alternatives designated as the comparator against which the intervention was evaluated?
4. Is the perspective stated?
   - Is WTP the public-sector WTP or the aggregated individual WTP? Has the WTP been recalibrated when the basis for its calculation has not coincided with the perspective being used?
5. Are all important and relevant costs and outcomes for each alternative identified?
   - Check to see if the study is of money costs and 'benefits' which are savings of future money costs.
6. Has effectiveness been established?
7. Are costs and outcomes measured accurately?
8. Are costs and outcomes valued credibly?
9. Have all important and relevant costs and outcomes for each alternative been quantified in money terms?
   - If not, state which items were not quantified, and the likely extent of their importance in terms of influencing the benefit:cost ratio.
10. Are costs and outcomes adjusted for differential timing?
11. Has at least one of Net Present Value, benefits:costs ratio, and pay-back period been estimated?
12. Were any assumptions of materiality made?
13. Were all assumptions reasonable in the circumstances in which they were made, and were they justified?
14. Were sensitivity analyses conducted to investigate uncertainty in estimates of cost or benefits?
15. How far do study results include all issues of concern to users?
16. Are the results generalizable to the setting of interest in the review?
    - Country differences.
    - Question of interest differs from the CBA question being reviewed.
17. Have equity considerations been addressed in any way?

Source: <https://www.nice.org.uk/article/pmg4/chapter/Appendix-I-Quality-appraisal-checklist-economic-evaluations#cba-checklist-for-compilers-of-nice-public-health-reviews> (Accessed 21 October 2018).

Chapter 10

Cost–consequence analysis of public health interventions

Ned Hartfiel and Rhiannon T. Edwards

10.1 Introduction

The *Encyclopaedia of Public Health* defines cost–consequence analysis (CCA) as:

> a form of health economic evaluation study in which all direct and indirect costs and a catalogue of different outcomes of all alternatives are listed separately. No specific preference for one costing approach or one outcome measure (as is the case for cost-effectiveness analysis or cost–utility analysis) is made. Consequently, the result is not a definite cost-outcome ratio. The reader or the decision maker has to form their own opinion concerning the relative importance of costs and outcomes. (Kirch, 2008, p. 30)

A pragmatic and transparent approach to economic evaluation, CCA presents a series of outcome measures alongside costs in the form of a cost–consequence balance sheet, enabling decision-makers to consider the outcomes most relevant to them (Herman, 2012; Drummond et al., 2015). CCA provides a clear descriptive summary for decision-makers that is often easier to interpret than cost-effectiveness, cost–utility, and cost–benefit analysis (Gage et al., 2006).

In the United Kingdom, the National Institute for Health and Care Excellence (NICE) has recommended CCA in addition to cost–utility analysis for evaluating public health interventions (PHIs) (NICE, 2012). CCA is sometimes referred to as a *disaggregated* approach because the benefits and costs are not combined in a single ratio such as incremental cost-effectiveness ratios (ICERs) in cost–utility analysis (see Chapter 2), cost–benefit ratios in cost–benefit analysis (see Chapter 9), and return on investment analysis (see Chapter 12).

A possible drawback of CCA is that it does not provide guidance as to how the different outcomes in the balance sheet should be weighed against each other. When some outcomes show benefits and others show disbenefits, it becomes necessary to ask about the relative value of these outcomes (Marsh et al., 2012). Decision-makers are required to devise their own system to appraise the results, and these decisions made at an individual level may not always be in the best interest of patients or society (Charles and Edwards, 2016).

Earlier chapters have outlined role of CCA in economic evaluation of PHIs in providing a clear descriptive summary of costs and benefits easily understood by stakeholders in both health and non-health sectors (Trueman and Anokye, 2013). This chapter offers a case study of CCA by comparing a yoga-based intervention with self-care for managing musculoskeletal conditions in the workplace.

10.2 **Case study**

This case study is based on a CCA conducted alongside a randomized controlled trial (Hartfiel, N., Phillips, C.J., and Edwards, R.T., 2017. Cost-effectiveness of yoga for managing musculoskeletal conditions in the workplace. *Occupational Medicine, 67*(9):687–95). The trial compared a yoga-based programme with self-care for managing musculoskeletal conditions in the workplace. The study population included 151 National Health Service (NHS) employees from three hospital sites in North Wales. Participants were randomly allocated to receive either an eight-week Dru Yoga programme, or self-care which consisted of two educational booklets for managing stress and back pain.

The 8-week yoga programme included weekly 60-minute classes held after work in the manual handling training rooms at each hospital site. In addition, yoga participants received an instructional DVD and illustrated booklet for home practice. Valid and reliable outcome measures for back pain, well-being, and health-related quality of life were assessed at baseline, eight weeks, and at six-month follow-up. Sickness absence data were also obtained from the employer at six months.

The CCA considered only those costs relevant to the employer. These costs were the direct intervention costs (i.e. cost of yoga instructors and equipment) and the production loss costs which were the number of sickness absence days due to musculoskeletal conditions.

10.2.1 **Background**

10.2.1.1 Musculoskeletal conditions in the workplace

Musculoskeletal conditions (MSCs) are the most common cause of chronic pain and disability in industrialized countries (Connelly et al., 2006; Ward et al., 2013). The four main musculoskeletal conditions include osteoarthritis, osteoporosis, rheumatoid arthritis, and back pain (Woolf and Pfleger, 2003; Ward et al., 2013).

Of these conditions, back pain is the most prevalent (Woolf and Pfleger, 2003). In both industrialized and developing countries, back pain is a major cause of sickness absence from work (Connelly et al., 2006). In the United Kingdom, most people (80 per cent) experience back pain at some point during their lifetime (Maniadakis and Gray, 2000), and about a third of the population (20 million people) experience back pain each year (National Institute for Health and Care Excellence, 2009). In 2013, musculoskeletal conditions and back pain resulted in more than 30 million sickness absence days (Office for National Statistics, 2014), costing British employers approximately £5.6 billion (Confederation of British Industry, 2013; Chartered Society of Physiotherapists, 2013).

To prevent back pain, NICE recommends effective early intervention strategies including structured exercise programmes designed to stretch/strengthen muscles and to improve posture (National Institute for Health and Care Excellence, 2016).

The NICE guidance suggests group exercise programmes of 8 sessions over a 12-week period, with class sizes of up to 10 people (National Institute for Health and Care Excellence, 2016).

Although research indicates that few workplace interventions are effective for preventing back pain and musculoskeletal conditions (van Poppel et al., 2004), the workplace provides an ideal setting for health promotion and physical activity (World Health Organization, 1997). For preventing back pain at work, systematic reviews report that exercise programmes are more effective than lumbar supports or education (van Poppel et al., 2004). Workplace exercise programmes are shown to have a positive effect in preventing back pain, although the evidence is limited due to a lack of high-quality studies (van Poppel et al., 2004; Luhman et al., 2006; Bell and Burnett, 2009).

10.2.1.2 Effectiveness of yoga for managing musculoskeletal conditions and back pain

Recent research suggests that yoga is one form of exercise that can reduce musculoskeletal conditions and back pain (Sherman et al., 2011; Tilbrook et al., 2011). Yoga is a popular form of exercise which usually includes four components: physical movement, breathing exercises, relaxation methods, and meditation/mindfulness techniques (Collins, 1998; Woodyard, 2011; Ward et al., 2011; National Institute for Health, 2013). Practised by approximately 30 million people worldwide, yoga is now commonplace in Western countries and taught in leisure centres, health clubs, schools, hospitals, and GP surgeries (National Institute for Health, 2013; Cramer et al., 2013b).

Two recent systematic reviews of yoga for musculoskeletal conditions found yoga to be a safe, acceptable, and feasible intervention, superior to usual care in reducing pain and improving functional outcomes (McCaffrey and Park, 2012; Ward et al., 2013). Five additional systematic reviews on yoga for back pain have found strong evidence of the effectiveness of yoga for relieving short-term back pain and moderate evidence of the effectiveness of yoga for reducing long-term back pain (Posadski and Ernst, 2011; Bussing et al., 2012; Cramer et al., 2013a; Holzman and Beggs, 2013; Hill, 2013).

10.2.1.3 Cost-effectiveness of yoga for managing back pain

Although these recent systematic reviews indicate that yoga can be effective for managing musculoskeletal conditions and back pain, few studies have explored the cost-effectiveness of yoga. Two recent studies suggest that yoga can be cost-effective for *patient populations* with chronic or non-specific low-back pain (Chuang et al., 2012; Aboagye et al., 2015).

The Chuang and Aboagye studies found that a series of 12 yoga classes had a favourable impact on sickness absence days for patients with low-back pain. Chuang reported that yoga participants missed an average of 3.8 days off work compared to 12.3 in a usual care group over a one-year period (Chuang et al., 2012). Similarly, Aboagye and colleagues reported that patients offered yoga treatment missed an average of 12.4 days of work over a one-year period compared to 29.6 days missed by patients offered self-care (Aboagye et al., 2015). Although these findings are promising for *patient populations* with chronic or non-specific low-back pain, further studies are needed to determine if yoga can generate cost savings for employers by preventing back pain and associated sickness absence in workplace settings with relatively healthy employee populations.

10.2.2 Methods

In this case study comparing yoga and self-care for managing musculoskeletal conditions, CCA was performed from the employer perspective, meaning that only those costs and consequences relevant to the employer were considered.

10.2.2.1 Relevant costs

Relevant costs from the employer perspective included both intervention costs and production loss costs. Intervention costs for the yoga group included the costs for the yoga equipment, learning materials (i.e. instructional video and illustrated booklet), instructors, and recruitment. Intervention costs for the self-care group consisted of the cost for two educational booklets: *The Back Book* and *How to Manage Stress*.

Production loss costs were the absenteeism costs attributed to musculoskeletal conditions during the eight-week yoga programme and six-month follow-up. The number of sickness absence days due to musculoskeletal conditions was compared between the yoga and self-care groups. To determine the production loss costs, the number of sickness absence days for each group during the six-month study was multiplied by the average daily wage rate for an NHS employee in 2013.

In this analysis, all costs were presented in 2013 British sterling prices. Discounting (discussed in Chapter 2 of this book) for changes in pricing over time was not necessary because the eight-week yoga programme and follow-up period were completed within one year.

Overhead costs and opportunity costs in this analysis were minimal, and therefore not included in this analysis. Yoga sessions did not compete with the working hours of employees or with any alternative uses of manual handling rooms where the yoga classes were held.

Overhead costs included electricity and heating for the manual handling rooms. These rooms were provided at no cost by the employer after working hours. These rooms were on pre-set heating, and the cost of lighting during the one-hour class was negligible.

10.2.2.2 Relevant consequences

The relevant outcomes of the eight-week yoga programme were measured at the six-month follow-up using valid and reliable measures that assessed:

◆ back pain,
◆ psychological well-being, and
◆ health related quality of life.

10.2.3 Findings of the study

10.2.3.1 Intervention costs

Intervention costs were presented in two scenarios: scenario 1 was the actual costs accrued during the eight-week programme when yoga instructors were paid £91 per

Table 10.1 Two cost scenarios for yoga classes

Cost scenarios	Description of costs
Scenario 1 (actual study cost scenario including instruction, travel, room set-up, and administration)	◆ Instruction costs at £91 per session ◆ Equipment costs at wholesale prices ◆ Recruitment costs at £19 ◆ No venue costs
Scenario 2 (instruction costs only at typical rates)	◆ Instruction costs at £64 per session ◆ Equipment costs at wholesale prices ◆ Recruitment costs at £19 ◆ No venue costs

session, which, under these specific arrangements, included the costs for instruction, travel, room set-up, and administration. Scenario 2 represented intervention costs when yoga instructors were paid at £64 per session which is a more typical rate in the United Kingdom (Table 10.1). According to the National Careers Service in the United Kingdom, the average wage rate for yoga teachers ranges between £35 and £60 per session (National Careers Service, 2015).

Intervention costs for the yoga and self-care groups consisted of:

(i) equipment costs

(ii) operational costs

The equipment costs were £7.26 per person for yoga participants and £2.00 per person for self-care (Table 10.2).

The operational costs ranged from £40.67 to £57.72 per person for yoga participants depending on the cost scenario (Table 10.3). There were no operational costs for self-care participants.

When both operational costs and equipment costs were considered, the difference in total intervention costs between the two groups ranged from £45.93 to £62.98 per person depending on the cost scenario (Table 10.4).

10.2.3.2 Production loss costs

Production loss costs can be defined as costs associated with lost or impaired ability to work due to sickness or illness (Brouwer et al., 1998). Production loss costs are conventionally calculated by multiplying the average daily wage rate by the number of sickness days (Drummond et al., 2015).

This calculation can be made with either the human-capital approach or the friction-cost method (McIntosh et al., 2010). The human-capital approach has been the conventional method in economic evaluation and takes the perspective of the sick leave employee by counting every day of sick leave as a day of productivity lost (van den Hout, 2010).

The friction-cost method, on the other hand, takes the perspective of the employer, counting every day of sick leave as a day of productivity lost until a replacement worker is found. Using the friction-cost approach, the value of production loss costs is usually less than the value using the human-capital approach. Research indicates

Table 10.2 Difference in equipment costs between groups

Yoga group	Units	Unit price £	Equipment cost/person £	Total equipment costs £
Yoga DVD	76	2.00	2.00	152.00
Illustrated booklet	76	1.00	1.00	76.00
Yoga mats	36	5.00	2.37	180.00
Yoga cushions	36	4.00	1.89	144.00
Total equipment costs			**£7.26**	**£552.00**
Self-care group	Units	Unit price £	Equipment cost/person £	Total equipment costs £
The Back Book	75	1.00	1.00	75.00
How to Manage Stress	75	1.00	1.00	75.00
Total equipment costs			**£2.00**	**£150.00**

that the friction cost approach generates between 18 per cent and 44 per cent of the costs calculated using the human-capital approach (Hanley et al., 2012). Thus, the two methods can produce widely different results (van den Hout, 2010).

In this case study, the human-capital approach was used to calculate the value of production loss costs from sickness absence days due to musculoskeletal conditions. NHS electronic staff records (ESR) showed that during the six-month study period, yoga group participants missed in total 2 calendar days, while the self-care group missed 43 days due to musculoskeletal conditions (Table 10.5).

The production loss costs for yoga participants were £3 per person compared with £65.27 per person for self-care participants. This difference in production loss costs between the two groups over the six-month study was £4,667.44 or £62.27 per person (Table 10.5).

10.2.3.3 Total costs

From the employer perspective, the yoga programme was slightly more costly than self-care in scenario 1 when yoga instructors were paid £91 per session. However, the yoga programme was substantially less costly per person in scenario 2 when yoga instructors were compensated at £64 per session (Table 10.6).

10.2.3.4 Total consequences

Mean scores between groups at baseline, eight weeks, and six-month follow-up were compared for relevant outcome measures (Table 10.7). The results showed that at the six-month follow-up, the yoga group had less back pain, more psychological well-being, and better health-related quality of life than the self-care group. Although the

Table 10.3 Difference in operational costs between groups

Yoga (n = 76)	Units	Scenario 1			Scenario 2		
		Unit price £	Cost per person £	Total costs £	Unit price £	Cost per person £	Total costs £
Recruitment	2 hours	9.50/hour	0.25	19.00	9.50/hour	0.25	19.00
Teaching	48 sessions	60.00/session	37.89	2,880.00	40.00/session	25.26	1,920.00
Travel	48 sessions	15.00/session	9.47	720.00	8.00/session	5.05	384.00
Room prep	48 sessions	10.00/session	6.33	480.00	10.00/session	6.32	480.00
Administration	48 sessions	6.00/session	3.79	288.00	6.00/session	3.79	288.00
Total Operational Costs (yoga)			£57.72	£4,387.00		£40.67	£3,091.00

Table 10.4 Differences in intervention costs between groups

Scenario	Equipment cost per yoga participant £	Operational cost per yoga participant £	Intervention cost per yoga participant £	Intervention cost per self-care participant £	Difference in intervention cost per participant between groups £
1	7.26	57.72	64.98	2.00	62.98
2	7.26	40.67	47.93	2.00	45.93

Table 10.5 Differences in production loss costs between groups

Group	NHS Band	Yoga classes attended	Sickness absence calendar days	Total cost (£113.84/day) £	Total cost per person £
Yoga	Band 2	7	2	227.68	3.00
Yoga total			2	227.68	3.00
Self-care	Band 4	0	5	569.20	7.59
Self-care	Band 5	0	1	113.84	1.52
Self-care	Band 7	0	29	3,301.36	44.02
Self-care	Band 6	0	3	341.52	4.55
Self-care	Band 4	0	5	569.20	7.59
Self-care total			43	4,895.12	65.27
Yoga total			2	227.68	3.00
Difference between groups			41	4,667.44	62.27

Table 10.6 Differences in costs between groups

	Scenario 1		Scenario 2	
	Yoga group £	Self-care £	Yoga group £	Self-care £
Intervention costs per person	64.98	2.00	47.93	2.00
Production loss costs per person	3.00	65.27	3.00	65.27
Employer perspective per person	**£67.98**	**£67.27**	**£50.93**	**£67.27**

Table 10.7 Mean scores (SD), mean differences, and p-values

Domains	Yoga group					Self-care group					Between groups			
	Baseline	End programme 8 weeks	Mean change 8 weeks	Follow-up 6 months	Mean change 6 months	Baseline	End programme 8 weeks	Mean change 8 weeks	Follow-up 6 months	Mean change 6 months	Mean difference 8 weeks	Mean difference 6 months	P-value 8 weeks	P-value 6 months
1. RDQ Back pain	2.09(2.44) n = 76	1.34(1.72) n = 56	-0.75	1.26 (2.05) n = 43	-0.83	1.93(2.97) n = 75	2.30(3.31) n = 53	0.37	2.03(3.30) n = 32	0.10	-1.12	-0.93	P = 0.035	P = 0.196
2. Keele Back pain	1.37(1.16) n = 76	0.76(0.77) n = 55	-0.61	0.95(1.17) n = 42	-0.42	1.41(1.40) n = 74	1.62(1.36) n = 53	0.21	1.50(1.30) n = 32	0.09	-0.82	-0.51	P < 0.001	P = 0.071
3. WHO-5 Well-being	13.45(4.44) n = 74	17.27(4.09) n = 55	3.82	16.42(4.54) n = 43	2.97	13.57(5.15) n = 75	15.29(4.26) n = 49	1.72	15.22(5.20) n = 32	1.65	2.1	1.32	P = 0.014	P = 0.132
4. EQ5D-5L Health-related quality of life	0.704(0.296) n = 75	0.780(0.224) n = 55	0.076	0.712(0.320) n = 42	0.008	0.677(0.309) n = 73	0.566(0.380) n = 52	-0.111	0.647(0.308) n = 31	-0.030	0.187	0.038	P = 0.001	P = 0.323

Table 10.8 Cost–consequence balance sheet at six-month follow-up

COSTS	Scenario 1 £	Scenario 2 £		
Employer perspective (yoga)	67.98	50.93		
Employer perspective (self-care)	67.27	67.27		
Mean difference in costs between groups	0.71	−16.34	v	
CONSEQUENCES	back pain (RDQ)	back pain (Keele)	wellbeing (WHO-5)	HRQOL (EQ5D-5L)
Mean difference between groups	−0.93	−0.51	1.32	0.038
***p*-value**	$p = 0.196$	$p = 0.071$	$p = 0.132$	$p = 0.323$

differences between the two groups for these outcome measures were statistically significant at eight weeks, they were not at six months, as shown in Table 10.7.

10.2.3.4 Cost–consequence balance sheet

The cost–consequence balance sheet showed that the yoga programme was more expensive by £0.71 per person than self-care in scenario 1 where yoga instructors were paid £91 per session. In scenario 2, the yoga programme was less costly than self-care by £16.34 per person where yoga instructors were compensated at more typical rates of £64 per session. On the consequence side, yoga participants at six months experienced less back pain, greater well-being, and better health-related quality of life (HRQoL) than self-care participants (Table 10.8).

10.2.4 Discussion

From the employer perspective, the yoga programme was less costly than self-care in scenario 2 when yoga instructors were paid £64 per session, but slightly more expensive in scenario 1 when they were paid £91 per session. On the consequences side, the yoga programme at six-months was more effective than self-care for reducing back pain, and for improving psychological well-being and health-related quality of life.

This CCA indicated that when instructors were compensated at rates more in-line with national averages (£35 to £60 per session), the yoga intervention was less costly than self-care. This was mainly due to lower production loss costs in the yoga group from fewer sickness absence days related to musculoskeletal conditions.

10.2.4.1 Limitations

Although the findings of this CCA seem favourable to yoga, the results need to be interpreted with caution due to the small sample size. During the eight-week yoga programme and six-month follow-up, only six participants missed working days due to musculoskeletal conditions. Five of these participants were in the self-care group

Table 10.9 Case study summary

Title	**Yoga for managing musculoskeletal conditions in the work-place: cost–consequence analysis alongside a randomized controlled trial**
Setting	North Wales
Participants	151 NHS employees (76 intervention, 75 control)
Recruitment	Occupational Health
Intervention	Eight-week yoga intervention comprising weekly one-hour classes, plus a DVD and illustrated booklet for home practice compared with self-care consisting of *The Back Book* and *How to Manage Stress*
Follow up period	6 months
Outcome measures	Health outcomes were measured at eight weeks and a six-month follow-up using valid and reliable measures assessing back pain, psychological well-being, and health-related quality of life.
Measurement of Costs	Health outcomes at six-months were compared with intervention and production loss costs from the employer perspective
Perspective	Employer
Study type	Cost–consequence analysis alongside a randomized controlled trial
Existing Evidence of Effectiveness	Two recent systematic reviews of yoga for musculoskeletal conditions found yoga to be a safe, acceptable, and feasible intervention, superior to usual care in reducing pain and improving functional outcomes (McCaffrey and Park, 2012; Ward et al., 2013). Five additional systematic reviews on yoga for back pain have found strong evidence of the effectiveness of yoga for relieving short-term back pain and moderate evidence of yoga's effectiveness for reducing long-term back pain (Posadski and Ernst, 2011; Bussing et al., 2012; Cramer et al., 2013a; Holzman and Beggs, 2013; Hill, 2013).
Existing Evidence of Cost-Effectiveness	Two recent studies suggest that yoga can be cost-effective from the employer perspective for patient populations with chronic or non-specific low-back pain (Chuang et al., 2012; Aboagye et al., 2015). The Chuang and Aboagye studies found that a series of 12 yoga classes had a favourable impact on sickness absence days for patients with both chronic low-back pain (Chuang et al., 2012) and non-specific low-back pain (Aboagye et al., 2015).
Objective	Although these findings are promising for *patient populations* with chronic and non-specific low-back pain, further studies with larger sample sizes are needed to compare the costs with the consequences of yoga in workplace settings with relatively healthy *employee populations*.

and only one was in the yoga group. Of these five self-care participants, one missed 29 days, which accounted for 67 per cent of the total sickness absence days due to musculoskeletal conditions.

Although it could be argued that participation in the yoga programme may have prevented these 29 days of sickness absence, such an outlier may have overinflated the cost savings attributed to yoga. High-quality investigations of yoga in workplace settings, with more robust sample sizes, are needed to verify these results.

Nevertheless, the sickness absence benefits reported in this case study are consistent with the results of the two previously mentioned yoga studies (Chuang et al., 2012; Aboagye et al., 2015), which also reported substantial savings from reduced absenteeism due to back pain. Taken together, these two studies, along with this case study, suggest that yoga can reduce production loss costs for back pain and musculoskeletal-related conditions.

Finally, future economic evaluations of yoga in the workplace will benefit not only from larger sample sizes but also by measuring presenteeism as well as absenteeism. Presenteeism refers to the loss of productivity when employees show up to work when unwell and consequently underperform (Ashby and Mahdon, 2010; Johns, 2010).

These costs were not included in this study because of the difficulty and lack of consensus in measuring presenteeism (Ashby and Mahdon, 2010; Braakman-Jansen et al., 2012). However, research suggests that the loss of productivity from presenteeism could be even greater than from absenteeism, especially in the field of health care (Aronson and Gustafsson, 2005; Phillips, 2005; Ashby and Mahdon, 2010).

Summary of Chapter 10

- ♦ CCA compares the costs of implementing an intervention with its consequences.
- ♦ It presents a 'balance sheet' by comparing monetary, quantitative, and descriptive consequences with the costs.
- ♦ CCA provides a clear descriptive summary for decision-makers about the costs of an intervention and the various outcomes from which value-for-money decisions can be made.
- ♦ CCA aims to consider all health and non-health outcomes and reports them in a disaggregated manner, accepting that different types of benefits cannot be measured using the same units.
- ♦ It is an appropriate method for interventions with a wide variety of health and non-health outcomes which are not easily measured by a common unit such as a quality-adjusted life year (QALY).
- ♦ The National Institute for Health and Care Excellence (NICE) recommends using CCA in addition to cost–utility analysis for evaluating public health interventions.
- ♦ Unlike cost-benefit analysis or cost-effectiveness analysis, CCA does not attempt to summarise outcomes in a single measure, a ratio or in financial terms.
- ♦ Outcomes are reported in their natural units, and decision-makers may want to devise a system for assigning monetary values to outcomes and deciding whether an intervention is worth implementing.

◆ The decision whether or not to implement an intervention may depend on the monetary values assigned by decision-makers to the outcomes and their willingness to pay.

References

Aboagye, E., Karlsson, M.L., Hagberg, J., and Jensen, I., 2015. Cost-effectiveness of early interventions for non-specific low back pain: A randomized controlled study investigating medical yoga, exercise therapy and self-care advice. *Journal of Rehabilitation Medicine*, 47(2): 167–73.

Aronsson, G. and Gustafsson, K., 2005. Sickness presenteeism: Prevalence, attendance-pressure factors and an outline model for research. *Journal of Occupational Environmental Medicine*, 47: 958–66.

Ashby, K. and Madon, M., 2010. *Why Do Employees Come to Work When Ill? An Investigation into Sickness Presence in the Workplace.* The Workplace Foundation. Available at: <http://www.istas.ccoo.es/descargas/FINAL%20Why%20do%20employees%20come%20to%20work%20when%20ill.pdf> (Accessed 22 October 2018).

Bell, J.A. and Burnett, A., 2009. Exercise for the primary, secondary and tertiary prevention of low back pain in the workplace: A systematic review. *Journal of Occupational Rehabilitation*, 19(1): 8–24.

Braakman-Jansen, L.M., Taal, E., Kuper, I.H., and van de Laar, M.A., 2012. Productivity loss due to absenteeism and presenteeism by different instruments in patients with RA and subjects without RA. *Rheumatology*, 51(2): 354–61.

Brouwer, W.B.F., Koopmanschap, M.A., and Rutten, F.F.H., 1998. Patient and informal caregiver time in cost-effectiveness analysis. *International Journal of Technology Assessment in Health Care*, 14(3): 505–13.

Bussing, A., Ostermann, R., Ludtke, R., and Michalsen, A., 2012. Effects of yoga interventions on pain and pain-associated disability: A meta-analysis. *Journal of Pain*, 13(1): 1–9.

Charles, J. and Edwards, R.T., 2016. *A Guide to Health Economics for those Working in Public Health.* Bangor: Public Health Wales.

Chartered Society of Physiotherapists. 2013. Physiotherapy works: occupational health. Available at: <http://www.csp.org.uk/publications/physiotherapy-works-occupational-health> (Accessed 15 October 2018).

Chuang, L.H., Soares, M.O., Tilbrook, H., Cox, H., Hewitt, C.E., Aplin, J., Semlyn, A., et al., 2012. A pragmatic multicentered randomized controlled trial of yoga for chronic low back pain: Economic evaluation. *Spine*, 37:1593–601.

Collins, C., 1998. Yoga: Intuition, preventive medicine, and treatment. *Journal Obstetric, Gynecologic and Neonatal Nursing*, 27(5): 563–8.

Confederation of British Industry. 2013. *Fit for Purpose: Absence and Workplace Health Survey.* Available at: <http://www.kmghp.com/assets/cbi-pfizer_absence___workplace_health_2013-(1).pdf> (Accessed 21 October 2018).

Connelly, L.B., Woolf, A. and Brooks P., 2006. In D.T. Jamieson, J.G. Breman, A.R. Measham, G. Alleyeyne, M. Claeson, D.B. Evans, and Jha, P., et al. (eds). *Disease Control Priorities in Developing Countries* (2nd edn). Washington, DC: World Bank, pp. 963–80.

Cramer, H., Lauche, R., Haller, H., and Dobos, G., 2013a. A systematic review and meta-analysis of yoga for low back pain. *Clinical Journal of Pain*, 29(5): 450–60.

Drummond, M.F., Sculpher, M.J., Claxton, K., Stoddart, G.L., and Torrance, G.W., 2015. *Methods for the Economic Evaluation of Health Care Programmes* (4th edn). Oxford: Oxford University Press.

Gage, H., Kaye, J., Thomas, C.O., Trend, P., and Wade, D. (2006). Evaluating rehabilitation using cost–consequences analysis: An example in Parkinson's disease. *Clinical Rehabilitation, 20*: 232–8.

Hanley, P., Timmons, A., Walsh, P.M., and Sharp, L., 2012. Breast and prostate cancer productivity costs: A comparison of the human capital approach and the friction cost approach. *Value Health, 15*(3): 429–36.

Hartfiel, N., Phillips, C.J., and Edwards, RT., 2017. Cost-effectiveness of yoga for managing musculoskeletal conditions in the workplace. *Occupational Medicine, 67*(9): 687–95.

Herman, P.M., 2012. *Evaluating the Economics of Complementary and Integrative Medicine.* Alexandria: Samueli Institute.

Hill, C., 2013. Is yoga an effective treatment in the management of patients with chronic low back pain compared with other care modalities—a systematic review. *Journal of Complementary and Integrative Medicine,* (1).

Holzman, S. and Beggs, R.T., 2013. Yoga for chronic back pain: A meta analysis of randomized controlled trials. *Pain Research and Management, 18*(5): 267–72.

Johns, G., 2010. Presenteeism in the workplace: A review and research agenda. *Journal of Organizational Behavior, 31*(4): 519–42.

Kirch, W. (ed.), 2008. *Encyclopedia of Public Health.* New York, NY: Springer.

Luhman, D., Stoll, S., Burkhardt-Hammer, T., and Raspe, H., 2006. Prevention of relapsing backache. *GMS Health Technology Assessment, 2*: 1–11.

Maniadakis, N. and Gray, A., 2000. The economic burden of back pain in the UK. *Pain, 84*(1): 95–103.

Maraschke, E. and Mujtaba, B.G., 2014. Creating a wellness culture through human resources. *Journal of Physical Education and Sports Management, 1*(1): 61–80.

Marsh, K., Phillips, C.J., Fordham, R., Bertranou, E., and Hale, J., 2012. Estimating cost-effectiveness in public health: A summary of modelling and valuation methods. *Health Economics Review, 2*(17). doi:10.1186/2191-1991-2-17.

McCaffrey, R. and Park, J., 2012. The benefits of yoga for musculoskeletal disorders: A systematic review. *Journal of Yoga Physical Therapy, 2*(5): 1–11.

McIntosh, E., Clarke, P., Frew, E., and Louivere, J., 2010. *Applied Methods of Cost-Benefit Analysis in Health Care.* Oxford: Oxford University Press.

National Careers Service, 2015. *Job Profiles: Yoga Instructor.* Available at: <https://nationalcareersservice.direct.gov.uk/job-profiles/yoga-teacher> (Accessed 22 October 2018).

National Institute for Health and Care Excellence, 2009. Low back pain: Early management of persistent non-specific low back pain. 2009. (Clinical guideline 88) <http://www.nice.org.uk/CG88> (Accessed 21 October 2018).

National Institute for Health and Care Excellence, 2012. *The NICE public health guidance development process (third edition).* Available at: <http://www.nice.org.uk/article/pmg4/resources/non-guidance-methods-for-the-development-of-nice-public-health-guidance-third-edition-pdf> (Accessed 15 October 2018).

National Institute for Health and Care Excellence, 2016. *Low back pain and sciatica in over 16s: assessment and management.* Available at: <https://www.nice.org.uk/guidance/ng59> (Accessed 15 October 2018).

National Institute for Health, 2013. *Yoga for Health.* Bethesda, MD: U.S. Department of Health and Human Sciences, National Institute of Health, National Center for Complementary and Alternative Medicine.

Office for National Statistics, 2014. *Full report: Sickness absence in the labour market.* London: Office for National Statistics.

Phillips, C., 2005. *Health Economics: An Introduction for Health Professionals.* Oxford: Blackwell Publishing Ltd.

Posadski, P. and **Ernst, E.,** 2011. Yoga for low back pain: A systematic review of randomized clinical trials. *Clinical Rheumatology, 30*: 1257–62.

Sherman, K.J., Cherkin, D.C., Wellman, R.D., Cook, A.J., Hawkes, R.J., Delaney, K., and **Deyo, R.A.,** 2011. A randomized trial comparing yoga, stretching and a self-care book for chronic low back pain. *Archives of Internal Medicine,171*(22): 2019–26.

Tilbrook, H.E., Cox, H., Hewitt, C.E., Kang'ombe, A.R., Chuang, L.H., Jayakody, S., Aplin, J.D., et al., 2011. Yoga for chronic low back pain: A randomized trial. *Annals of Internal Medicine, 155*(9): 569–78.

Trueman, P. and **Anokye, N.K.,** 2013. Applying economic evaluation to public health interventions: The case of interventions to promote physical activity. *Journal of Public Health,* March, **35**(1): 32–9. doi:10.1093/pubmed/fds050. Epub 2012 Jul 2.

van den Hout, W.B., 2010. The value of productivity: Human-capital versus friction-cost method. *Annals of the Rheumatic Diseases, 69*(1): i89–i91.

van Poppel, M.N., Hooftman, W.E., and **Koes, B.W.,** 2004. An update of a systematic review of controlled clinical trials on the primary prevention of back pain at the workplace. *Occupational Medicine, 54*: 345–52.

Ward, L., Treharne, G.J., and **Stebbings, S.,** 2011. The suitability of yoga as a potential therapeutic intervention for rheumatoid arthritis: A focus group approach. *Musculoskeletal Care, 9*(4): 211–21.

Ward, L., Stebbings, S., Cherkin, D., and **Baxter, G.D.,** 2013. Yoga for functional ability, pain and psychological outcomes in musculoskeletal conditions: A systematic review and meta-analysis. *Musculoskeletal Care, 11*(4): 203–17.

Woodyard, C., 2011. Exploring the therapeutic effects of yoga and its ability to increase quality of life. *International Journal Yoga, 4*(2): 49–54.

Woolfe, A.D. and **Pfleger, B.,** 2003. Burden of major musculoskeletal conditions. *Bulletin of the World Health Organization, 81*(9): 646–56.

World Health Organization. 1997. *WHO's Global Healthy Works Approach.* Geneva: WHO, Division of Health Promotion, Education & Communication and Office of Occupational Health.

Chapter 11

The use of modelling approaches for the economic evaluation of public health interventions

Hazel Squires and Kathleen Boyd

11.1 Introduction

Typically, economic evaluation has been applied to assess medications and health care technologies, as the majority of the health care budget is spent treating disease rather than on prevention, as discussed in Chapter 1 of this book. However, in recent years the spectrum for economic evaluation has broadened to include public health interventions (PHIs) due to growing interest in initiatives which can prevent disease, for example, in areas such as obesity, oral health, smoking and alcohol, as well as reduce health inequalities and health care costs. PHIs tend to be preventative in nature so while costs are incurred upfront, they can often offset long-term health problems and potentially improve patients' lives and save costs in the long run. With the emergence of novel PHIs, it is essential to evaluate whether these (and those currently being funded) are worthwhile, or whether the money could be better spent on alternative programme(s).

Owen and colleagues recently reviewed the literature and highlighted a lack of economic evidence on PHIs, yet they note that those that have been assessed are shown to be highly cost-effective (Owen et al., 2012, see also Chapter 8). However, these PHIs are predominantly compared against a 'do nothing' alternative, which could potentially inflate the case for support by overlooking routine initiatives that are already underway. Care needs to be taken when evaluating PHIs, not only to ensure the relevant comparators are used but also to ensure the methods for analysis adequately capture the important aspects of the public health intervention (Weatherly et al., 2009). Traditional economic evaluation methods are well established, yet they are insufficient for capturing the broad spectrum of costs and outcomes relevant to the assessment of PHIs (Marsh et al., 2012) and often raise additional methodological challenges (Weatherly et al., 2009). Economic modelling has been put forward as a tool to ensure a robust analysis which captures all costs and outcomes, ensuring a full picture of the potential gains from investing in PHIs (Marsh et al., 2012).

Economic evaluation using modelling techniques can provide insight into the value of public health investments to the entire health system, exploring incremental effects of novel initiatives and programmes as well as the population impacts of changes in policies. Such a 'systems' approach is in line with the recommendations of Smith and Petticrew (2010) to conduct macro-level evaluations of PHIs at a societal level where possible. Most recently, modelling has been used to explore the impact of changes in government policies to address rising costs related to alcohol consumption (Brennan et al., 2014), smoking (Jones et al., 2011) and obesity (Trueman and Anokye, 2012). Brennan and colleagues used economic modelling to assess the impact of proposed minimum alcohol pricing and a ban on promotion policies on the UK population (Brennan et al., 2014). Their modelling work highlighted the policies that are effective and cost-effective, which in turn have informed government decision-makers for public health policy development. With rising costs for treating preventable diseases and increasing pressure to shrink health budgets around the globe, there is a need for economic evidence to support the case for investing in PHIs. Economic modelling is an ideal tool for assessing PHIs, but with it come challenges.

In this chapter we consider the use and challenges of economic modelling of PHIs. Section 11.2 describes the use of decision analytic modelling within health economics more generally. We then identify the key challenges associated with the development of health economic models of PHIs within section 11.3, highlighting the features of public health systems which create the challenges, current practice for dealing with them, and the latest methodological research. Section 11.4 describes early-stage decision modelling and its benefits for evaluation of PHIs, showcased by a case study assessing foster care interventions. Finally, within section 11.5 we set out four key principles of good practice for developing the structure of public health economic models.

11.1 Modelling for economic evaluations

11.1.1 What is a decision analytic model?

A decision analytic model in health economics refers to a mathematical decision-making tool which structures evidence on costs and outcomes to inform decisions regarding health care resource use in public health services and clinical practices (Weinstein et al., 2003). A decision model is a framework for undertaking an economic evaluation which can be structured in different ways. The role of a model is used to synthesize evidence on costs and outcomes from a variety of sources. Models can vary substantially with regards to structure and complexity, some being nothing more than extended spreadsheet calculations, while in recent years more complex and detailed models have emerged as computing capacity has increased.

Decision analysis has been adopted as a robust framework for conducting economic evaluations of health technologies and PHIs (Briggs et al., 2006). An economic evaluation can be designed to compare two or more interventions using a decision model based entirely on previously published evidence, or it can be built using purposely collected data from a trial. This could be supported by a wider range of data beyond the trial time frame on costs and effects from other sources, such as observational studies and meta-analysis (Kuntz and Weinstein, 2001) to be synthesized within the model in order to derive cost-effectiveness outcomes. In this case, the model uses mathematical relationships to synthesize input information (such as clinical and cost inputs) from numerous sources and defines a series of possible consequences depending on the options being compared (Briggs et al., 2006).

11.1.2 **Decision analytic modelling: Basic steps**

As just set out, decision analysis represents a technique for structuring decision problems. It is an approach that has been used in a range of disciplines such as engineering, law and business (Raffia and Schlaifer, 1959), and more recently environmental remediation. It has also been adopted in health care as a framework for making decisions under uncertainty (Goldie and Corso, 2003).

The basic steps for building a decision analytic model (Briggs et al., 2006) involve (i) understanding and specifying the decision problem, (ii) defining the boundaries, (iii) specifying the model structure, (iv) identifying and synthesizing evidence, and (v) dealing with uncertainty. An additional step involves (vi) using value of information (VOI) techniques to explore potential value of further research (Briggs et al., 2006). These key components are discussed in turn, although they would not necessarily be undertaken in a linear fashion in practice.

11.1.2.1 Understanding and specifying the problem

This stage requires a thorough understanding of the decision problem so that an appropriate and clear objective for the evaluation is set. This will help clearly define the relevant aspects of the question that need to be addressed by the analysis. The alternative health care interventions or technologies being evaluated need to be specified, which is likely to be the new intervention compared to a control or current practice. However, the evaluation may involve more than two alternatives depending on the decision problem. The outcome measures should be defined: what will be the primary measure of effectiveness? Additionally, the relevant health care area and population should be specified. Other aspects to be included are the setting (e.g. community health services, primary care) and the perspective of the analysis. The perspective will tend to be determined by who is funding the research or who it will be used by; that is, a National Health Service- (NHS) funded research project may request a NHS perspective, as opposed to a societal perspective which could incorporate 'indirect' costs incurred by patients and carers. In PHIs a broader perspective, beyond that of the NHS, is likely to be of importance as there may be a significant cost burden (or saving) for patients and carers or other sectors. As discussed in Chapter 3 of this book, recent National Institute for Health and Care Excellence (NICE) guidance recommends adopting a broad enough perspective to capture costs borne by patients and carers that are not reimbursed by the public sector, as well as the traditional NHS and Social Service costs (National Institute for Health and Care Excellence, 2014a).

11.1.2.2 Defining boundaries

This stage involves considering what time horizon is relevant to the model and what range of impacts we are interested in. Should the outcomes be modelled over the patient's lifetime or is a shorter duration more appropriate to answer the research question? This will relate to the health care area and outcome of interest. For example, are short-term intervention specific health outcomes of relevance, such as improvements in mental health, or are longer-term outcomes of more relevance such as life expectancy or quality-adjusted life years (QALYs)? With respect to recommended guidelines, different countries have differing preferences for outcome measurement in economic evaluations. As discussed in Chapter 8 of this book, the UK decision-making body, NICE, has a preference for using QALY outcomes to inform their decision-making (Latimer, 2013). However, the most recent NICE guidelines recognize that a QALY outcome may not adequately capture the most important benefits from a PHI (National Institute for Health and Care Excellence, 2014a). The guidance still advises on cost–utility analyses but gives more weighting to cost–consequence analyses which can consider a wide range of health and non-health outcomes that may be more appropriate. It is therefore advisable to consider both short- and longer-term outcomes for PHIs and attempt to meet the decision-maker's requirements for a QALY as well as considering specific outcome measures relevant to the public health situation.

Defining boundaries also relates to the potential impacts of the interventions under evaluation and whether they need to be included in the model. For example, it is usually important to incorporate negative side-effects from interventions as well as the potential benefits. If the intervention was an intensive service to promote smoking cessation amongst pregnant women, use of nicotine replacement therapy (NRT) alongside cognitive behavioural therapy could potentially have negative impacts on the unborn baby which should be considered as well as the benefits for both mother and child from quitting smoking. In defining boundaries for this example, consideration should be given to the positive and negative impacts for the mother and for the child, and whether the boundary should include both individuals or just focus on the mother, who is the target of the intervention. As this example highlights, careful consideration should be given to defining the boundaries of the model so that all important consequences relevant to the decision problem are incorporated. Researchers could ask, 'do the consequences impact on the costs or quality of life of the target population within the time horizon relevant to the model?' In some cases, consequences or side-effects may be negligible and not be expected to have a large impact on the model population; alternatively, there may be longer-term impacts outwith the relevant model time frame. In such cases it may be appropriate to consider such impacts to be beyond the boundaries of the model.

Defining boundaries ensures that the model is an appropriate (yet simplified) reflection of real life. It is important that the model adheres to quality assurance in that the boundaries are not so restrictive that they bias the analysis by excluding important factors.

11.1.2.3 Specifying the model structure

An appropriate structure for a model should be determined based on the problem specification and defined boundaries. A model can be as simple or as complex as required, as long as it is fit for purpose. The most commonly employed model structures for health care evaluations are now outlined.

Decision trees are a common structure used for simple analyses or those with short time horizons. A decision tree is a model which maps the patient pathway, assigning cost and outcomes to alternative pathways or 'branches' throughout the tree (Barton et al., 2004). Decision trees are popular due to their simple structure and the transparent nature of the tree; however, they are less valuable for modelling complicated interventions or over long time durations as they can become 'bushy' very quickly if there are numerous decision options (decision nodes) at different stages in the model, and they lack an explicit time variable (Petrou and Gray, 2011).

Markov models are more useful for analyses over a longer duration, involving transitions between various health states and outcomes over time (Sonnenberg and Beck, 1993). The main limitation with Markov models is that they do not account for the history of progression in the model. This is known as the Markovian assumption (Briggs and Sculpher, 1997) and means that transition probabilities between health states are independent of the history of the patient and depend only on the current health state. This also means that it is difficult to incorporate individual characteristics which may affect outcomes. Despite these limitations, Markov models remain a common structure for modelling lifetime outcomes, however, in recent years more complex forms of modelling have become ever more popular (Caro et al., 2012).

Over the last decade, discrete event simulations (DES) (Karnon et al., 2012) have grown in popularity, simulating the progress of individuals through a health care system. The nature of DES permits more flexible modelling, allowing programming of individual characteristics and patient history to affect outcomes and interaction between patients over long time durations, thereby overcoming some of the restrictions of Markov modelling (Brennan et al., 2006). However, they require specialist software and programming skills to develop and run (Barton et al., 2004). Other more complex modelling approaches include agent-based modelling (ABM) an individual-level simulation approach (which allows interaction and special aspects to be modelled more easily) and system dynamics (a cohort approach which allows dynamic processes to be modelled using stocks and flows and feedback loops). Dynamic models are popular for modelling infectious diseases and may be appropriate for use in modelling PHIs (Squires et al., 2016) as they can capture relevant complex relationships and feedback loops.

The choice of model structure depends on various factors but they are predominantly determined by the decision-makers' requirements, the complexity of the disease or health care area, and the modellers expertise or preference (Brennan et al., 2006). It is important to note that a simple model structure does not necessarily imply a simple analysis, and indeed some complex models may not address the research question appropriately. The key issue is not the complexity of a model but that the model structure chosen is appropriate to meet the needs of and address the decision problem under consideration. The type of model used is subjective to the modeller, but as different modelling approaches can produce different results and have different levels of transparency, it is important for researchers to be explicit in the reasoning for choice of model structure.

11.1.2.4 Identifying and synthesizing evidence

This stage involves the systematic combination of evidence from a range of sources (literature, professional expert opinion and statistical analysis) in order to structure and populate the decision model. There needs to be a systematic approach taken to identifying all the relevant evidence for the model (Paisley, 2016). The model input evidence is classified into functions and parameters which are used to reflect the data on events, effectiveness, utility information, resource use, and unit cost information. For example, quality of life and utility data for the population may be derived from a survey or from an observational study; the probability of different delivery options for a public health service may be informed by a combination of published national guidelines or health professional expert opinion, while effectiveness data may be derived from one or more community or randomized trials.

The synthesis of data from various sources can give rise to potential issues, such as no direct comparisons from randomized controlled trials (RCTs) for the interventions of interest, different follow-up times from different studies, multiple endpoints, and heterogeneity. Heterogeneity issues are common in PHIs which have differing patient characteristics between trials and also tend to suffer from poorly described interventions, short follow-up durations, and inconsistent analyses. Issues with heterogeneity can be dealt with through a variety of methods including indirect and mixed treatment comparisons and meta-regression (Glenny et al., 2005; Ades et al., 2006). However, better designed PHIs to generate higher quality primary data are required, as discussed further in section 11.3.

11.1.2.5 Dealing with uncertainty

Regardless of whether an economic evaluation is undertaken based on a decision analytic model, or based on a single well-designed RCT, it will be subject to uncertainty. With regards to decision modelling, uncertainty can pertain to sampling variation, heterogeneity, methodological uncertainty, structural uncertainty, parameter uncertainty and decision uncertainty, each of which requires to be dealt with differently (Briggs, 2000, 2001; Briggs et al., 2006)

In trials, variability between individual patients is normally addressed through randomization and analysis of baseline statistics. Sensitivity analysis can be undertaken with access to patient level data, but in a model where the data have been derived from published evidence, this may or may not have been addressed by those reporting the evidence, and it cannot be addressed through collection of more data (Briggs et al., 2006). Assessing heterogeneity requires consideration of various study population subgroups to assess whether other factors inherent in these groups influence the study outcomes by confounding or overriding the actual treatment effects; that is, different age groups, differences in gender or socio-economic background. NICE recognizes the importance of heterogeneity and specifically recommends subgroup analysis in all technology and public health intervention appraisals submitted for its consideration (Latimer, 2013; National Institute for Health and Care Excellence, 2014a). Despite this, reporting on subgroups is particularly poor in studies on PHIs. Section 11.4 of this chapter describes using early decision modelling which could help facilitate the identification of appropriate subgroups upon which to collect primary data.

Parameter uncertainty refers to uncertainty in the point estimates used to reflect the specific parameters in the model, that is, uncertainty in the mean utility value assigned to a specific group of individuals, or uncertainty in the probability of an event. Parameter uncertainty can be dealt with deterministically through univariate and multivariate sensitivity analysis, however, probabilistic sensitivity analysis (PSA) is recommended best practice (Caro et al., 2012; Husereau et al., 2013) as it accounts for the uncertainty around each of the model input parameters, and is used to demonstrate how this impacts on the expected outcomes and uncertainty in the final cost, effect, and cost-effectiveness outcomes (Claxton, 1999b; Briggs, 2000).

Methodological uncertainty refers to uncertainty regarding whether the methods used were the most appropriate. Methodological uncertainties can be dealt with through the use of a benchmark approach or reference case for appropriate methodology, that is, by following good practice guidelines for undertaking modelling (Philips et al., 2006; Caro et al., 2012). The generalizability of model results can be explored by altering parameters in the model that may have been specific to a particular setting.

Uncertainty around the most appropriate model structure may be dealt with retrospectively following model implementation by expressing the impact of uncertainties upon the model results and/or prospectively by considering the process through which decisions are made around the conceptualization, structuring, and implementation of the model. Uncertainty regarding the structure of the model is most commonly dealt with by one-way sensitivity analyses and scenario analyses, modifying one or more structural aspects or assumptions of the model, and determining the impact on outcomes. More recently, it has been suggested that a formal framework is required to address structural uncertainty, both prospectively (Squires et al., 2016) and retrospectively (Bojke et al., 2009; Jackson et al., 2011).

Finally, decision uncertainty should also be explored. Decision uncertainty refers to the level of uncertainty in the cost-effectiveness outcome from the model, and is typically illustrated by plotting the outcomes from the PSA on a cost-effectiveness plane (Fenwick and Byford, 2005; Barton et al., 2008). If there is considerable decision uncertainty and it is unclear whether an intervention should be adopted, an exploration can be undertaken to assess whether further evidence is required to support this decision in the future.

11.1.2.6 Exploring the value of further information

Value of information analyses (VOI) can be undertaken to help deal with decision uncertainty. VOI is based on the rationale that decisions based on existing information will be uncertain, and given this uncertainty, there is a chance that the wrong decision will be made which will have a cost in terms of health (and public health) implications for individuals receiving suboptimal care or services and inefficient use of health care resources (Claxton et al., 2004). VOI analyses value further research for its potential ability to reduce the expected costs of uncertainty surrounding the cost-effectiveness decision, rather than deciding on further research through arbitrary means (Claxton, 1999a; Claxton 1999b). VOI can be of particular use for informing the design of PHIs and also when used as part of an 'early-stage' decision model, undertaken prior to a large-scale primary public health trial, as discussed further in section 11.4.

11.1.3 **Best practice for modelling in healthcare evaluation**

Brennan and Akehurst (2000) discuss the many roles of economic modelling, while others (Brennan et al., 2006) classify various model structures to indicate the range of modelling approaches and their structural relationships. The authors also provide some guidance on choice of model structure, and highlight the fact that different modelling approaches can produce very different results. As computing capacity has increased over the last few decades, so too have the variety of modelling methods available and therefore best practice guidelines are regularly updated to reflect the variety of model forms and promote robust methods and guidance on choice of model (Caro et al., 2012). The guidance promotes a systematic, rigorous, and transparent approach to data collection, synthesis of cost and effect data, analysis, reporting of outcomes, and exploration of uncertainty and heterogeneity. Reporting guidelines have also been consolidated and updated to promote transparent reporting of the methods employed (Husereau et al., 2013).

11.3 **Key challenges for modelling PHIs**

There are a number of modelling challenges when undertaking economic evaluations of PHIs which are not necessarily a concern when modelling clinical interventions. Table 11.1 shows an overview of these key challenges, together with current practice and the latest methodological research associated with each. They are discussed in detail throughout this section. A model assessing the cost-effectiveness of interventions to encourage young people to use contraceptives and contraceptive services will be used as a case study example throughout.

Contraception case study

NICE commissioned an evidence review and model of interventions to encourage young people to use contraceptives and contraceptive services (National Institute for Health and Care Excellence, 2014b).

The choice of interventions to assess within the model was based upon discussions with a Programme Development Group (PDG) according to the evidence reviews and their expertise. Interventions assessed were: the dispensing of condoms within schools, the dispensing of hormonal contraception within schools, intensive case management to prevent repeat teenage pregnancies, advanced provision of emergency hormonal contraception provided to those young people who attend a clinic for contraceptive services, and usual current practice.

A conceptual model was developed of the relationships between factors which might be included within a health economic model. Literature searches were undertaken to facilitate decisions about what to include and exclude. In particular, a search for econometric studies around the causal relationship between teenage pregnancy and associated short- and long-term outcomes (including low birth weight, education, employment, government-funded benefits).

A model was developed in Excel to follow an imaginary cohort of 100,000 young people over a lifetime from the age at which the intervention is provided. There is a probability of becoming pregnant at each age and, following conception, dependent on age, there is a probability of the female having a birth, an abortion, a miscarriage, an ectopic pregnancy, or a stillbirth. The model calculates the costs and consequences associated with these pregnancy outcomes and the cost of the intervention and associated contraceptive services. The model also calculates the impact of any changes in condom use upon sexually transmitted infection (STI) rates.

Costs were calculated from a public sector perspective. Model outcomes are presented in terms of the cost per age-specific pregnancy averted and the cost per abortion averted. It was not feasible or considered appropriate to calculate results in terms of a cost per QALY gained. An elicitation technique was used with members of the PDG at NICE to try and establish a valuation of delaying pregnancy for interventions falling in the north-east quadrant.

Table 11.1 Key modelling challenges in public health and current practice and research

Feature of public health systems	Modelling challenge	Current practice	Latest methodological research
The aim of public health is to be equitable rather than to maximize cost-effectiveness.	The extent that equity considerations should be incorporated within a model. More complex modelling approaches may be required to capture individual characteristics.	Cost-effectiveness over the entire population of the model is typically reported and equity considerations are not often incorporated within the model.	Cookson and colleagues have recently proposed practical options for including health equity concerns in cost-effectiveness analyses (Cookson, et al., 2017).
Interventions are often multi-component.	Extrapolating intervention effectiveness beyond study data. However, the solution is better primary data rather than the development of modelling methods.	Simple methods of extrapolation are often used such as linear regression. Methods of extrapolation are well developed, but studies of PHIs are generally inconsistent, with short follow-up and poorly described interventions.	The MRC has produced guidance for developing and evaluating complex interventions (Medical Research Council, 2008). Early-stage decision modelling can be used to guide primary data collection (see section 11.4).
The system is often dynamically complex.	Models must capture relevant complex relationships and feedback loops.	Often simple cause-and-effect is modelled using decision trees and Markov models with little transparency over decisions about the model boundary.	A conceptual modelling framework has been developed which proposes using a systems approach (Squires et al., 2016). Also, more use could be made of econometric methodology (Kelly et al., 2005; Weatherly et al., 2009).

Table 11.1 Continued

Feature of public health systems	Modelling challenge	Current practice	Latest methodological research
Human behaviour is a key driver of outcomes.	Modelling human behaviour.	A large majority of models developed to assess PHIs are cohort models which do not attempt to capture the interventions' mechanism of action. Individual-level simulations that have been developed are generally informed via large datasets.	There are hundreds of models of human behaviour within psychology, sociology, and behavioural economics which could be useful. Additional research would be required to employ them within a health economic model.
The social determinants of health affect intervention effectiveness.	Capturing relevant non-health costs and outcomes and the relationship between individual and social determinants.	A large majority of models developed to assess PHIs are cohort models and many of them focus upon health costs and outcomes.	A conceptual modelling framework has been developed to help modellers identify and choose relevant costs and outcomes to include within the decision-analytic model (Squires et al., 2016). Methods are also being developed for presenting model results in alternative formats to help decision-makers understand where costs and outcomes are incurred (Kelly et al., 2005; Claxton et al., 2007).

Challenge 1: Incorporating equity

One of the key aims of the discipline of public health is to promote equity and work towards improving the health of the worst-off in society. This is arguably at variance with the implicit goal of maximizing cost-effectiveness across the entire population, the latter being the premise upon which standard health economic modelling is based. Thus, to handle this, cost-effectiveness is typically reported over the entire population of the model with equity considerations often omitted (West et al., 2003; Rush et al., 2004; McDaid and Needle, 2009). The different options for considering equity are discussed as one of the challenges facing health economists in Chapter 15 of this book. Cookson and colleagues have recently proposed some practical options for including health equity concerns in cost-effectiveness analyses (Cookson, et al., (2019)) and indeed it is the focus of the 6th book in this OUP series. In order for equity to be included quantitatively within a model, ideally intervention effectiveness evidence would be available by relevant subgroups and individual characteristics would be modelled. Established individual simulation methods exist including DES and agent-based modelling (ABM) (Pidd, 2009; Macal and North, 2010; Chhatwal and He, 2015). There is a growing recognition that such modelling methods are well suited to the economic evaluation of PHIs. DES is a top-down approach which involves assigning individual characteristics to entities which determine their pathways within the system. ABM is a bottom-up approach which involves defining 'rules' for the behaviour of the individuals and their interaction with the system (Siebers et al., 2010). DES may be appropriate when the interaction between the individual and their environment is important (e.g. a person attends cancer screening which changes the probability of subsequent outcomes); whilst ABS may be preferable when the interactions between heterogeneous agents are important in addition to their interactions with the environment (e.g. infectious disease modelling). ABS allows the analyst to capture spatial aspects more easily in order to model appropriate interactions (e.g. family and friend networks) (Siebers et al., 2010). The merits of both approaches have recently been recognized by the health economics community (Karnon et al., 2012; Marshall et al., 2015) and the application of DES is growing within health economic modelling (Karnon et al., 2012). Training for health economic modellers and publishing case studies using these methods should increase their adoption within the health and public health economics community.

Contraception case study

Within the contraception case study, the project scope was to assess contraceptive interventions for young people, especially socially disadvantaged young people. No evidence was identified around specific subgroups of people that might be considered to be socially disadvantaged; however, since the proportion of socially disadvantaged people having teenage pregnancies is greater than the proportion of teenage pregnancies within the general population, those teenagers becoming pregnant within the model will predominantly consist of socially disadvantaged young people.

The model submitted to NICE could have been improved by using an individual-level simulation to capture outcomes according to individual characteristics such as social class and education level. This would allow variation between individuals to be captured. An example of an individual-level simulation schematic is shown within Figure 11.1. It should be noted that the modelling would be limited by the data

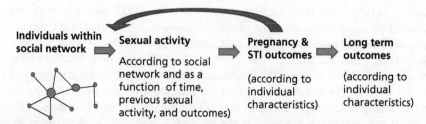

Figure 11.1 Example of an individual-level model.

available, and hence in the absence of effectiveness data by these individual characteristics the analysis would need to be exploratory.

Additional advantages of an individual-level simulation for this case study are:

—The spread of STIs could be modelled dynamically, allowing the infections to be passed to more than one individual to avoid systematically underestimating costs and effects (see Challenge 3).

—Individual learning could be captured following an unintended pregnancy, affecting future behaviour (see Challenge 3).

Challenge 2: Extrapolating multi-component intervention effectiveness beyond study data

PHIs are complex interventions by definition and as such, tend to be made up of multiple components. This makes extrapolation beyond study data problematic if the mechanism of action is unknown. Methods of extrapolation are well developed (Latimer, 2013; Collett, 2015), but studies of PHIs are generally inconsistent, with short follow-up and poorly described interventions (West et al., 2003; Rush et al., 2004; McDaid and Needle, 2009). The short follow-up, often of a year or less, usually means that long-term outcomes must be predicted using a series of intermediate outcomes which do not generally have well-described relationships. In addition, randomized controlled trials are often not feasible or inappropriate due to the nature of the interventions.

Better primary data collection would help to address this challenge. This could be done by obtaining health economic modelling expertise at the design stage so that relevant outcomes are collected within an appropriate design. Section 11.4 describes the process and benefits of early-stage decision modelling. In addition, the Medical Research Council (MRC) has produced guidance for developing and evaluating complex interventions (Medical Research Council, 2008). Finally, modelling assumptions should be described transparently within the report.

Contraception case study

Within the effectiveness studies identified there was wide variation in intervention delivery, results were reported at 3, 6, or a maximum of 12 months, and the reported outcomes varied between studies (including pregnancy, contraceptive use, contraceptive knowledge, access to services).

We do not know:

- How the different components of the interventions contribute to the outcomes;
- Whether the effectiveness of the interventions continues beyond the last point of follow-up;
- Whether the pregnancies which are prevented by the interventions are unwanted or mistimed (i.e. whether it has led to fewer pregnancies and what the counterfactual is);
- If the interventions are more effective for one age group than another, or for females compared with males;
- Precisely how immediate outcomes such as access to services are related to pregnancy outcomes and how this is related to longer-term outcomes such as educational attainment, employment status, and quality of life.

There are also issues with the generalizability of the studies, with many undertaken in other countries, leading to uncertainty around the effectiveness of the interventions in the United Kingdom.

Due to the extensive heterogeneity between studies, each intervention assessed within the model was based upon a specific study, chosen to be of the highest quality and the most representative for a UK analysis. Within the model, a large number of assumptions were made in order to deal with these issues and these were described transparently within the accompanying report (Pilgrim et al., 2010). Alternative structural assumptions around whether pregnancies were prevented or mistimed were incorporated into the model and then included within the probabilistic sensitivity analysis via a probability parameter. In addition, one-way sensitivity analysis was undertaken to assess the impact of alternative assumptions where possible.

Challenge 3: Models must capture relevant complex relationships and feedback loops of a dynamically complex system

Public health systems are generally dynamically complex. The characteristics of this sort of system are shown in Table 11.2, illustrated by the contraception case study.

Tools which can help us to understand these complex systems are required for public health economic modelling. A systems approach takes a holistic way of thinking about complex systems, and focuses upon the interactions between the entities and between entities and their environment, rather than assuming that a system can be understood by breaking it down into its individual entities and studying each part separately (Miller and Page, 2007). The system of interest is subjectively defined and there is always a higher level system within which it belongs and a lower level system which describes detailed aspects. It is not feasible to take a completely systemic approach as this would involve modelling the whole world, and it is thus important to understand the most appropriate boundary around the model in order to avoid excluding important consequences of an intervention. Smith and Petticrew (2010) advocate such a systems approach and there have been a number of case studies within public health which adopt this systems approach, to attempt to handle the complexity of the systems (McPherson et al., 2007; National Cancer Institute, 2007); however, this is not currently standard practice within health economic modelling.

Key systems approaches are shown in Table 11.3 based upon the four-volume *Systems Thinking* by Midgley (2003) and *Total Systems Intervention* by Flood and Jackson (1991).

A conceptual modelling framework has been developed which recommends using a systems approach for public health economic modelling, including drawing upon problem structuring methods, considering the use of individual-level simulation and network analysis, and having stakeholder input throughout model development (Squires et al., 2016).

There are a number of existing approaches to facilitate understanding of causal relationships including econometric methodology and causal mapping (Kelly et al., 2005; Weatherly et al., 2009).

Table 11.2 Aspects of a dynamically complex system

Key aspects of a dynamically complex system	Contraception case study example
Interactions between the individuals and their environment are important in defining outcomes.	The rate of pregnancies and STIs is dependent upon the sexual interactions between people.
Characterized by feedback loops (non-linearity). The dynamics of complex systems arise from the interaction between positive feedback loops (where an increase [decrease] in one factor leads to an increase [decrease] in another, which in turn causes the first factor to increase [decrease], which would lead to exponential growth [decay] if no other factors were present) and negative feedback loops (where an increase [decrease] in one factor leads to a decrease [increase] in another, which in turn causes the first factor to decrease [increase], which often leads to self-correcting behaviour) (Sterman, 2000). The interaction between these feedback loops often produces counter-intuitive behaviour, particularly where there are long time delays between cause and effect, and this makes it difficult to predict the behaviour (Sterman, 2000).	*Positive:* An unintended teenage birth is thought to be associated with an increased probability of the child having a disadvantaged background which is associated with unintended pregnancy in later life. *Negative:* Poor contraceptive use may lead to the development of a STI which may lead to better contraceptive use.
Variability between individuals is important, which may result in emergent behaviour. Modelling the 'average' person would be misleading in these cases (Miller and Page, 2007).	The decision of one person to use contraception might just be sufficient to encourage another person to use contraception and so on until there is a general change in attitudes and behaviour.
Timing and time delays are important. Factors within the system change over time at different rates and outcomes may be affected by when particular events happen (Miller and Page, 2007). Time delays within feedback loops mean that long term outcomes are often incorrectly predicted by policy-makers due to the interactions between feedback loops, the limited learning cycles available as a result of changing policies, and the difficulty of holding other variables within the system constant within trials for longer time periods (Sterman, 2000).	The time at which a person has a baby during their lifetime may affect outcomes. In addition, differences in socio-economic outcomes may not be seen for a number of years.
Characterized by self-organization, dependent upon networks. Each individual does not understand the behaviour of the system as a whole (Sterman, 2000). Individuals may organize themselves so that those with similar preferences group together (Miller and Page, 2007; Kelly et al., 2009).	The sexual activity and contraceptive behaviour of young people is not centrally organized. The groups young people associate with will influence their sexual activity, their contraceptive use and attitude towards STIs and pregnancy.

(*continued*)

Table 11.2 Continued

Key aspects of a dynamically complex system	Contraception case study example
There may be unintended consequences of the interventions. Policy-makers may not appreciate the impact of time delays, non-linearity, variability, and social networks. In addition, outcomes are often unanticipated because of the responses of people within the system who the intervention is not aimed at and who have different aims to the policy-makers (Sterman, 2006).	Encouraging young people to use intrauterine devices may decrease the number of pregnancies but increase the number of STIs, as well as condom companies potentially increasing advertising.
No clear boundary around the system. All systems are subsystems of a bigger system, and it is important to define the system of interest at a level where all important interactions between the individuals for the purpose of the model are captured (Flood and Jackson, 1991).	Interventions to reduce initial disadvantage may have impacts in addition to reducing unintended teenage pregnancies such as decreasing crime rates.
Individuals may learn over time and change their behaviour accordingly. Individual behaviours also tend to reinforce one another through their interactions (Miller and Page, 2007).	Young people may change their contraceptive use over time. For example, after having a STI a person may be more likely to use condoms in the future.

Table 11.3 Systems approaches

Approach	Description
Critical systems heuristics and boundary critique	A qualitative approach which involves the analyst identifying the boundary judgements (what is included in the system and what is part of its external environment), questioning the practical and ethical implications of those judgements with all relevant stakeholders (the choice of stakeholders being part of the boundary judgement in itself), and challenging claims of the stakeholders using factual knowledge.
Problem-structuring methods	Qualitative techniques to draw out the structure and nature of a problem situation from all stakeholders' perspectives in an exploratory and transparent manner, acknowledging uncertainties.
Network analysis	Qualitatively mapping and measuring relationships between entities including people and groups.
Cybernetics	Quantitatively describing the flow of information around a system, and the way in which this information is used by the system as a means of controlling itself.
System dynamics modelling	A quantitative cohort simulation modelling approach which captures the stocks and flows and positive and negative feedback loops within the system over time.
Individual-level modelling (including DES and ABM)	Quantitative modelling which captures individual characteristics and their impact upon outcomes.

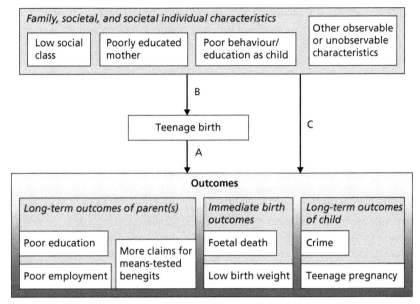

Figure 11.2 Relationship between individual characteristics, teenage birth and outcomes.

Contraception case study

Studies which compare long-term outcomes of people who had a teenage pregnancy with those who had an older pregnancy suggest that teenage pregnancy is associated with negative long-term outcomes (relationship A in Figure 11.2). However, it may be that there are underlying characteristics which affect both the likelihood of teenage pregnancy (relationship B in Figure 11.2) and long-term outcomes (relationship C in Figure 11.2).

A literature review was undertaken of studies using econometric techniques, such as family-fixed effects, instrumental variable techniques, and propensity score matching, to understand these causal relationships. The results of these studies were used within the model.

One way in which systems thinking was used within the contraception case study was involving all relevant stakeholders throughout the model development process via workshops, facilitating the development of a valid and useful model. The model could have been improved by using some of the systems approaches outlined within Table 11.3, including social network analysis and individual-level simulation (as described within Challenge 2).

Challenge 4: Modelling human behaviour

Human behaviour is often a key driver of outcomes of complex PHIs. Within psychology, hundreds of models of human behaviour have been developed which provide an understanding of the individual factors required for the adoption of a specified behaviour. However, only a small number of these have had empirical applications. A review by Taylor and colleagues identified the 'Health Belief Model', the 'Theory of Reasoned Action', the 'Theory of Planned Behaviour', and the 'Trans-Theoretical Model' as the most commonly used cognitive models within health promotion (Taylor et al., 2006). However, none of these four models adequately capture social, economic, or environmental factors as predictors and determinants of health behaviour (Taylor et al., 2006). Recently, case studies have been undertaken to consider incorporating human behaviour into mathematical models of public health (Brailsford and Schmidt, 2003; Hu and Puddy, 2011; Kruger et al., 2013). However, there were difficulties with parameterization in these cases. Whilst theoretically, all four of the above behavioural models could be used to model quantitatively how behaviour changes within public health, this requires substantial methodological research both in terms of practical implementation and in terms of methods for parameterization. Currently, the incorporation of psychological models has been largely overlooked and this could be an important area of further research in public health economic modelling. Similarly, research around the potential benefits of employing behavioural economics, which integrates psychology with neoclassical economics, may be useful (Thaler and Mullainathan, 2008).

Sociology seeks to provide insights into the many forms of relationships between people (including cultural, economic, and political) to understand how society works (McKie and Ryan, 2016). It has the potential to provide tools for modelling the impact of interactions within society upon outcomes. Within the last decade, sociology has been linked with dynamically complex systems (see Challenge 3) to form a discipline defined as sociology and complexity science (SACS) (Castellani and Hafferty, 2009). Both sociology and complexity science follow a non-reductionist, subjective approach, making use of qualitative research methods (as well as quantitative methods in the case of complexity science). One of the biggest areas of work within SACS is complex social network analysis (Castellani and Hafferty, 2009) which involves the use of a range of techniques including ABM and social network analysis (mapping social networks to understand who is at the hub of the network) (Siebers et al., 2010). Social network analysis could be applied within ABMs (Christakis and Fowler, 2008). Methods for both of these are well established, although they have rarely been employed for public health economic evaluation models. Currently, a large majority of models developed to assess PHIs are cohort models, and the small number of individual-level simulations that have been developed have generally been informed via large datasets (West et al., 2003; Rush et al., 2004; McDaid and Needle, 2009). There is enormous scope for advancing modelling methods within public health economic evaluation through collaboration with the disciplines of psychology and sociology.

Contraception case study

Sexual behaviour and sexually transmitted infections are affected by social groupings and environmental factors. Since this modelling project was undertaken, there has been some research into adolescent sexual behaviour using social network analysis which could be incorporated into future models by assigning probabilities for sexual interaction for each individual within the model (Brakefield et al., 2014). There may also be existing models of sexual behaviour from psychology or sociology which could be incorporated into a health economic model.

Challenge 5: Capturing relevant non-health costs and outcomes and the relationship between individual and social determinants

The determinants of health are individual-, community-, and population-level factors (Kelly et al., 2009), and they need to be sufficiently considered to identify all relevant costs and outcomes of PHIs. In addition, the broader determinants of health relating to the community and the population create dynamic complexity (see Challenge 3) due to the interactions between individuals and their social structure. Health economic models help to make predictions about the future and it is not possible to do this well without an understanding of underlying mechanisms.

There are many different classifications of the determinants of health and the determinants of health inequities. Dahlgren and Whitehead's model, reproduced in Figure 1.1 of this book, developed perhaps the most well-known model within a document for the World Health Organization which aimed to describe the determinants of health inequities (Dahlgren and Whitehead, 1991), including inherent characteristics, lifestyle factors, social and community networks, living and working conditions, and the structural environment.

There may often be discrepancies between the data provided by intervention effectiveness studies and the evidence required for models in relation to the determinants of health. Intervention effectiveness studies may capture all or some of the effects of the broader determinants of health and their interactions within the outcomes presented. However, they tend not to report how the determinants of health impact upon outcomes, making extrapolation of the outcomes over the long term or to other contexts challenging (see Challenge 2). Capturing the heterogeneity between individuals within the model in terms of the broader determinants of health is likely to be important because it is this heterogeneity that impacts upon the effectiveness of the interventions. In addition, the modeller should be aware that the determinants may impact upon overall health and health inequities in different ways (see Challenge 1).

There is an abundance of literature around the causal relationships between the determinants of health within the public health literature (Kelly et al., 2009); however, Kelly and colleagues suggest that whilst much is known about the general relationship between health and social factors, the precise causal pathways are not yet fully understood. Little consideration is currently given to the broader determinants of health within the health economics literature. A large majority of models currently developed to assess PHIs are cohort models and many of them focus upon health costs and outcomes (West et al., 2003; Rush et al., 2004; McDaid and Needle, 2009). A conceptual modelling framework has recently been developed which aims to help modellers identify and choose relevant costs and outcomes to include within the model and to describe the causal relationships between them (Squires et al., 2016). The key principles of good practice underlining this are described within section 11.5. In addition, methods are being developed for presenting model results in alternative formats to help decision-makers understand within which sectors costs and outcomes are incurred (Kelly et al., 2005; Claxton et al., 2007; Weatherly et al., 2009).

Contraception case study

Within the contraception case study, sexual activity is affected by social networks and the choice of partner may impact upon contraceptive use. There is also a complex relationship between socio-economic status and teenage pregnancy and abortion. Teenage pregnancy is associated with a range of outcomes including poorer living and working conditions, although the causal relationships are not well described. During a conceptual modelling process stage we attempted to map out the potential causal relationships and identify evidence which attempts to describe those relationships.

Two approaches for attempting to address the challenges identified within this section are set out within sections 11.4 and 11.5; Section 11.4 describes early-stage decision modelling which could be used to guide primary data collection within the context of an iterative approach to evaluating PHIs, whilst Section 11.4 sets out four key principles of good practice when developing public health economic model structures, taken from a recently developed conceptual modelling framework for constructing such models.

11.4 Early-stage decision modelling for health economics and public health economics

11.4.1 Early-stage decision modelling

An 'early-stage' decision model, undertaken prior to primary research, allows explorative evaluation of cost-effectiveness based on existing evidence and can be used to help inform the design of a future study or trial, based on an assessment of current uncertainty surrounding the cost-effectiveness decision (Fenwick et al., 2000; Claxton et al., 2005). Early-stage modelling is based within the framework of an iterative approach to economic appraisal (Sculpher et al., 2006). The iterative framework that has been proposed as best practice (Sculpher et al., 1997; Sculpher et al., 2006) for evaluating health care technologies, can be applied to PHIs which are often complex. The framework proposes that the process of health care evaluation should begin with an explorative 'early-stage' modelling approach using indicative studies and information from health professionals and experts to assess cost-effectiveness based on existing information, and progress to more rigorous assessments, updating a decision model over time as more data becomes available (Sculpher et al., 1997; Sculpher et al., 2006). The iterative approach to evaluation provides a structure in which evidence from a range of sources can be synthesized and continually updated in order to answer cost-effectiveness decision problems for a defined context and population. The premise is that rather than using economic evaluation as a restrictive, one-off analysis, it should be an iterative process conducted alongside all stages of health care research.

Adopting an iterative approach to economic evaluation through building early-stage decision models prior to the design of public health intervention trials would also promote the good practice recommended in section 11.5 of this chapter.

The iterative approach to economic evaluation is now discussed within the context of evaluating PHIs.

11.4.2 **Iterative approach to economic evaluation of PHIs**

The iterative framework to economic evaluation has five main stages and utilizes the key methodologies for decision analytic modelling which were outlined in section 11.1 of this chapter. The five stages of the iterative approach are: (i) identify decision problem, (ii) synthesis and modelling given available evidence, (iii) setting research priorities, (iv) primary research, and (v) synthesize and modelling. Figure 11.3 (Boyd, 2012) illustrates the five-stage iterative approach initially illustrated by Sculpher and colleagues (Sculpher et al., 2006) and adapted to present the economic tools and decision modelling processes undertaken at each stage (Boyd, 2012).

This section uses a case study of a novel foster care intervention to demonstrate the advantages of adopting an iterative approach to economic appraisal for PHIs.

11.4.2.1 Stage 1—Identify decision problem

This is an explorative stage, focusing on identifying potentially important decision problems for different populations and sub-populations within the identified health care area in order to formulate an appropriate (economic) question. The iterative process therefore begins by exploring the literature, existing information, and consulting stakeholders to identify the decision problem and specify the details. The decision problem may well have been predetermined, for example by a public funding body using their own research, stakeholders, and agendas. If the interventions of interest and patient/population groups have also been predefined, caution should be applied as a set decision question may be too narrowly defined and not necessarily be appropriate. The stage of identifying the decision problem in itself may involve an iterative process where exploration of the literature leads to updating and redefining of the research question itself.

Foster care case study

Services for maltreated children are insufficient in many parts of the world, yet intervening with vulnerable children in their early life can have vast benefits for the child, their family, and society as a whole. Despite this knowledge, infant mental health services in the United Kingdom are poor and none are aimed specifically at maltreated infants. There are also problems in securing permanent placements for abused and neglected children. To explore this decision problem, a wide array of local and international stakeholders and local foster care services were consulted, an audit of local foster care services was undertaken as well as a comprehensive literature review (Scott et al., 2001; Minnis et al., 2010; Boyd et al., 2015) to define an appropriate research question and identify appropriate interventions that would address both the permanency/adoption problem and the mental health issues faced by maltreated children.

11.4.2.2 Stage 2—Synthesis and modelling given current information

Once a specific decision problem has been identified and an appropriate question defined, existing information and evidence can be used to develop and populate an early stage economic model. Evidence from systematic reviews and meta-analyses on effectiveness can be utilized as well as broader evidence from a range of sources

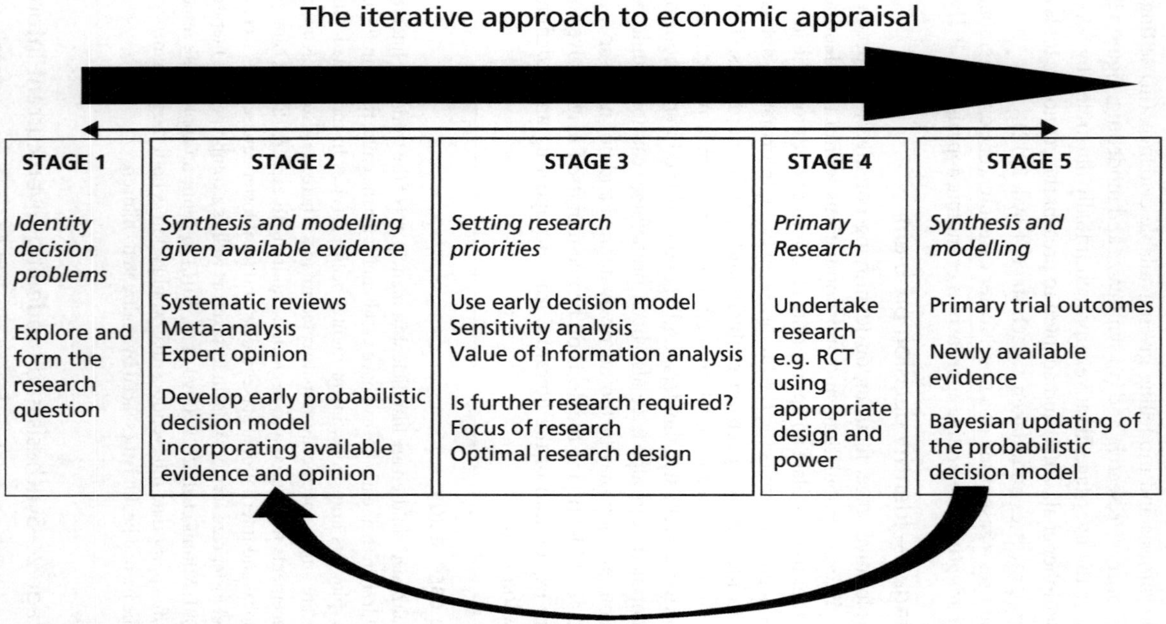

The iterative approach to economic appraisal

STAGE 1	STAGE 2	STAGE 3	STAGE 4	STAGE 5
Identify decision problems	*Synthesis and modelling given available evidence*	*Setting research priorities*	*Primary Research*	*Synthesis and modelling*
Explore and form the research question	Systematic reviews Meta-analysis Expert opinion Develop early probabilistic decision model incorporating available evidence and opinion	Use early decision model Sensitivity analysis Value of Information analysis Is further research required? Focus of research Optimal research design	Undertake research e.g. RCT using appropriate design and power	Primary trial outcomes Newly available evidence Bayesian updating of the probabilistic decision model

Figure 11.3 The iterative approach to economic appraisal.

including expert opinion, can generate evidence for use in a probabilistic decision model. Developing an early-stage model can provide an indication of whether the new intervention is likely to be cost-effective and help define the associated uncertainty.

Foster care case study

An exploratory model of the proposed new intervention and how it could operate in the local context was developed in comparison to the existing local foster care service. It was decided that a formal economic evaluation through a cost-effectiveness analysis was not appropriate as the existing foster care service was not clearly defined and there was no direct clinical evidence on health outcomes in this system or on the proposed new system. Instead a cost–consequence framework was adopted to define and measure the existing local services and compare this with a hypothetical model for the potential new intervention, allowing decision-makers to compare the potential costs and consequences of these two approaches and form their own view of the importance of the different outcomes. The early-stage model highlighted the fact that the proposed intervention for maltreated children in foster care would most likely shift resources from social services on to the NHS. The resource-intensive nature of the new intervention would most likely increase the cost of an episode in care; however, the probability of repeated episodes in care would be likely to fall substantially, thereby reducing the cost per child over the five-year time horizon (Boyd et al., 2015). The proposed new intervention would also be likely to require a much greater time input from birth parents than the current system and would have consequences for the legal system.

11.4.2.3 Stage 3—Setting research priorities

This is a formal process of research prioritization determined by the current evidence and outcomes from the early decision modelling undertaken in stage 2. If a cost-effectiveness analysis has been undertaken using a probabilistic decision model then VOI analysis (Claxton, 1999b) is an ideal tool for setting research priorities and informing whether further research is potentially worthwhile, and in particular which parameters (or groups of parameters) require further evidence. Where VOI is not undertaken, key evidence on outcomes and the associated uncertainty from the decision model in stage 2 can still be used by researchers and policy-makers to inform research priorities and the design of further research.

Foster care case study

Even though a cost-effectiveness analysis and VOI techniques were not undertaken in the early modelling of this study, the early-stage cost–consequence model was extremely helpful for informing local and national policy-makers about the potential resource use and cost impacts in a way that was digestible and useable. It provided policy-makers and service managers with some insight as to the problems (and the associated costs) in existing services and how the system could change with the proposed new intervention from the perspectives of the NHS, social services, and birth families.

The evidence from the early-stage model helped build a case for funding and design of a phase II explorative RCT of the proposed foster care intervention (Pritchett et al., 2013) which then led onto a full phase III RCT (Minnis, et al., 2016) and associated health economic analysis protocol (Deidda et al., 2018).

11.4.2.4 Stage 4—Primary research

Trials in this stage, whether they be exploratory or definitive, should have been designed and powered appropriately to detect a difference in the key parameter driving the primary research, based on the stage 2 early model outcomes and the research priorities established in stage 3. Attempts should be made to adhere to the gold standard practices for economic evaluations within trials (Petrou and Gray, 2011; Glick et al., 2014;) to strengthen the design of the research and improve the quality of the economic evaluation.

Foster care case study

An explorative phase II randomized trial of the proposed foster care intervention was undertaken to evaluate the feasibility of the intervention, assess the process of the new service, and explore the potential cost-effectiveness of this in comparison to current service (Pritchett et al., 2013). This helped inform whether a large-scale definitive RCT was viable and feasible, and then helped inform the design of a definitive trial (Minnis, et al. 2016). The early modelling work also helped inform the design of the explorative phase II trial. In particular, it helped identify important primary and secondary outcomes as well as quality of life outcomes that could be of use to future economic analyses. This explorative trial provided important evidence on both the current system and the new intervention, on which a rigorous economic evaluation can be undertaken. This in turn informed the design of further primary research (Minnis, et al. 2016), including the design of a detailed health economic protocol for the definitive phase III trial (Deidda, et al. 2018).

11.4.2.5 Stage 5—Synthesis and modelling

In this stage, new evidence is incorporated into the information set used within the model; that is, the early decision model from stage 2 is amended and updated with the data generated in the primary trial undertaken in stage 4 and any other evidence published during the interim. The structure of the model may be modified to reflect the decision question rather more effectively, as well as updating the data for the parameter inputs. This is based on a Bayesian concept whereby evidence or knowledge about each parameter in the model can be updated by new information as it becomes available (Claxton, 1999a). Having synthesized the primary research outcomes with any other relevant data in stage 5 (see also Chapter 4), the iterative process can then loop back to stage 2 again if further evidence is required (see Figure 11.3).

Foster care case study

The economic evaluation undertaken alongside the exploratory trial in stage 4, used probabilistic sensitivity analysis. This enables VOI techniques to be used to assess uncertainty in the cost-effectiveness decision based on the trial results. VOI can help inform the value of further research and identify particular areas of uncertainty which still exist that could require further and more rigorous evidence. The outcomes from the exploratory trial were used to update the early-stage model from stage 2, synthesizing the evidence in a robust decision model to make an informed decision about whether a definitive large-scale RCT is needed.

Within this section, we have highlighted the process and advantages of using early modelling and adopting an iterative approach to economic evaluation of PHIs which are often complex, have multiple components, and are less well defined than standard clinical interventions. This iterative approach is also consistent with the systems approach recommended in section 11.3, and aligns with the key principles of good practice which are now set out in section 11.5 for developing public health economic model structures.

11.5 Developing the structure of public health economic models

Decisions about the structure of public health economic models are often more difficult than for models of clinical interventions due to the key challenges described in section 11.3. A conceptual modelling framework to help modellers develop the structure of public health economic model structures has been developed by one of the authors which attempts to address some of these challenges (Squires et al., 2016). The full framework is not described here; however, four key principles of good practice which underlie the framework are set out.

11.5.1 Key principles of good practice

(1) A systems approach to public health modelling should be taken

As described within section 11.3, a systems approach, or systems thinking, is a holistic way of thinking based on the philosophy that to understand a problem it is important to understand the interactions between parts within a system and with its environment (Von Bertalanffy, 1969). The challenge within health economic modelling is to determine an appropriate model boundary to capture all important consequences of the interventions by having sufficient knowledge about the higher-level system (the broader understanding of the problem), and subsequently to be able to define an appropriate level of detail for the system of interest. Within systems thinking, the importance of not considering one aspect of a system in isolation is emphasized to avoid ignoring unintended consequences.

(2) Developing a thorough documented understanding of the problem is imperative prior to and alongside developing and justifying the model structure

As also proposed by Kaltenthaler and colleagues within the context of clinical economic modelling, it is recommended that the model structure be developed in two phases: (i) an understanding of the decision problem which should not be limited by what empirical evidence is available; and (ii) to specify a model structure for the decision problem that is feasible within the constraints of the decision-making process (Kaltenthaler et al., 2011). Documenting an understanding of the problem prior to analysing available datasets allows that understanding to be reflected upon and shared. This reduces the risk of ignoring something which may be important to the model outcomes, which is particularly important given the potential dynamic complexity of the system. It also reduces the risk of developing an inappropriate model structure. Documenting an understanding of the problem (the higher-level system) allows the modeller to be able to define and justify the boundary of the system of interest for modelling (see key principle of good practice 1). It also enables communication with stakeholders and the project team (see key principle of good practice 3), and it will enable researchers and policy-makers who are not involved within the project to understand the problem, and it will form the basis for decisions about the model structure. This links in with stages 1 and 2 of the iterative approach discussed in section 11.4, where identification of the decision problem, interaction with stakeholders, and early-stage modelling can aid identification of further primary research.

(3) Strong communication with stakeholders and members of the team throughout model development is essential

Literature suggests that stakeholders can encourage learning about the problem (including geographical variation of health care provision and stakeholders' values and preferences), help to develop appropriate model objectives and requirements, facilitate model verification and validation, help to develop credibility and confidence in the model and its results, guide model development and experimentation, and encourage creativity in finding a solution and facilitate model reuse (Vennix and Gubbels, 1992; Rodriguez-Ulloa and Paucar-Caceres, 2005; Fernández and Kekäle, 2008; Howick et al., 2008; Kaltenthaler et al., 2011; Robinson, 2011; Roberts et al., 2012). Thus stakeholders should be involved throughout model development.

(4) A systematic consideration of the determinants of health is central to identifying all key impacts of the interventions within public health economic modelling

The determinants of health include inherent characteristics, individual lifestyle factors, social and community networks, living and working conditions, and general socio-economic, cultural, and environmental conditions (Dahlgren and Whitehead, 1991). Individual behaviours impact upon the broader determinants of health, which in turn impact upon individual behaviours (Kelly, 2009). It would not be appropriate or feasible to include all of the determinants of health within a model; however, they should be systematically reflected upon during the understanding of the problem phase to consider which determinants it might be important to include within the model so that all important mechanisms and outcomes of the interventions can be captured.

Summary of Chapter 11

This chapter considered the use of decision analytic modelling for public health economic evaluation. It highlights key challenges for public health economic modelling which can and should be addressed. They are as follows:

♦ Incorporating equity.

♦ Extrapolating multi-component intervention effectiveness beyond study data.

♦ Capturing relevant complex relationships and feedback loops of a dynamically complex system.

♦ Modelling human behaviour.

♦ Capturing relevant non-health costs and outcomes and the relationship between individual and social determinants.

It also described two general approaches which could help to address these challenges:

◆ Adopting an iterative approach to the evaluation by using early-stage decision modelling to guide primary data collection.

◆ Using a conceptual modelling framework to guide the model development process.

References

Ades, A.E., Sculpher, M., Sutton, A., Abrams, K., Cooper, N., Welton, N., and Lu, G., 2006. Bayesian methods for evidence synthesis in cost-effectiveness analysis. *Pharmacoeconomics*, *24*(1): 1–19.

Barton, G.R., Briggs, A.H., and Fenwick, E.A., 2008. Optimal cost-effectiveness decisions: The role of the cost-effectiveness acceptability curve (CEAC), the cost-effectiveness acceptability frontier (CEAF), and the expected value of perfection information (EVPI). *Value in Health*, *11*(5): 886–97.

Barton, P., Bryan, S., and Robinson, S., 2004. Modelling in the economic evaluation of health care: Selecting the appropriate approach. *Journal of Health Services Research & Policy*, *9*(2): 110–18.

Bojke, L., Claxton, K., Sculpher, M., and Palmer, S., 2009. Characterizing structural uncertainty in decision analytic models: A review and application of methods. *Value in Health*, *12*(5): 739–49.

Boyd, K.A., 2012. *Employing early decision analytic modelling to inform economic evaluation in health care: Theory & practice.* PhD thesis University of Glasgow.

Boyd, K.A., Balogun, M.O., and Minnis, H., 2015. Development of a radical foster care intervention in Glasgow, Scotland. *Health Promotion International*, *31*(3): 665–73.

Brailsford, S. and Schmidt, B., 2003. Towards incorporating human behaviour in models of health care systems: An approach using discrete event simulation. *European Journal of Operational Research*, *150*(1): 19–31.

Brakefield T., Mednick S., Wilson H.W., De Neve J-E., Christakis N.A., and Fowler J.H., 2014. Same-Sex Sexual Attraction Does Not Spread in Adolescent Social Networks. *Archives of Sexual Behavior*, *43*(2);335–44.

Brennan, A. and Akehurst, R., 2000. Modelling in health economic evaluation. What is its place? What is its value? *Pharmacoeconomics*, *17*(5): 445–59.

Brennan, A., Chick, S.E., and Davies, R., 2006. A taxonomy of model structures for economic evaluation of health technologies. *Health Economics*, *15*(12): 1295–310.

Brennan, A., Meng, Y., Holmes, J., Hill-McManus, D., and Meier, P.S., 2014. Potential benefits of minimum unit pricing for alcohol versus a ban on below cost selling in England 2014: Modelling study. *British Medical Journal*, *349*: g5452.

Briggs, A.H., 2000. Handling uncertainty in cost-effectiveness models. *Pharmacoeconomics*, *17*(5): 479–500.

Briggs, A.H., 2001. Handling uncertainty in economic evaluations and presenting the results. In: M. Drummond and A. McGuire, (eds), *Economic Evaluation in Health Care: Merging Theory with Practice.* Oxford: Oxford University Press, pp. 172–214.

Briggs, A.H., Claxton, K., and Sculpher, M.J., 2006. *Decision Modelling for Health Economic Evaluation.* Oxford: Oxford University Press.

Briggs, A. and Sculpher, M., 1997. Commentary: Markov models of medical prognosis. *British Medical Journal*, *314*(7077): 354.

Caro, J.J., Briggs, A.H., Siebert, U., and Kuntz, K.M., 2012. Modeling good research practices—overview. A report of the ISPOR-SMDM modeling good research practices task force-1. *Medical Decision Making, 32*(5): 667–77.

Castellani, B. and Hafferty, F.W., 2009. *Sociology and Complexity Science: A New Field of Inquiry*. Berlin: Springer Science & Business Media.

Chhatwal, J. and He, T., 2015. Economic evaluations with agent-based modelling: An introduction. *Pharmacoeconomics, 33*: 423–33.

Christakis, N.A. and Fowler, J.H., 2008. The collective dynamics of smoking in a large social network. *New England Journal of Medicine, 358*(21): 2249–58.

Claxton, K., Sculpher, M., and Culyer, A., 2007. *Mark versus Luke? Appropriate Methods for the Evaluation of PHIs* (No. 031cherp). York: Centre for Health Economics, University of York.

Claxton, K., 1999a. Bayesian approaches to the value of information: Implications for the regulation of new pharmaceuticals. *Health Economics, 8*(3): 269–74.

Claxton, K., 1999b. The irrelevance of inference: A decision-making approach to the stochastic evaluation of health care technologies. *Journal of Health Economics, 18*(3): 341–64.

Claxton, K., Cohen, J.T., and Neumann, P.J., 2005. When is evidence sufficient? *Health Affairs, 24*(1):93–101.

Claxton, K., Ginnelly, L., Sculpher, M., Philips, Z., and Palmer, S., 2004. A pilot study on the use of decision theory and value of information analysis as part of the NHS Health Technology Assessment programme. *Health Technology Assessment, 8*(31): 1–103.

Collett, D., 2015. *Modelling Survival Data in Medical Research* (3rd edn). CRC Press.

Cookson, R., Griffin, S., Norheim, O.F., and Culyer, A.J., (forthcoming). *Distributional Cost-Effectiveness Analysis: A Handbook of Equity-Informative Health Economic Evaluation.* Oxford: Oxford University Press.

Cookson, R., Mirelman, A. Griffin, S., Asaria, M., Dawkins, B., Norheim, O., Verguet, S., et al., 2017 Using cost-effectiveness analysis to address health equity concerns. *Value in Health,* **20**(2): 206–12.

Cookson, R., Griffin, S., Norheim, and Culyer, A.J., 2019. Distributional Cost- Effectiveness Analysis: A Handbook of Equity- Informative Health Economic Evaluation. Oxford: Oxford University Press.

Dahlgren, G. and Whitehead, M., 1991. *Policies and Strategies to Promote Social Equity in Health*. Stockholm: Institute for Future Studies.

Deidda, M., Boyd, K.A., Minnis, H., BeST study team, et al., 2018. Protocol for the economic evaluation of a complex intervention to improve the mental health of maltreated infants and children in foster care in the UK (The BeST? services trial). *British Medical Journal Open, 8*: e020066. doi:10.1136/bmjopen-2017-020066.

Fenwick, E. and Byford, S., 2005. A guide to cost-effectiveness acceptability curves. *British Journal of Psychiatry, 187*(2): 106–8.

Fenwick, E., Claxton, K., Sculpher, M., and Briggs, A., 2000. *Improving the Efficiency, and Relevance of Health Technology Assessment: The Role of Iterative Decision Analytic Modelling* (No. 179chedp). York: Centre for Health Economics, University of York. Available at: <https://www.york.ac.uk/che/pdf/DP179.pdf> (Accessed 12 November 2018).

Fernández, I. and Kekäle, T., 2008. Better models with Delphi and analytic hierarchy process approaches: The case of reverse logistics. *International Journal of Logistics Systems and Management, 4*(3): 282–96.

Flood R. and Jackson M., 1991. *Creative Problem Solving: Total Systems Intervention*. Chichester: Wiley.

Glenny, A.M., Altman, D.G., Song, F., Sakarovitch, C., Deeks, J.J., D'Amico, R., Bradburn, M., et al., 2005. Indirect comparisons of competing interventions. *Health Technology Assessment (Winchester, England)*, 9(26): 1–134.

Glick, H.A., Doshi, J.A., Sonnad, S.S., and Polsky, D., 2014. *Economic Evaluation in Clinical Trials*. Oxford: Oxford University Press.

Goldie, S. and Corso, P., 2003 Decision Analysis. In: A.C. Haddix, S.M. Teutsch, and P.S. Corso (eds), *Prevention Effectiveness: A Guide to Decision Analysis and Economic Evaluation* 2nd edn. Oxford: Oxford University Press, pp. 103–26.

HM Treasury, 2015. *Spending Review and Autumn Statement 2015*. Available at: <https://www.gov.uk/government/uploads/system/uploads/attachment_data/file/479749/52229_Blue_Book_PU1865_Web_Accessible.pdf> (Accessed 16 October 2018).

Howick, S., Eden, C., Ackermann, F., and Williams, T., 2008. Building confidence in models for multiple audiences: the modelling cascade. *European Journal of Operational Research*, 186(3): 1068–83.

Hu, X. and Puddy, R., 2011. Cognitive modeling for agent-based simulation of child maltreatment. In: J. Salerno, S.J. Yang, D. Nau, and S.K. Chai (eds), *International Conference on Social Computing, Behavioral-Cultural Modeling, and Prediction*. Berlin: Springer, pp. 138–46.

Husereau, D., Drummond, M., Petrou, S., Carswell, C., Moher, D., Greenberg, D., Augustovski, F., et al., 2013. Consolidated health economic evaluation reporting standards (CHEERS)—explanation and elaboration: A report of the ISPOR health economic evaluation publication guidelines good reporting practices task force. *Value in Health*, 16(2): 231–50.

Jackson, C.H., Bojke, L., Thompson, S.G., Claxton, K., and Sharples, L.D., 2011. A framework for addressing structural uncertainty in decision models. *Medical Decision Making*, 31(4): 662–74.

Jones, A., Laporte, A., Rice, N., and Zucchelli, E., 2011. *A Model of the Impact of Smoking Bans on Smoking with Evidence from Bans in England and Scotland*. Health, Econometrics & Data Group. WP 05.11.: Health, Econometrics & Data Group, University of York.

Kaltenthaler, E., Tappenden, P., Paisley, S., and Squires, H., 2011. Identifying and reviewing evidence to inform the conceptualisation and population of cost-effectiveness models. National Institute for Health and Care Excellence (NICE) DSU Technical Support Documents. London: NICE.

Karnon, J., Stahl, J., Brennan, A., Caro, J.J., Mar, J., and Möller, J., 2012. Modeling using discrete event simulation: A report of the ISPOR-SMDM Modeling Good Research Practices Task Force–4. *Medical Decision Making*, 32(5): 701–11.

Kelly, M.P. 2009. The individual and the social level in public health. In: A. Killoran and M.P. Kelly (eds), 2010. *Evidence-Based Public Health: Effectiveness and Efficiency*. Oxford: Oxford University Press, pp. 425–35.

Kelly, M.P., McDaid, D., Ludbrook, A., and Powell, J., 2005. *Economic Appraisal of PHIs*. London: Health Development Agency.

Kelly, M.P., Stewart, E., Morgan, A., Killoran, A., Fischer, A., Threlfall, A., and Bonnefoy, J., 2009. A conceptual framework for public health: NICE's emerging approach. *Public Health*, 123(1): e14–e20.

Kruger, J., Brennan, A., Thokala, P., Cooke, D., Clark, M., Bond, R., and Heller, S., 2013. Modelling the potential cost-effectiveness of a targeted follow-up intervention to improve glycaemic response following structured training in flexible intensive insulin therapy. HEDS Discussion Paper 13.10. Available at: <https://www.sheffield.ac.uk/polopoly_fs/1.283936!/file/1310.pdf> (Accessed 12 November 2018).

Kuntz, K.M. and Weinstein, M.C., 2001. Modelling in economic evaluation. In: M. Drummond and A. McGuire (eds), *Economic Evaluation in Health Care: Merging Theory with Practice*. Oxford: Oxford University Press, pp. 141–71.

Latimer, N.R., 2013. Survival analysis for economic evaluations alongside clinical trials—extrapolation with patient-level data: Inconsistencies, limitations, and a practical guide. *Medical Decision Making*, 33(6): 743–54.

Macal, C.M. and North, M.J., 2010. Tutorial on agent-based modelling and simulation. *Journal of Simulation*, 4(3): 151–62.

Marsh, K., Phillips, C.J., Fordham, R., Bertranou, E., and Hale, J., 2012. Estimating cost-effectiveness in public health: A summary of modelling and valuation methods. *Health Economics Review*, 2(1):17.

Marshall, D.A., Burgos-Liz, L., Ijzerman, M.J., Crown, W., Padula, W.V., Wong, P.K., Pasupathy, K.S., et al., 2015. Selecting a dynamic simulation modeling method for health care delivery research—Part 2: Report of the ISPOR Dynamic Simulation Modeling Emerging Good Practices Task Force. *Value in Health*, 18(2): 147–60.

McDaid, D and Needle, J., 2009. What use has been made of economic evaluation in public health? A systematic review of the literature. In: S. Dawson and Z.S. Morris (eds), *Future Public Health*. Basingstoke: Palgrave Macmillan, pp. 248–64.

McKie, L. and Ryan, L. (eds), 2016. *An End to the Crisis of Empirical Sociology? Trends and Challenges in Social Research*. London: Routledge.

McPherson, K., Marsh, T., and Brown, M., 2007. *Tackling Obesities: Future Choices: Modelling Future Trends in Obesity and the Impact on Health*. Foresight, Government Office for Science. Available at: <https://www.gov.uk/government/publications/reducing-obesity-modelling-future-trends (Accessed 12 November 2018).

Medical Research Council, 2008. *Developing and Evaluating Complex Interventions: New Guidance*. Available from: <https://www.mrc.ac.uk/documents/pdf/complex-interventions-guidance/> (Accessed 16 October 2018).

Midgley, G., 2003. *Systems Thinking*. London: Sage Publications.

Miller, J.H. and Page, S.E., 2007. *Complex Adaptive Systems: An Introduction to Computational Models of Social Life*. Princeton, NJ: Princeton University Press.

Minnis, H., Bryce, G., Phin, L., and Wilson, P., 2010. The 'Spirit of New Orleans': Translating a model of intervention with maltreated children and their families for the Glasgow context. *Clinical Child Psychology and Psychiatry*, 15(4): 497–509.

Minnis, H., Boyd, K.A., Fitzpatrick, B., Forde, M., Gillberg, C., Henderson, M., McMahon, L., et al., 2016 Protocol 15PRT/6090: The Best Services Trial (BeST?): Effectiveness and cost-effectiveness of the New Orleans Intervention Model for Infant Mental Health. *Lancet*. Available from: <http://www.thelancet.com/doi/story/10.1016/html.2016.11.15.4368> (Accessed 16 October 2018).

National Institute for Health and Care Excellence, 2014a. *Developing NICE Guidelines: The Manual. Process and Methods [PMG20]*. Available from: <https://www.nice.org.uk/process/pmg20> (Accessed 16 October 2018).

National Institute for Health and Care Excellence, 2014b. *Contraceptive Services for Under 25s. Public Health Guideline [PH51]*. Available from: <https://www.nice.org.uk/guidance/ph51> (Accessed 16 October 2018).

Owen, L., Morgan, A., Fischer, A., Ellis, S., Hoy, A., and Kelly, M.P., 2012. The cost-effectiveness of PHIs. *Journal of Public Health*, 34(1): 37–45.

Paisley, S., 2016. Identification of evidence for key parameters in decision-analytic models of cost effectiveness: A description of sources and a recommended minimum search requirement. *Pharmacoeconomics*, 34(6): 597–608.

Petrou, S. and Gray, A., 2011. Economic evaluation using decision analytical modelling: Design, conduct, analysis, and reporting. *British Medical Journal*, **342**, (1766): 1195–8.

Philips, Z., Bojke, L., Sculpher, M., Claxton, K., and Golder, S., 2006. Good practice guidelines for decision-analytic modelling in health technology assessment. *Pharmacoeconomics*, 24(4): 355–71.

Pidd, M., 2009. *Tools for Thinking; Modelling in Management Science*. Chichester: John Wiley and Son Ltd.

Pilgrim, H., Payne, N., Chilcott, J., Blank, L., Guillaume, L., and Baxter, S., 2010. Modelling the cost-effectiveness of interventions to encourage young people, especially socially disadvantaged young people, to use contraceptives and contraceptive services. Sheffield: School of Health and Related Research (ScHARR), University of Sheffield. Available from: <https://www.nice.org.uk/guidance/ph51/evidence/health-economics-pdf-431662573> (Accessed 12 November 2018).

Pritchett, R., Fitzpatrick, B., Watson, N., Cotmore, R., Wilson, P., Bryce, G., Donaldson, J., et al., 2013. A feasibility randomised controlled trial of the New Orleans intervention for infant mental health: A study protocol. *The Scientific World Journal*, (ID 838042) 1–6. Available from: <http://www.hindawi.com/journals/tswj/2013/838042/> (Accessed 16 October 2018).

Raffia, H. and Schlaifer, R., 1959. *Probability and Statistics for Business Decisions*. New York, NY: McGaw-Hill.

Roberts, M., Russell, L.B., Paltiel, A.D., Chambers, M., McEwan, P., and Krahn, M., 2012. Conceptualizing a model a report of the ISPOR-SMDM modeling good research practices task force–2. *Medical Decision Making*, 32(5): 678–89.

Robinson, S., 2011. *Conceptual Modeling for Simulation*. New York, NY: Wiley.

Rodriguez-Ulloa, R. and Paucar-Caceres, A., 2005. Soft system dynamics methodology (SSDM): Combining soft systems methodology (SSM) and system dynamics (SD). *Systemic Practice and Action Research*, 18(3): 303–34.

Rush, B., Shiell, A., and Hawe, P., 2004. A census of economic evaluations in health promotion. *Health Education Research*, 19(6): 707–19.

Scott, S., Knapp, M., Henderson, J., and Maughan, B., 2001. Financial cost of social exclusion: Follow up study of antisocial children into adulthood. *British Medical Journal*, 323(7306:191.

Sculpher, M.J., Claxton, K., Drummond, M., and McCabe, C., 2006. Whither trial-based economic evaluation for health care decision making? *Health Economics*, 15(7): 677–87.

Sculpher, M., Drummond, M., and Buxton, M., 1997. The iterative use of economic evaluation as part of the process of health technology assessment. *Journal of Health Services Research*, 2(1): 26–30.

Siebers, P.O., Macal, C.M., Garnett, J., Buxton, D., and Pidd, M., 2010. Discrete-event simulation is dead, long live agent-based simulation! *Journal of Simulation*, 4(3): 204–10.

Smith, R.D. and Petticrew, M. 2010. Public health evaluation in the twenty-first century: Time to see the wood as well as the trees. *Journal of Public Health*, 32: 2–7.

Sonnenberg, F.A. and Beck, J.R., 1993. Markov models in medical decision making a practical guide. *Medical Decision Making, 13*(4): 322–38.

Squires, H., Chilcott, J., Akehurst, R., Burr, J., and Kelly, M.P., 2016. A framework for developing the structure of public health economic models. *Value in Health, 19*(5): 588–601.

Sterman, J.D., 2000. *Business Dynamics: Systems Thinking and Modeling for a Complex World.* Singapore: McGraw-Hill Higher Education.

Sterman, J.D., 2006. Learning from evidence in a complex world. *American Journal of Public Health, 96*(3): 505–14.

Taylor D., Bury M., Campling N., Carter S., Garfield S., Newbould J., and Rennie T., 2006. *A review of the use of the Health Belief Model (HBM), the Theory of Reasoned Action (TRA), the Theory of Planned Behaviour (TPB) and the Trans-Theoretical Model (TTM) to study and predict health related behaviour change.* School of Pharmacy, University of London. Available from: <https://www.nice.org.uk/guidance/ph6/resources/behaviour-change-taylor-et-al-models-review2> (Accessed 16 October 2018).

Thaler, R.H. and Mullainathan, S., 2008. Behavioral economics. *The Concise Encyclopedia of Economics, 2.* Liberty Fund.

Trueman, P. and Anokye, N.K., 2013. Applying economic evaluation to PHIs: The cases of interventions to promote physical activity. *Journal of Public Health, 35*(1): 32–9.

National Cancer Institute, 2007, April. *Greater Than the Sum: Systems Thinking in Tobacco Control. Tobacco Control Monograph No. 18.* Bethesda, MD: U.S. Department of Health and Human Services, National Institutes of Health, National Cancer Institute. NIH Pub. No. 06-6085.

Vennix, J.A. and Gubbels, J.W., 1992. Knowledge elicitation in conceptual model building: A case study in modeling a regional Dutch health care system. *European Journal of Operational Research, 59*(1): 85–101.

Von Bertalanffy, L., 1969. *General System Theory: Foundations, Development, Applications.* New York, NY: George Brazillier, Inc.

Weatherly, H., Drummond, M., Claxton, K., Cookson, R., Ferguson, B., Godfrey, C., Rice, N., et al., 2009. Methods for assessing the cost-effectiveness of PHIs: Key challenges and recommendations. *Health Policy, 93*(2): 85–92.

Weinstein, M.C., O'Brien, B., Hornberger, J., Jackson, J., Johannesson, M., McCabe, C., and Luce, B.R., 2003. Principles of good practice for decision analytic modeling in health-care evaluation: Report of the ISPOR Task Force on Good Research Practices—Modeling Studies. *Value in Health, 6*(1): 9–17.

West, P., Sanderson, D., Redmond, S., Taylor, M., and Duffy, S., 2003. *A critique of the Application of Cost-Effectiveness Analysis to Public Health.* Report to inform the Wanless team at HM Treasury (accessed through personal communication with the authors).

Chapter 12

Return on investment, social return on investment, and the business case for prevention

Joanna M. Charles, Alice Jones,
and Huw Lloyd-Williams

12.1 Social return on investment

Social return on investment (SROI) assesses the value created as a result of inter-ventions and services, and compares this to the money invested in such services. As outcomes are typically allocated a financial value rather than being valued using pref-erence based welfare economic methods, SROI can be considered a less theoretical but, some may argue, more pragmatic form of cost–benefit analysis (CBA) (discussed in Chapter 9 of this book). SROI is based on the concept of return on investment (ROI) largely used in the world of finance to measure the efficiency of investments. SROI takes this concept a step further and takes into account the social impacts of projects by endeavouring to include all relevant stakeholders in the allocation of resources. The method results in a ratio of benefits to costs, estimating the value created for every £1 invested. The central purpose of SROI is to address the challenge of measuring a wider concept of value, capturing aspects across the 'triple bottom line' of economic, social, and environmental value. SROI can therefore be employed as a method of understanding how effectively and efficiently money is spent. SROI is concerned with the impact that an intervention or service has, defined as the outcomes (benefits and changes) that matter to stakeholders (i.e. those who are directly affected by the inter-vention or service). There are, however, a number of criticisms of the SROI approach, not least its approach to valuing outcomes, and these are also outlined in this chapter. A recent systematic review of ROI in PHIs reported that local and national PHIs are highly cost-saving. The review noted that cuts to public health budgets in high income countries represent a false economy, and are likely to generate billions of pounds of additional costs to health services and the wider economy (Masters et al., 2017).

12.1.2 How does SROI differ from CBA?

Both CBA and SROI analysis place monetary values on all costs and benefits from an intervention or service. CBA is a long-established technique used by econo-mists (Mishan, 1971), whilst SROI is still in its infancy (Cabinet Office, 2009;

<http://www.neweconomics.org/>). Although SROI is seen by some as an extension of CBA, Arvidson and colleagues highlight a few main differences between the two methods (Arvidson et al., 2010). CBA can include stakeholder involvement as part of its methods and principles but tends to present this as a societal perspective with different perspectives reported (which may be linked to stakeholders) as and when required. SROI is based around clear involvement of stakeholders throughout the process of analysis. CBA is designed to be comparable across different activities. However, SROI guidance warns against comparing SROI analyses across activities. The reasons for this lie with the high level of stakeholder engagement, which can result in different indicators and outcomes being measured, therefore making comparisons difficult. CBA uses the underlying principles of welfare economics to value outcomes (e.g. contingent valuation (Ryan et al., 2007) as discussed in Chapter 9 of this book). SROI also advocates the use of such methods but in addition allows for a range of other methods and working assumptions to assign values to outcomes. SROI practitioners have developed knowledge banks of proxy values that can be used to help monetize those outcomes difficult to state in financial terms (Fujiwara, 2013).

12.2 **SROI principles and key stages**

The Cabinet Office outlines seven key principles that underpin an SROI analysis (Cabinet Office, 2009). These are:

1. Involve stakeholders
2. Understand what actually changes (for the stakeholder/s)
3. Value the things that matter
4. Only include what is material
5. Do not over-claim
6. Be transparent
7. Verify the result

12.2.1 **The stages of SROI**

SROI is conducted in six stages as described by the Cabinet Office Guide to SROI (2009).

12.2.2 **Stage 1—Setting the scope**

A general question to consider during this stage is what is the purpose of the SROI? There are two types of SROI. The first, an evaluative analysis, is carried out after an intervention has taken place and retrospectively measures to what extent outcomes have actually been achieved. This helps inform decision-makers as to whether an intervention has delivered on its intended outcomes and whether it is deemed to be cost effective using SROI criteria. The second type is a forecast SROI, which aims to estimate how much value would be created by an activity or intervention if the intended outcomes were achieved. This may be motivated by strategic planning or to help a policy-maker establish whether a service or intervention would be considered a good use of resources to warrant investment.

The evaluator should also consider who the audience is and how findings will be articulated and disseminated. What activities will you focus on? If a service provides multiple activities, will you assess all activities or focus on specific ones? Will the activities be separated by a particular source of funding, specific outcomes of interest, or priority service areas for the organization?

To illustrate each of the key stages a worked example is provided entitled 'Improving health through investment in housing improvement'. The following case study is included to demonstrate the application of SROI analysis to a programme relating to public health outcomes. The programme was run by Nottingham City Homes and was called 'Decent Homes', in which improvements were made to substandard housing in order to bring them up to government standards and improve the health outcomes of tenants.

The main findings of the Decent Homes impact study were reported under four separate headings (Jones et al., 2016):

12.2.2.1 Crime and security

Compared with a reduction in burglary of 21 per cent in the city during the period 2007 and 2010, two sample areas, where 'Secured by Design' double glazing was fitted, experienced a reduction in burglary of 42 per cent. Tenants in this area reported that they felt safer and experienced less in the form of dampness, condensation, draughts, and external noise.

12.2.2.2 Energy efficiency and fuel poverty

The average energy efficiency rating in homes where the work was carried out rose from 60 to 68 points out of 100, measured by the Standard Assessment Procedure (SAP) (UK Government, 2014). This is equivalent to a reduction in carbon emissions of 15,500 tonnes per year or to planting 360,000 trees. Fuel poverty has also reduced among tenants. According to the Energy Saving Trust, new windows can save between £95 and £223 per year while a new boiler can save up to £225 in fuel costs which equates to a total saving for tenants who have received the work of around £3.5 million a year.

12.2.2.3 Health and well-being

It has been estimated that the Decent Homes initiative could potentially save two lives per year by protecting tenants from the effect of cold temperatures. It could also improve the respiratory health of around 1000 children locally. By relieving excess cold and fuel poverty, it could improve the mental health of around 1400 tenants. Making houses safer would also prevent twelve admissions a year into hospital as a result of falls.

12.2.2.4 Local economy and employment

The programme has provided direct employment to carry out the work and 560 people have been employed, with one-third of them living within the city and one-half living within Nottinghamshire.

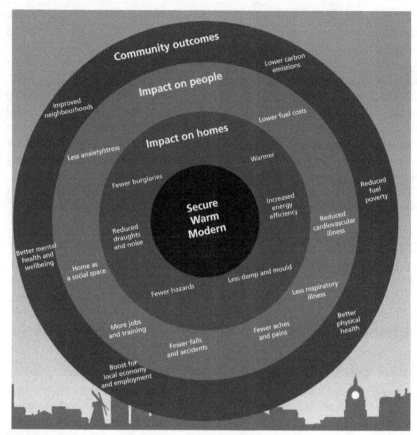

Figure 12.1 Ripple effect diagram of impact from secure, warm homes.
Reproduced with permission from Jones, A., Valero-Silva, N., Lucas, D., 2016. The effects of 'Secure, Warm, Modern' homes in Nottingham: Decent Homes Impact Study, Nottingham City Homes. Copyright © 2016 Nottingham City Homes and Nottingham Business School at Nottingham Trent University.

The Decent Homes case study example highlights the application of aspects of the SROI process throughout the chapter. This case study is reproduced with permission from Nottingham City Homes and Nottingham Trent University for whom the original SROI analysis was undertaken (Jones et al., 2016). Figure 12.1 shows the ripple effects of the impact from secure, warm homes.

Identifying stakeholders is also a key consideration in this first stage. Stakeholders are those who are *directly* impacted by the intervention or service. A list should be drawn up of all the people who are likely to be affected by the intervention or service. To help decide whether a stakeholder is material to the evaluation, the following definition may be helpful—'Stakeholders are people or organizations that experience change, or are directly affected by the intervention or service. This change or effect can be positive, negative, intended or unintended'. Asking the following two questions also helps to appraise each stakeholder; 'Is the change the stakeholder experiences relevant? Is the change significant?'

Box 12.1 Case study: Improving health through investment in housing improvement—Stage 1, Setting the scope

In 2000 the government introduced the Decent Homes standard for social housing, which set out a minimum standard that all socially rented properties are required to meet. The government at the time recognized that '[d]ecent housing strengthens communities and provides a better setting in which to raise families. It improves health and educational achievements and provides a long-term asset that can be passed on to future generations' (Department for the Environment, Transport and the Regions, 2000, p. 7). The Decent Homes programme was centrally funded to meet the backlog of investment required to bring the national social housing stock up to this standard.

In Nottingham, the Decent Homes standard has been met through a programme of housing investment known locally as 'Secure, Warm, Modern'. Under the programme, improvements were made to the 29,000 council-owned homes, such as the installation of new double-glazed windows, heating systems and boilers, and kitchen and bathroom facilities.

Existing evidence shows a clear relationship between housing and health, particularly the harmful effects of poor housing on both physical and mental health. The World Health Organization has collated this evidence (Braubach et al., 2011), and demonstrates the links between cold, damp housing, and poor cardiovascular and respiratory health. Around a third of all excess winter deaths in the United Kingdom are thought to be caused by poor housing (Braubach et al., 2011). Other hazardous conditions in the home can also cause accidental injuries, such as trips, falls, burns, and electric shocks. Living in poor housing conditions is also linked to lower well-being and poorer mental health (Barnes et al., 2013).

It was therefore anticipated that there would be a significant positive health impact, as well as other social and environmental benefits, from improving council housing in Nottingham through the Decent Homes programme. The housing provider, Nottingham City Homes, together with Nottingham Trent University, therefore decided to carry out an SROI evaluation on the programme (Jones et al., 2016). The research focused on one area of the city (Aspley) where the properties had already been improved in the pilot stages of the investment programme.

The Cabinet Office states that the list of stakeholders should be kept as a record of the process of the analysis (Cabinet Office, 2009). Also, the reason for why a particular person or organization was excluded or included as a stakeholder should also be contained in this record.

12.2.3 Stage 2—Mapping outcomes

Outcomes are the changes resulting from an activity or intervention and can be identified in a number of ways. Engagement with stakeholders through interviews

Box 12.2 Case study: Identifying stakeholders

The first step for the Decent Homes SROI was to establish a list of stakeholders and consult with them, to describe the impact on them from the programme. Some examples are given in Table 12.1.

Table 12.1 List of stakeholders developed for the Nottingham improving homes case study SROI analysis

Stakeholder	Outcomes	Type of outcome
Social housing tenants	Better health, as housing conditions prevent and/or relieve relevant health conditions and prevent accidents in the home.	Positive, expected
	Reduced fear of crime, as homes are made more secure.	Positive, expected
	Increased stress as a result of construction work in the home.	Negative, expected
	Better educational attainment for children, from having warm, comfortable, personal space away from the main living area in which to do homework.	Positive, unexpected
NHS	Fewer tenants requiring treatment with GPs and hospitals.	Positive, expected
Housing Repairs Service	Fewer repairs require to properties with new fixtures and fittings.	Positive, expected

Nottingham tenants were the primary stakeholder group affected by the programme. The health outcomes for this group were considered to be highly material to the SROI evaluation, because:

♦ This stakeholder group are the main recipients of the intervention, and the primary aim of the evaluation is to establish whether the intended improvements to their quality of life have been achieved.

♦ The changes experienced are also significant, as a considerable proportion of tenants affected by health conditions that can be improved through better housing (e.g. higher levels of COPD amongst Nottingham residents than the national average).

However, in the final SROI analysis the outcomes for the Housing Repairs Service were considered to be non-material to the SROI evaluation. This was because:

♦ The reduction in the number of repairs was lower than expected, as tenants' expectations were raised and therefore made more callouts for other minor repairs not previously reported

♦ The internal, cost-saving impacts of the Decent Homes programme were not considered relevant to the scope of the evaluation, given the focus of the SROI on social outcomes.

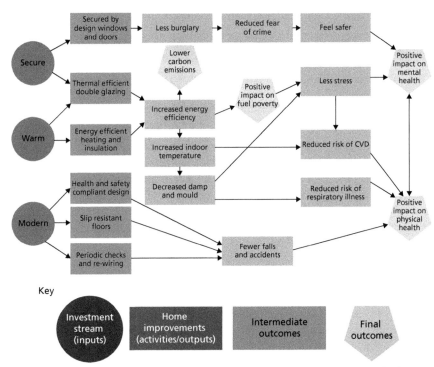

Figure 12.2 Theory of change map for the Decent Homes (Secure, Warm, Modern) programme in Nottingham.

Reproduced with permission from Jones, A., Valero-Silva, N., Lucas, D., 2016. The effects of 'Secure, Warm, Modern' homes in Nottingham: Decent Homes Impact Study, Nottingham City Homes. Copyright © 2016 Nottingham City Homes and Nottingham Business School at Nottingham Trent University.

or focus groups can help identify what the stakeholders believed changed for them because of the intervention or service. This evidence can then be used to map outcomes, using a theory of change (or impact) map. This sets out the story of how the change was created; starting with the initial investment and activities carried out, then showing the measurable outputs from these activities, and finally mapping this onto the resulting outcomes that stakeholders experience. Some outcomes may be achieved through a chain of events that may include some intermediate outcomes. When exploring such a chain of events, this raises the possibility of double counting outcomes. This is avoided by only including the final outcome in the analysis. However, outcomes can be attributed to more than one group of stakeholders. Also, outcomes attributed to one group of stakeholders may lead to the identification of 'knock-on' outcomes (e.g. employment opportunities) for other stakeholders. It is also important to check back with your stakeholders if the outcomes identified are plausible and sensible before proceeding with the next stages.

Box 12.3 Case study: Stage 2—Mapping the theory of change

The basic framework for the theory of change is to map the inputs, activities, outputs, and outcomes:

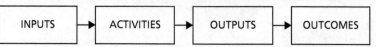

However, a 'real-life' theory of change can be more complex than this basic, linear presentation of the theory, and involve complexities such as intermediate outcomes in a chain of events, and knock-on effects on other outcomes. Figure 12.2 illustrates the theory of change map for the Decent Homes (Secure, Warm, Modern) programme in Nottingham, showing health outcomes as well as other social, economic, and environmental outcomes achieved:

12.2.4 Stage 3—Establish indicators

Indicators tell you whether or not outcomes have been achieved, and the magnitude to which they have been achieved. It is advised that outcomes be identified before thinking about indicators to measure them; that is, the primary consideration is to get the right measure of change rather than jumping straight to thinking about where there may already be readily available data. The data for indicators may be available from existing sources or new data may need to be collected from stakeholders as part of the SROI analysis. The SROI approach is non-prescriptive regarding the way that indicators are measured, allowing for a number of methods (including those established and tested in the health field) to be used. For example, these could include: methods used by health economists (as outlined in Chapter 6), which include preference-based health-related quality of life measures (e.g. EQ-5D, EuroQol Group, 1990); standardized well-being scales such as the Warwick–Edinburgh Mental health and Wellbeing Scale (Tennant et al., 2007), and self-reported happiness scales such as the Oxford Happiness Questionnaire (Hills and Argyle, 2002); or a specifically prepared survey or questionnaire to indicate changes in outcomes because of an intervention or service. Magnitude of change may be assessed by administering measures on a number of occasions; for example, pre- and immediately post intervention or at pre-intervention, 6 months post intervention, and 12 months post intervention.

12.2.5 Stage 4—Value change

In SROI analysis, financial proxies are used to estimate the social value of non-traded goods to different stakeholders. Financial proxies can be derived from either stated preference, using techniques such as willingness to pay and willingness to accept compensation or revealed preference, using techniques such as the travel cost method and hedonic pricing as discussed in Chapter 6 of this book. An alternative method that has been developed more recently is the 'well-being valuation' approach (also outlined in

Box 12.4 Case study: Stage 3—Outcomes, indicators, and methods for data collection

Table 12.2 describes examples of outcomes, indicators, and data collection methods to illustrate the process of establishing and measuring indicators of change in the case study.

Table 12.2 Outcomes, indicators, and data collection methods utilized in the Nottingham improving homes case study SROI analysis

Outcome	Indicator	Source
Reduced fear of crime.	Change in number of tenants who felt safe at home alone after dark, before and after home improvements.	Tenant surveys.
Decreased fuel bill and fuel poverty.	Average fuel savings from installation of new heating system and double-glazed windows.	Data provided by Energy Savings Trust.
Tenants have better health, as internal conditions prevent/ improve management of relevant health issues and prevent accidents in the home.	Reduction in harms from physiological, psychological, infection, and accident hazards.	Modelling of health outcomes, based on property surveys (health and safety risks) and local health data.

Table 12.2 shows how outcomes can be measured in a range of ways. In this case, some primary data were collected through direct surveying of tenants before and after the work. A standardized questionnaire was sent to tenants before and after the works, including a question asking 'how safe do you feel at home alone after dark?' Prior to the home improvements, 31 per cent replied that they felt 'safe' or 'very safe', and after the works this increased to 37 per cent, an increase of 6 per cent following the improvements. This was applied to the number of homes in the area that were improved to give a total number of tenants who felt safer in their homes following the improvements.

Changes in health outcomes were modelled rather than measured directly in this case, due to limited resources and timescales, which precluded a full-scale health assessment. Instead, a method developed by Building Research Establishment (BRE) (Davidson et al., 2010) was applied to model the reduction in risks of harms to health as a result of property improvements. This used actual property survey data from the homes that highlighted health and safety hazards in each home prior to improvements (using the government's Housing Health and Safety Rating System), and estimated the type of harm and the likelihood

---

Box 12.4 Case study: Stage 3 (continued)

of it arising from each type of hazard. The hazards covered a range of issues and risks to health, such as:

- ◆ Excess cold and its impact on cardiovascular and respiratory health
- ◆ Damp and mould and its effect on respiratory outcomes, including childhood asthma
- ◆ Accident hazards, such as trip or fall hazards, electrical, and scald/burn hazards

Serious hazards were addressed in 367 homes in the pilot area of the scheme. The model estimated that this would result in thirteen fewer moderate harms to health to these residents each year.

Chapter 6). Well-being valuation aims to value non-market goods and services. This approach is championed by Dolan and Peasgood and Fujiwara to value aspects that affect people's quality of life, such as fear of crime, pollution, and increased sense of safety (Dolan and Peasgood, 2008; Fukiwara, 2013). Well-being valuation uses large datasets that include questions on a range of life circumstances as well as subjective well-being scores. It uses statistical or econometric techniques to assess how different life events affect subjective well-being, and compare this to the amount of income needed to achieve the same effect on well-being (Fujiwara, 2013). Using subjective well-being techniques reduces the likelihood of bias when asking people to assess how different health conditions or situations would affect their lives (Dolan and Peasgood, 2008). This is because well-being valuations are based on people's actual life experiences, rather than their perception of them. For example, when we ask people what they would feel in different health states (such as in willingness-to-pay exercises), they typically overestimate the impact as they are unlikely to have direct experience of that health state; for example, asking a mobile adult how they would assess the hypothetical impact on their lives of needing to use a wheelchair due to mobility problems.

The valuation is considered from the perspective of the stakeholder to whom the outcome is assigned. Valuation can be straightforward in some cases, and in other cases may need some ingenuity to establish a suitable financial proxy for the outcome where a direct measure of value of the outcome is not available. For example, the value of improved physical health to the health service could be valued at the costs saved to the National Health Service (NHS) through reduced GP visits, for which unit costs are readily available through Curtis and Burns (2017). However, valuing the improvement in health from the individual's perspective can be more challenging, as the value of 'good health' is less readily valued than cost savings. In such cases some assumptions may need to be made, such as substituting the direct value for the value of preventing the loss of that outcome, or the cost achieving that outcome in another way. For example, the value of 'good health' to the individual could be arrived at by researching the cost of health insurance (i.e. assuming this is a representation of how much people are willing to pay to avoid the loss of good health). It could potentially also be proxied by the value that individuals spend on social or leisure activities (e.g. gym membership), assuming that this is what they are willing to pay to achieve good health.

Box 12.5 Case study: Stage 4—Valuing change

The research estimated that there would be thirteen fewer harms to health as a result of the home improvements, such as burns/scalds, falls, and treatment for respiratory conditions linked to damp and mould or excess cold. In the theory of change model, the improvement in health as a result of housing improvements is an outcome for two stakeholders: the tenants themselves as well as the health service. The outcome, therefore, has to be valued from both these perspectives.

The value of the outcome from the health service perspective is actually a cost saving i.e. the reduction in use of health services. The model produced by BRE and Warwick University used to estimate the changes in health also included an estimate of the costs of treatment that were therefore avoided, which range from £100 for a moderate injury/illness to £50,000 for a severe injury/illness. The total costs saved for the health services from avoiding thirteen incidents of moderate harm (valued at £100) therefore amounted to £1,300 per year.

For the tenants, the value of this outcome is in avoiding ill-health and the associated discomfort and disruption to daily life from being unwell. In this SROI, the proxy value was derived from the assumption that this would also avoid individuals having to take sick leave from work, with the associated loss of income. As the injuries/illnesses were categorized as 'moderate', the assumption was made that this would prevent the loss of one week's wages through being unable to work while unwell. The average weekly wage in Nottingham is £481, giving a total proxy value for this outcome (thirteen incidents of injury/illness avoided) of £7,904.

There are a range of possible alternative proxies that could have been used in this case. For example, Fujiwara (2013) provides a well-being valuation associated with improvements in chest/breathing problems, asthma, or bronchitis of £2,230 per year, or alternatively an overall value for 'good' health of £6,310 per year. As part of the SROI process, alternative proxies should be tested to see how sensitive the final SROI ratio is to individual assumptions, such as the choice of proxy (see later section on sensitivity analysis).

Resources to assist valuation include the Global Value Exchange established by Social Value UK, Personal Social Services Research Unit (PSSRU), unit costs of health and social care (Curtis and Burns, 2017), and the Family Spending Survey (Office for National Statistics, 2014). Stakeholders can also be used as a resource for checking that the chosen method of valuation is sensible (i.e. a sense check).

12.2.6 Stage 5—Understanding impact

The final stage is to calculate the impact of the intervention or service, which specifically refers here to the cumulative benefits or changes created that are directly attributable to the intervention, over the period of time that they are anticipated to last. Therefore, as part of the analysis, assumptions need to be made to ensure that only the benefits that can be directly attributed to the intervention are counted. The following considerations are required to calculate impact: deadweight, displacement, attribution, and projecting into the future (i.e. benefit period, drop-off, and discounting).

Deadweight—refers to the amount of the outcome that would have been achieved anyway as a result of the status quo, without the intervention. The assessment of deadweight ascertains whether changes that have occurred are a consequence of the intervention or service, or whether this would have happened anyway. The best practice method is to compare outcomes for stakeholders with a control group. In the absence of a control group, national data can be used as a substitute to determine impact. Ideally, the comparison group would be as similar to the intervention group as possible, matched in terms of age, ethnicity, geographical area, and income. The proportion of what would have happened anyway (i.e. the deadweight) is expressed as a percentage and subtracted from the overall estimated outcome.

Displacement—refers to outcomes of the intervention that are moved from one place to another, displacing other outcomes. This 'displaced' value must be removed from the SROI calculation. Displacement does not occur in all cases, and is most common in interventions aimed at reducing crime. For example, crime may decrease when the local council installs additional street lighting in an area, but if this results in higher crime in other, less well-lit areas, the problem has simply been displaced to another area of town rather than solved.

Attribution—is expressed as a percentage and states the amount of credit that factors, other than the intervention or service (e.g. other organizations or individuals), can assume for the impact experienced by the stakeholders. The percentage of attribution involves an estimation process, based upon the theory of change and understanding of impact. Stakeholders can also be consulted to help with attribution estimation, using questionnaires to help arrive at an estimate of overall attribution.

Projecting into the future—the benefit period is the length of time that outcomes from the intervention or service are expected to endure. In addition, 'drop-off' accounts for a potential reduction in the outcome in future years. This can occur either where the outcome diminishes over time (e.g. first-time offenders re-offend), or through attribution drop-off, where the credit taken for an outcome by the original intervention or service reduces (e.g. further training through a different organization or service has more impact on the outcome). The benefit period and drop-off may be informed by the intervention developers, theory of change, longitudinal data, or by previous research conducted using the same intervention or service.

In order to take account of differential timing, as discussed in Chapter 2 of this book, discounting should be applied to the value of future benefits. Discounting recognizes that individuals would prefer to receive money today rather than in the future. In the United Kingdom, it is recommended that the public health economic evaluation discount rate of 1.5 per cent be applied to costs and benefits each year after the initial investment in the programme (<http://www.NICE .org>). The annual rate of 1.5 per cent should be applied to both costs and effects, but an annual rate of 1.5 per cent for health benefits and 3.5 per cent for costs should routinely be used in sensitivity analysis, as should 3.5 per cent for both costs and benefits. (National Institute for Health and Care Excellence, 2013).

The final calculation of the impact takes into account all of the above consid-erations. The value of the benefits is calculated for the first time period after the intervention (T_1)

$$\text{Value of benefits in } T_1 = (\text{Quantity of change} \times \text{financial proxy}) - \% \text{ attribution} \\ - \% \text{ deadweight} - \% \text{ displacement}$$

The cumulative benefits are then added up over the benefit period that the outcomes are expected to last $(T_2 \dots T_x)$. In all future time periods, the drop-off for each period is subtracted from the total. The benefit is also discounted at the standard rate (r) in each time period.

$$\text{Value of benefits in } T_x = \frac{(\text{Value of benefits in } T_{x-1} - \% \text{ drop-off})}{(1+r)^x}$$

Adding up all the value of benefits in T_1 to T_x gives the total present value of the benefits.

The SROI calculation summarized below is arrived at by dividing the Present Value of benefits calculated in the previous stage by the total investment.

$$\text{SROI ratio} = \frac{\text{Present Value of benefits}}{\text{Investment}}$$

Sensitivity analyses allow the analyst to assess the sensitivity of the final SROI ratio to individual assumptions made during the process. It is carried out by varying deadweight, attribution, drop-off, financial proxies, outcomes, discount rate, and monetized inputs within appropriate ranges, and observing the effect on the overall SROI ratio.

Box 12.6 Case study: Stage 5—Calculating the SROI ratio of improving health through investment in housing improvement

The example outcome explored previously is now fully worked through to dem-onstrate all the stages and assumptions to calculate the value of this one outcome.

Assumptions

Attribution: Some of the more specialist home improvements required were car-ried out by the City Council's Occupational Health (OT) team; for example, hand rails, level access showers. NCH's project management records show that around 5 per cent of the total works were carried out by the OT team, and so this proportion is deducted from the total impact.

Box 12.6 Case study: Stage 5 (continued)

Table 12.3 Worked example calculation of one outcome from indicator to total present value from the Nottingham improving homes case study SROI analysis

Outcome	Indicator	Quantity of change	Financial proxy	Attribution	Dead-weight	Impact (Year 1)
Tenants have better health, as internal conditions prevent/ improve management of relevant health issues and prevent accidents in the home.	Reduction in harms from physiological, psychological, infection, and accident hazards.	13	£481	5%	14%	£5,109

Duration (benefit period)	Drop-off	Impact (Year 2)	Impact (Year 3)	Impact (Year 4)	Impact (Year 5)	Total Present Value (3.5% discount)
5 years	20%	£4087	£3,270	£2,616	£2,093	£15,741

Deadweight: Local health statistics show that health in the area is generally improving over time. Therefore, some of the improvements in health would have occurred without the intervention. Data for the area from the Indices of Multiple Deprivation's Health Index show a 14 per cent improvement in the area population's health over the same time period that the home improvements were carried out. This is therefore deducted from the total.

Benefit period: The decision was taken to measure the impact over the five years following the housing improvements. Although the life expectancy of the capital investments is much longer than this period (e.g. boilers are expected to have a serviceable lifetime of fifteen years), the guidance for SROI makes clear that the duration of the benefits of capital investments is not necessarily the same as the life expectancy of those elements. Over such long periods of time, there would be not only be some level of drop-off in the outcome, but attribution drop-off would certainly be high due to changing contextual circumstances and the role of other stakeholders in affecting the long-term trajectory of measured outcomes. Therefore, in line with the principle of SROI of 'do not overclaim', the duration of each outcome was estimated up to a maximum of five years into the future.

Drop-off: A drop-off of 20 per cent is included to account, first, for the depreciation of capital (i.e. accounting for wear and tear on the installations); and second, for attribution drop-off as the way in which the home is used (i.e. whether it is maintained at safe standards) or other lifestyle factors that also affect heath gradually outweigh the effect of housing improvements.

> **Box 12.6** Case study: Stage 5 (continued)
>
> ## Overall SROI ratio
>
> The same calculation process was carried out for each outcome identified in the theory of change. The present value of each of the outcomes was then added up to give the Total Present Value of the scheme, which amounted to £24.3 million over the five years following the improvements. The total invested in home improvements in this pilot area was £16.6m. Therefore, the SROI ratio was calculated as follows:
>
> $$\text{SROI ratio} = \frac{\text{Total present value}}{\text{Total investment}} = \frac{£24.3m}{£16.6m} = £1.46$$
>
> This shows that **every £1 invested in improving homes in the pilot area generates £1.46 in social value**.

12.2.7 **Stage 6—Reporting**

The audience of the report should be clear before writing the report. It is important to report results in a way that is relevant to stakeholders. For example, a more technical audience (such as other analysts or sector organizations) may require a detailed description of the methods and process to derive at the final SROI calculation, whereas other stakeholders, such as service users, may require a headline summary of the results. A report should be made available that contains enough information on the methods and assumptions in order for others to replicate results.[1] Stakeholders may wish to receive pictorial infographics alongside the full report to put up on websites or distribute at events as a platform to relay the key messages from the SROI analysis. The main cornerstone of SROI reporting is known as the 'impact map'. It relates a theory of change to the actual data collected for any given project. There are five sections to any impact map that include: identifying changes expected for stakeholders, identifying and valuing inputs and outputs, putting a value on outcomes, measuring deadweight, attribution, and drop-off, and, finally, calculating the SROI ratio itself. The results can be presented in a pre-prepared spreadsheet template which can be adapted for a given project and offers a framework that provides transparency on the results of any SROI analysis (<http://www.socialvalueuk.org/resource/blank-value-map/>).

12.3 **Increased use of SROI in public health and use of the business case for prevention through social impact bonds**

SROI is more commonly used in the United States than in Europe. For example, Washington state has used SROI extensively to explore topics of legislative interest.

---

[1] SROI reports can be submitted for external accreditation to Social Value UK, in which case a full technical report is required for the auditors.

The Washington State Institution for Public Policy has calculated the return on investment to taxpayers from evidence-based prevention and intervention programmes and policies (Lee et al., 2012). The Washington State Institute for Public Policy has also published SROI analyses of youth crime prevention programmes (Aos, 2010). Further, researchers from the United States are beginning to publish the results from SROI analyses, with particular reference to public health (Eckermann et al., 2014). SROI analysis is becoming of interest in the United Kingdom; policy-makers, local authorities, and charities are now regularly commissioning SROI analyses to demonstrate the impact of their activities. The King's Fund has compiled SROI evidence from a range of PHIs including smoking cessation, contraception to reduce teenage pregnancy, enabling disadvantaged groups to gain employment, cycle or walk to work schemes, improving home environments, and increasing green spaces (Buck and Gregory, 2013).

> The highest rate of return in early childhood development comes from investing as early as possible, from birth through age five, in disadvantaged families. Starting at age three or four is too little too late, as it fails to recognize that skills beget skills in a complementary and dynamic way. Efforts should focus on the first years for the greatest efficiency and effectiveness. The best investment is in quality early childhood development from birth to five for disadvantaged children and their families. James J. Heckman (2012, p. 1).

Benjamin Franklin said an 'ounce of prevention is worth a pound of cure' (Franklin, 1735). This concept is gathering steam in public health, particularly in developed countries where poor health can be related to lifestyle choices. Concerns about the cost of health care has led policy makers in developed countries such as the United States and the United Kingdom to turn their attention to instilling good habits early on such as healthy eating, regular exercise, and not smoking in order to prevent poor health in later life. The increased focus on prevention creates a need for an economic argument to support the funding and roll-out of such programmes. In order to demonstrate the effect of prevention, the analyses need to capture the full value of prevention now and into the future and thus SROI analyses are being employed for this purpose.

As discussed in Chapter 2 of this book, the nature of preventive goods and services is such that they will be underprovided by the free market. By preventive goods and services, we mean government policies, education and information, and environments that prevent ill-health and promote healthy behaviours. Such service provision is discussed in detail by Edwards and colleagues, particularly relating to prevention in the early years of life (Edwards et al., 2016).

This market failure in preventive activity, and the reasons behind it, leads to the need for consideration of different forms of evaluation on behalf of the government or other payers for preventive services. In this context, therefore, it is often the case that SROI techniques are recommended for analysing the case for prevention. As health economists, we might favour the use of theory-driven CBA, and it is interesting that there are still relatively few full CBAs undertaken when compared with other evaluative methods used in health economics.

The government has recognized the potential for SROI to support delivery of publicly funded services by the free market, by correcting for potential market failures. The government introduced social impact bonds (SIB) in 2010, under which providers of publicly funded services are paid on the basis of evidence of social outcomes achieved as a result of service delivery. The aim of SIBs is to redirect funding towards preventive services, by recognizing the full social value of an outcome rather than just the financial costs. In this model, investors pay for a set of interventions that improve outcomes of interest to the government. If social outcomes are shown to improve above a certain level, investors are repaid their costs (plus a return of the risks that they took) by a government commissioner. SIBs have been deployed across a range of services, including prisoner rehabilitation, homelessness services, and support for vulnerable children (UK Government, 2017). SROI supports the delivery of SIBs by providing a framework for valuing social outcomes and providing evidence as to whether or not that value has been achieved.

12.4 Future directions for those applying SROI in public health

Methods of ROI and SROI as practical tools informing the business case for prevention have their advocates and critics. Shiell and Hawe (1995) advocate the use of SROI in economics, arguing that conventional cost-effectiveness analyses cannot gauge the expected long-term effects of health promotion and prevention programs in community settings. Stone shares the view that SROI is an appropriate economic tool, particularly under circumstances in which there are budgetary constraints or limited funds (Stone, 2005). Stone also states that the method is advantageous; as outcomes are valued strictly in monetary terms, councils, policy-makers, and government officials do not need to understand economic terms and concepts such as QALYs in order to understand the relevance of results to them and the services they provide (Stone, 2005). In the current economic climate, service funders increasingly want to invest in programmes that are evidence based and shown to be effective, as budgets become more constrained.

However, one should be mindful that SROI, as a pragmatic version of CBA, is a method is still in its infancy and is not yet standardized. The main criticism is in regards to the extensive use of assumptions required to value outcomes and inform the analyses. The subjective elements of the analysis mean that SROI ratios are not considered to be comparable across different services. Another note of caution is in regards to the use of a single financial estimate (the SROI ratio) to summarize the impact of complex interventions, but this is no different from the use of cost–benefit ratios. Whilst it is sometimes beneficial to have a simple measurable figure such as the SROI ratio to estimate the ballpark return on investment of the programme, this can often hide the complexities of delivering interventions in reality, and it disguises the fact that 'value' is not always one dimensional, quantifiable, or comparable (Mulgan, 2011). Valuing social outcomes still requires an understanding of the specific context and character of the programme and its impact on stakeholders. Further criticism of the method has been provided by Fujiwara (2015). His seven principle problems associated with SROI have been reproduced in Table 12.4.

SROI analysis, therefore, may not be appropriate to use in all circumstances. Health economists may feel more comfortable with the four or five familiar methods of

Table 12.4 Seven principle problems of SROI as argued by Fujiwara

Number	Principle Problem
1.	SROI lacks a clear, principled, normative approach.
2.	SROI is silent on the issue of interpersonal comparisons and it can be argued that it places greater weight on the outcomes of the rich.
3.	SROI's views on stakeholders can be too narrow.
4.	The ratio calculation is susceptible to biases.
5.	Statistical methods for inferring causality are problematic in SROI.
6.	Valuation theory and methodology in SROI are outdated and incomplete.
7.	The meaning of the SROI ratio is vague.

As argued by Fujiwara. Fujiwara, D., 2015. The Seven Principle Problems of SROI. *Simetrica*. Available at: <http://www.simetrica.co.uk/single-post/2015/08/11/The-Seven-Principle-Problems-of-SROI> (Accessed 16 October 2018).

evaluation (including the recently recommended role of cost–consequence analysis for public health economic evaluation). For central and local government who, through legislation or otherwise, have some responsibility for and impact on public health, a pound-for-pound estimate of return on investment is the language that is understood. When deciding whether or not SROI is an appropriate method of evaluation of an intervention or service, the evaluator should consider how the evaluation will be used and who the main audience is. The main difference between SROI and other evaluation methods is that it is strongly stakeholder led, providing a detailed insight into *how* the intervention or service creates change, rather than simply the observable outcomes at the end. At the heart of SROI is the process of developing a theory of change model that encompasses the views of all who are affected (health economists deal with this by using different perspectives). In a public health setting, this means that the shape of the evaluation and the outcomes measured could be driven by patients or services users, their friends and family, and other service providers, as well as by clinical professionals and commissioners. Whilst this provides a holistic view of the value created, this may not be an appropriate form of evaluation in cases where the audience (such as commissioners) are only concerned with a predetermined set of clinical health outcomes. SROI sits well with the concept of asset-based public health, particularly through the importance given to stakeholder involvement in the analysis of ROI, as discussed in our section on health assets in Chapter 9 of this book.

12.5 **UK government ROI tools**

SROI is becoming more commonly used as a method of evaluation, particularly in public health and preventive medicine. A number of tools have been developed to support analysts with an SROI analysis, for example by the National Institute for Health and Care Excellence (NICE) and the Housing Associations' Charitable Trust (HACT), a housing think-tank (HACT, 2014). These tools assist the process by providing some of the assumptions and financial proxies available, based on the latest evidence from the sector. However, it should be noted that because the primary principle of SROI is to engage stakeholders directly, such tools can only be used to assist certain aspects of the SROI process rather than providing a direct route to complete a full SROI.

For example, the NICE and Public Health England (PHE) have recently developed ROI Tools, which are available on their websites for local authorities to use: (<https://www.nice.org.uk/about/what-we-do/into-practice/return-on-investment-tools> and <https://www.gov.uk/guidance/health-economics-a-guide-for-public-health-teams>). These tools are intended to aid decision-makers and local commissioners in local authorities and the NHS to make investment decisions. They are considered ROI tools rather than SROI tools due to the limited stakeholder engagement and social outcomes; instead, the focus is upon cost savings. There are an increasing number of ROI tools available, particularly in the areas of smoking, physical exercise, caries prevention, cardiovascular disease and alcohol misuse, and each tool allows the user to model packages of interventions and to assess the economic returns from each package of intervention; see the UK's PHE webiste and also: <https://www.nice.org.uk/about/what-we-do/into-practice/return-on-investment-tools>. Interventions can be customized if there are data on the costs and effects of the intervention in question. Users must first choose a geographic area or a clinical commissioning group (CCG) (in England) for which the tools have already inputted local population data along with prevalence of smoking, physical activity, and alcohol consumption. This population composition is then used to model the impact of interventions aimed at reducing the prevalence of smoking and alcohol consumption and increasing the prevalence of physical activity. If we take smoking as an example of how these NICE tools can be useful, then we see that the first step is to choose, using a drop-down menu, the area of interest. The tool will then estimate, based on up-to-date statistics, the prevalence of smokers and ex-smokers in the population. It is possible then for the user to mix and match different interventions to see which package of interventions provide the best 'value for money' compared with 'no services' or any other package of interventions. Four pay-back timescales are included in the tool—2, 5, 10 years, and lifetime, enabling the analyst to calculate how ROI changes over time. For advanced users it is also possible to conduct a deterministic sensitivity analysis to assess uncertainty by making assumptions to vary certain parameters to see what effect this has on the ROI metric. The ROI figures include cost savings from the perspective of the NHS and other sectors (e.g. social care) and some quasi-social benefits such as productivity gains and value of health benefits to the individual (NICE 2014).

Summary of Chapter 12

- ROI and SROI are pragmatic forms of CBA that allow an evaluator to assess the 'triple bottom line' of an intervention or service, and to give a ratio of value given from each £1 invested.

- The method is based upon a set of seven principles that underpin the analysis, with guidance and banks of valuation data available.

◆ The method has begun to be used more widely for evaluating PHIs in the United Kingdom. Internationally, the bulk of cost–benefit and ROI analysis of public health prevention initiatives has been generated by economists in the United States.

◆ SROI allows an evaluator to assess wider benefits of an intervention or service by measuring changes in outcomes and assigning them a proxy financial value, and can show the value of benefits accrued over a number of years.

◆ The case for use of SROI is particularly strong when it comes to supplying preventive goods, which would be under-supplied by the free market and therefore require government intervention in their provision.

◆ SROI aims to capture the full social value of an intervention rather than just its cost, and therefore helps avoid under-supply of publicly valuable goods. However, those interested in the method should keep in mind the limitations, for example, lack of comparability, subjectivity of assumptions used, and the relative infancy of the method compared to more established methods such as CBA.

References

Aos, S., 2010. Fight Crime and Save Money: Development of an investment tool for states to study sentencing and corrections public policy options—progress report. Washington State Institution for Public Policy. Document Number 10-04-1201. Available at: <http://www.wsipp.wa.gov/rptfiles/10-04-1201.pdf> (Accessed 16 October 2018).

Arvidson, M., Lyon, F., McKay, S., and Moro, D., 2010. The ambitions and challenges of SROI. Working Paper. TSRC, Birmingham. Available at: <https://eprints.mdx.ac.uk/7104/1/The_ambitions_and_challenges_of_SROI.pdf> (Accessed 16 October 2018).

Barnes, M., Cullinane, C., Scott, S., and Silvester, H., 2013. People living in bad housing – numbers and health impacts. NatCen Social Research. Available at: <https://england.shelter.org.uk/__data/assets/pdf_file/0010/726166/People_living_in_bad_housing.pdf> (Accessed 16 October 2018).

Braubach, M., Jacobs, D.E., and Ormandy, D., 2011. The Environmental Burden of Disease Associated with Inadequate Housing. Available at; <http://www.euro.who.int/__data/assets/pdf_file/0003/142077/e95004.pdf> (Accessed 16 October 2018).

Buck, D. and Gregory, S., 2013. Improving the public's health—A resource for local authorities. The Kings Fund. Available at: <http://www.kingsfund.org.uk/sites/files/kf/field/field_publication_file/improving-the-publics-health-kingsfund-dec13.pdf> (Accessed 16 October 2018).

Cabinet Office, 2009. A Guide to Social Return on Investment. Available at: <http://www.bond.org.uk/data/files/Cabinet_office_A_guide_to_Social_Return_on_Investment.pdf> (Accessed 16 October 2018).

Curtis, L., and Burns, A., 2017. Unit Costs of Health and Social Care. Available at: <https://www.pssru.ac.uk/project-pages/unit-costs/unit-costs-2017/> (Accessed 16 October 2018).

Davidson, M., Roys, M., Nicol, S., Ormandy, D., and Ambrose, P., 2010. The Real Cost of Poor Housing. Bracknell: IHS BRE Press.

Department for the Environment, Transport and the Regions, 2000. Quality and Choice: A Decent Home for All. London: The Stationery Office.

Dolan, P., and Peasgood T., 2008. Measuring well-being for public policy: preferences or experiences. *Journal of Legal Studies, 37*:S5–S31.

Eckermann, S., Dawber, J., Yeatman, H., Quinsey, K., and Morris, D., 2014. Evaluating return on investment in a school based health promotion and prevention program: the investment multiplier for the Stephanie Alexander Kitchen Garden National Program. *Social Science and Medicine, 114*: 103–12.

Edwards, R.T., Bryning, L., and Lloyd-Williams, H., 2016. Transforming Young Lives across Wales: The Economic Argument for Investing in Early Years. Centre for Health Economics and Medicines Evaluation, Bangor University. Available at: <http://cheme.bangor.ac.uk/reportspublications.php.en> (Accessed 16 October 2018).

EuroQoL Group. 1990. EuroQoL—a new facility for the measurement of health related quality of life. *Health Policy, 16*: 199–208.

Franklin, B., 1735. Protection of Towns from Fire. The Pennsylvania Gazette.

Fujiwara, D., 2013. The social impact of housing providers. *HACT.* Available at: <http://www.hact.org.uk/sites/default/files/uploads/Archives/2013/02/The%20Social%20Impact%20of%20Housing%20FINALpdf.pdf> (Accessed 16 October 2018).

Fujiwara, D., 2013. Centre for Economic Performance Discussion Paper Number 1233 A General Method for Valuing Non-Market Goods Using Wellbeing Data: Three-Stage Wellbeing Valuation. Available at: <http://cep.lse.ac.uk/pubs/download/dp1233.pdf> (Accessed 16 October 2018).

Fujiwara, D., 2015. The Seven Principle Problems of SROI. *Simetrica.* Available at: <http://www.simetrica.co.uk/single-post/2015/08/11/The-Seven-Principle-Problems-of-SROI> (Accessed 16 October 2018).

HACT, 2014. Value Calculator. Available at: <http://www.hact.org.uk/value-calculator> (Accessed 16 October 2018).

Heckman, J.J., 2012. Nobel Prize Winning Economist Professor James Heckman Releases Statement on Investing in Early Learning. Available at: <http://ffyf.org/nobel-prize-winning-economist-professor-james-heckman-releases-statement-on-investing-in-early-learning/> (Accessed 16 October 2018).

Hills, P. and Argyle, M., 2002. The Oxford Happiness Questionnaire: a compact scale for the measurement of psychological well-being. *Personality and Individual Differences, 33*: 1073–82.

Jones, A., Valero-Silva, N., and Lucas, D., 2016. *The Effects of 'Secure, Warm, Modern' Homes in Nottingham: Decent Homes Impact Study.* Nottingham: Nottingham City Homes.

Lee, S., Aos, S., Drake, E., Pennucci, A., Miller, M., and Anderson, L., 2012. Return on investment: Evidence-based options to improve statewide outcomes (Document No. 12-04-1201). *Olympia: Washington State Institute for Public Policy.* Available at: <http://www.wsipp.wa.gov/ReportFile/1102/Wsipp_Return-on-Investment-Evidence-Based-Options-to-Improve-Statewide-Outcomes-April-2012-Update_Full-Report.pdf> (Accessed 16 October 2018).

Masters, R., Anwar, E., Collins, B., et al., 2017. Return on investment of public health interventions:a systematic review. *J Epidemiol Community Health, 71*: 827–34.

Mishan, E.J., 1971. *CBA.* London: Allen & Unwin.

Mulgan, G., 2011. Effective supply and demand and measurement of public and social value In: J. Benington and M. Moore (eds), *Public Value: Theory and Practice.* Basingstoke: Palgrave Macmillan, pp. 212–24.

National Institute for Health and Care Excellence, 2013. *Guide to the Methods of Technology Appraisal*. London: National Institute for Health and Care Excellence.

National Institute for Health and Care Excellence, 2014. *Return on Investment Tools*. Available at: <https://www.nice.org.uk/about/what-we-do/into-practice/return-on-investment-tools> (Accessed 16 October 2018).

Office for National Statistics, 2014. Family Spending Survey. Available at: <http://www.ons.gov.uk/ons/rel/family-spending/family-spending/2014-edition/index.html> (Accessed 16 October 2018).

Ryan, M., Gerard, K., and Amaya-Amaya, M., 2007. *Using Discrete Choice Experiments to Value Health and Health Care*. Dordrecht: Springer Science & Business Media.

Shiell, A. and Hawe, P. 1995. Health promotion community development and the tyranny of individualism. *Health Economics*, 5:241–7.

Stone, P.W., 2005. Return on investment models. *Applied Nursing Research*, *18*: 186–9.

Tennant, R., Hiller, L., Fishwick, R., Platt, S., Joseph, S., Weich, S., Parkinson, J., et al., 2007. The Warwick–Edinburgh mental well-being scale (WEMWBS): development and UK validation. *Health and Quality of Life Outcomes*, *5*(1):63.

UK Government, 2014. Guidance Standard Assessment Procedure. Available at <https://www.gov.uk/guidance/standard-assessment-procedure> (Accessed 31 October 2018).

UK Government, 2017. Guidance Social Impact Bonds. Available at <https://www.gov.uk/guidance/social-impact-bonds> (Accessed 31 October 2018).

Chapter 13

The role of multi-criteria decision analysis (MCDA) in public health economic evaluation

Huw Lloyd-Williams

13.1 Introduction

Benjamin Franklin (1706–1790), a Founding Father of the United States, was one of the first proponents of multi-criteria decision analysis (MCDA). He devised a simple paper-based system of making important decisions. Whenever he had to decide on an important issue he would write down the arguments for on one side of a piece of paper and against on the other side. He would then strike out those arguments on each side of the paper that had relatively equal importance, and when all arguments were eliminated on one side he would look at the other side. If there were any arguments left on the other side, he would veer his decision towards that option (Köksalan et al., 2013).

This simple exercise shows a feature that is central in MCDA, namely that decisions are typically based on a series of criteria rather than one single criterion or measure of effectiveness, which is often the case in most types of economic evaluation. As discussed in the introductory chapters of this book, in the United Kingdom, the National Institute for Health and Care Excellence (NICE) makes recommendations to the National Health Service (NHS) based on the calculation of a single or suite of incremental cost-effectiveness ratios (ICERs) (National Institute for Health and Care Excellence, 2014). This has recently come into question as it is commonly accepted that the ICER or cost per quality-adjusted life year (QALY) does not capture all the decision-making criteria that commissioners of health care deem to be relevant to their decisions, particularly in public health, as discussed in Chapter 3 of this book. Although NICE considers other criteria (e.g. whether a new drug is for the treatment of a very rare disease or end of life care), it does not explicitly account for multiple criteria when evaluating health technologies. It is argued by commentators such as Baltussen and Nielsen that there is a real need for MCDA, particularly in evaluating public health interventions (PHIs) (Baltussen and Nielsen, 2006). However, one must add a cautionary note: there is general consensus that MCDA requires further refinement before use in economic evaluation (Marsh et al., 2014). Critics of MCDA argue that fundamental gaps in the method require further research (Ciomek et al., 2017), and it needs preference-based valuation methods which use trade-offs to weight 'criteria' akin to methods such as stated preference discrete choice experiment (SPDCE) (see Chapter 9) before MCDA is useful for the purposes of economic evaluation. See Kujawski for a generic range of limitations pitfalls and practical limitations of MCDA (Kujawski, 2003).

The roots of MCDA lie in early development of utility theory (introduced in Chapter 2 of this book) and decision analysis and the later development of multi-objective mathematical programming. Early work on utility theory was proposed by Ramsey (Ramsey, 1928), and von Neumann and Morganstern formalized the study of utility (Von Neumann and Morganstern, 1947). The earliest work on utility can be traced back to Edgeworth (Edgeworth, 1881) with his work on indifference curves. Howard Raiffa, Robert Schlaifer (Raiffa and Schlaifer, 1961), and Ron Howard (Howard et al., 1977) were early proponents of decision analysis and their work paved the way for what we understand as decision analysis today. At the time they undertook their research, the field of multi-objective mathematical modelling diverged from utility theory and decision analysis in that the former addressed deterministic problems while the latter addressed decision-making under uncertainty. It is the former that has led to what we know of today as MCDA, a branch of multi-criteria analysis (MCA).

13.2 **Theory**

13.2.1 **Multi-criteria analysis (MCA)**

The bedrock of multi-criteria analysis (MCA) is the performance matrix in which each row describes the option to be evaluated and each column refers to a criterion by which the option can be measured in which to facilitate comparison of the different options. Each entry into the matrix then allows the decision-maker to assess how well each option performs with respect to each criterion. Techniques are then applied to analyse numerically the performance matrix using scoring and weighting. Mathematical methods are then used, by means of computer programming, to combine these elements in order to provide an overall assessment of each option being considered. This approach is often referred to as the 'compensatory MCA technique' as a high score on one criterion may offset a low score on another. The way one combines scores and weights is to use simple weighted averages which assumes the 'mutual independence of preferences' (Abbas & Sun, 2015). This is so that the strength of preference on one criterion will be independent of the strength of preference on another.

There are many different types of MCA; listed in the following are three of the most commonly used.

13.2.1.1 Direct appraisal of the performance matrix

The performance matrix can be used as a basic tool to guide decisions on the choice between different options or, in our case, PHIs. The main way of doing this is to establish some kind of dominance by looking at the data within the matrix. According to the manual on MCA by the Department for Communities and Local Government: 'Dominance occurs when one option performs at least as well as another on all criteria and strictly better than the other on at least one criterion' (Department for Communities and Local Government, 2009, p. 24).

In practice, however, since it is unlikely that one single option will strictly dominate, this technique allows decision-makers to eliminate options that are dominated.

13.2.1.2 Multi-attribute utility (MAU) theory

Multi-attribute utility (MAU) theory derives from the pioneering work of von Neumann and Morganstern (1947) which provides a formalized approach to the study of utility. The breakthrough came with the work of Keeney and Raiffa where they developed a set of procedures that would allow the evaluation of options using multiple criteria (Keeney and Raiffa, 1993). Their main contribution was the enabling of the development of a single index, *U*, to express the decision-maker's overall valuation of an option based on the value of its performance on each criterion. They were the first formally to include the possibility of accounting for uncertainty. The MAU is the basis for research into estimating the utilities associated with health states such as is found in health economic instruments such as the EQ-5D (introduced in Chapter 2 of this book).

13.2.1.3 Linear additive models

This model can be applied if it can be proved that the assumption of mutual independence of preferences holds and that uncertainty is not considered. Here the option's value on different criteria can be additively combined into one single value. This is done by multiplying the value score on each criterion by the weight of that criterion and then adding all those weighted scores together into an overall value. Most MCA techniques use this additive model, and this is the basis of MCDA, which is discussed in the section 13.2.2.

13.2.2 **Multi-criteria decision analysis (MCDA)**

MCDA is a branch of MCA that helps decision-makers evaluate alternative courses of action that require consideration of multiple criteria, some of which may be conflicting. It is defined, in a paper by Devlin and Sussex, as 'a set of methods and approaches to aid decision making, where decisions are based on more than one criterion, which make explicit the impact on the decision of all the criteria applied and the relative importance attached to them' (Devlin and Sussex, 2011, p.1).

Keeney and Raiffa define MCDA as being 'an extension of decision theory that covers any decision with multiple objectives. A methodology for appraising alternatives on individual, often conflicting criteria, and combining them into one overall appraisal' (Keeney and Raiffa, 1993).

The first two steps of MCDA are to identify: (i) the alternatives to be appraised and (ii) the criteria against which the alternatives are to be assessed. This is known as problem structuring and is performed by the stakeholders involved through a process of decision conferencing. Decision conferencing involves gathering together the key stakeholders and, through an impartial facilitator, iteratively and interactively structuring the problem at hand using on-the-spot computer modelling. The final two stages involve (iii) scoring each alternative's expected performance on each criterion and then (iv) using weights to adjust the importance of each criterion and deliver a ranking of the alternatives. Perhaps a simpler way to describe the process of MCDA is to think about it in the following way:

◆ Identifying interventions to evaluate.
◆ Identifying criteria against which to evaluate the interventions.

- ◆ Measuring the interventions against the criteria.
- ◆ Combining the criteria scores to produce a ranking of each intervention.

The traditional way of thinking about decision-making has been by recourse to a single objective function whereby the decision-makers seek to maximize (or minimize) this function (e.g. profit maximization, see Figueira et al., 2005). Most of the techniques of priority setting such as evidence-based medicine, burden of disease analysis, cost-effectiveness analysis, and equity analysis, are based on a single criterion.

Baltussen and Nielsen argue that PHIs need to be evaluated in a broader context (Baltussen and Nielsen, 2006). For example, the need to meet several policy goals such as improved overall population health and reduced inequalities in health and to undertake these activities within a constrained budget.

MCDA is not confined to simple weighting and scoring approaches; other approaches are available that are more relevant to NICE's health technology evaluation process (National Institute for Health and Care Excellence, 2014). According to Devlin and Sussex: 'it is *inevitable* that NICE decisions will be based on multiple criteria—they already are. The question is not whether multiple criteria should be taken into account in these decisions, but what those criteria should be and how best to incorporate them in decision-making' (Devlin and Sussex, 2011, p. 2).

It can be seen that the first step of MCDA, problem structuring, is akin to the scoping stage in health technology assessment (HTA). Where the two methods differ is in the decision-making stage. With the NICE approach, the ICER, which is a calculation, is used to capture and evaluate the evidence, whereas with the MCDA approach this evidence is put into mathematical models to identify the best alternatives. The difference in the approaches that can be used is accounted for in the way these models are specified.

Another approach is to look at the MCDA process in terms of following eight steps as identified by the International Society for Pharmacoeconomics and Outcomes Research (ISPOR) who, in 2014, established an MCDA Emerging Good Practice Taskforce. The taskforce defines MCDA and provides good practice guidelines for conducting MCDA in the arena of health care decision-making also relevant in the context of this book to public health. In the first ISPOR paper, (Thokala et al., 2016) the following steps are identified:

1. Defining the decision problem
   This is the first step of any MCDA and involves understanding and defining the research problem. It also involves identifying the appropriate stakeholders. These may be patients, clinicians, payers, regulators, or the general population, and are usually those providing preferences. This step also requires the analyst to identify the alternatives under consideration.

2. Selecting and structuring the criteria
   Once the research problem is defined, one can then select the criteria against which alternatives can be measured. This is akin to the 'problem structuring' stage mentioned earlier. Criteria can be identified by means of focus groups or workshops, for example.

3. Measuring performance

   This is where we measure the performance of the alternatives on each of the criteria. These data can be gathered by means of a systematic review or meta-analysis, for example, or by expert opinion.

4. Scoring alternatives

   Alternatives are then scored according to stakeholders' preferences for change within each criteria. Performance measurements are converted into scores using certain mathematical functions or rules. There are two methods of scoring broken down as they are to compositional and decompositional methods. The first type calculates separate estimates of scores and weights before combining them, while the decompositional method, which includes discrete choice experiments (DCE) and conjoint analysis, involves ranking two or more alternatives and then, using regression methods, estimates how the utility associated with each alternative varies with changes in performance against each criterion.

5. Weighting criteria

   Stakeholders' preference between criteria are then given weights. These weights represent 'trade-offs' between criteria and the scores on individual criteria, once the weights have been applied to them are converted into a measure of 'total value'.

6. Calculating aggregate scores

   For compositional methods each alternative's score on each criterion is multiplied by their respective weight to give a 'total value' for each alternative. For decompositional methods, such as Stated Preference Discrete Choice Experiments (SPDCE) (see Chapter 9) or conjoint analysis, the data on the alternatives are inputted into a valuation function derived from the regression analysis to estimate the utility of each alternative.

7. Dealing with uncertainty

   Each aspect of MCDA is subject to uncertainty. This includes criteria selection and the weighting/scoring of criteria. We can address parameter uncertainty by techniques such as probabilistic sensitivity analysis.

8. Interpretation and reporting the results

   The results of MCDA can be reported in graphical or tabular form. Alternatives are usually ranked according to their importance or at least to provide a measure of value for each alternative. The total scores of alternatives can also be monetized in order to provide an estimate of value for money associated with each alternative in order to guide resource allocation decisions.

13.3 Three approaches to MCDA

There are three main approaches within the technique of MCDA which are classified as value measurement models, outranking models, and goal, aspiration, or reference models.

13.3.1 Value measurement models

The first approach uses and compares numerical scores to assess the degree to which one option is preferred over another. It is based within the theory of utility. In economics, a number of assumptions are made about human behaviour, and rationality is one of these key assumptions. Rationality entails that individual agents have consistent preferences (as introduced in Chapter 2 of this book). In more technical terms, these preferences are said to be complete and transitive. In terms of complete preferences, any pairwise comparison, for example, between intervention a and b, either one must be preferred over the other or there is indifference between them ($a > b$, $b > a$, or $a \sim b$). If preferences are transitive then for any three alternatives a, b, and c if a is preferred to b, and b preferred to c, then a must be preferred to c. In order for a decision-maker to compare alternatives, a value must be placed on these alternatives $V(a)$. The decision-maker can then produce a preference ordering of the alternatives consistent with his/her value judgement. Alternative a is preferred to b only if $V(a) > V(b)$. Also, if $V(a) = V(b)$ there is said to be indifference between the two options. Keeney and Raiffa extended these axioms to consider decisions with multiple objectives (Keeney and Raiffa, 1993). Therefore, for each criterion, a score is developed followed by a weighting of these scores to arrive at a sum of scores for each alternative. These overall scores are then compared in order to decide on the preferred alternative. One of the main advantages of the value measurement model is its simplicity and this has led to the technique being the most frequently used within MCDA.

This approach is also the basis for the programme budgeting and marginal analysis (PBMA) method which is discussed in Chapter 14 of this book.

PBMA is a process that helps decision-makers maximize the impact of health care resources on the health needs of a local population or meet other specified goals such as equity considerations.

See Chapter 14 for an example of how PBMA has been used to review spending on public health in Wales (Edwards et al., 2014). As shown in the case study in Chapter 14, the stakeholders can be asked to vote electronically in order to establish which criteria carry more weight and then the alternative PHIs are assessed based on these weights (Edwards et al., 2014) see Figure 13.1.

13.3.2 Outranking models

The outranking approach compares alternatives pairwise in terms of each criterion. This is to establish the preference for each alternative for each specific criterion. The preference information is then aggregated in order to arrive at the total preference for each alternative. It is therefore based on the general principle of dominance. Consider the following example in Figure 13.2.

The results are then aggregated into what is known as the concordance index, which can be calculated as follows:

$$\text{Concordance Index}\,(\text{CI}) = \frac{\text{Sum of criteria weights where x is better}}{\text{Total sum of weights}}$$

Treatment A has a CI of $3 + 3 + 1 + 1/20 = 0.4$, while treatment B has a CI of $10 + 2/20 = 0.6$. If the predefined threshold is less than 0.6 we can say that treatment B is

Criteria	Percentage vote	n
Stakeholder views	20%	2
Presence and robustness of evidence of effectiveness	34%	4
Presence and robustness of evidence of cost-effectiveness	27%	3
Impact or potential impact on reducing inequalities in health	19%	2

Results of the electronic vote for the top 4 criteria for the health improvement review from 12 PBMA panel members.

Figure 13.1 An example of criteria for PBMA.
Reproduced from Edwards, R.T., et al. A national Programme Budgeting and Marginal Analysis (PBMA) of health improvement spending across Wales: disinvestment and reinvestment across the life course. *BMC Public Health*. 14(837). Copyright © Edwards et al.; licensee BioMed Central Ltd. 2014. Open Access.

preferred. The defining of this threshold is largely arbitrary and left to the judgment of the decision-maker.

13.3.3 Goal, aspiration, or reference models

The third method involves setting predetermined levels of achievement for each criterion and identifying those alternatives that are closest to matching these. An example of this approach is in value-based pricing where drugs/treatments are priced in order for the ICER to come under willingness-to-pay thresholds. The purpose of this method is to broaden the scope of NICE appraisals in the United Kingdom so that wider benefits of drugs are captured (Parliamentary Office of Science and Technology, 2015). The idea is based on a concept of 'satisficing' whereby 'goals' are predefined and linear programming is used to identify the interventions that satisfy these goals in the correct order. This approach is not based on value functions, as is the case with the previous two approaches, but rather on the attributes themselves, or at least the goals associated with those attributes. The relationship between the attribute value and the

Criterion	Weight	Treatment A	Treatment B
Cost Effectiveness	10		√
Equity	3	√	
Innovation	3	√	
Quality of Evidence	2		√
Compliance	1	√	
Mortality	1	√	

Figure 13.2. Example of outranking approach to MCDA.

goal can be maximizing, minimizing, or attaining; that is, the attribute can specify the minimum amount needed to satisfy the goal, or the maximum amount, or the intervention's attribute must be as close to the goal as is possible. The difference then between the attribute and its goal is seen as 'goal deviation'. For example, if one of the attributes of an intervention was equity and for intervention A this was 0.15 and B was 0.25. If the goal was set at 0.2 then only the attribute of intervention B would satisfy this goal. The goal deviation would be –0.05 for intervention A and +0.05 for intervention B. The aim of goal programming is to minimize these goal deviations, in order to achieve an outcome as close to the original policy goal as possible.

13.4 Availability of MCDA guidelines for use in health economics

As discussed earlier, there are a number of MCDA methods available and to choose between them can be a daunting task for the analyst. The updated ISPOR paper (Marsh et al., 2014) identifies good practice guidelines for conducting MCDA along with a checklist to support the design, implementation and review of MCDA. These guidelines assist decision-makers in the task of determining which method of MCDA to use in different circumstances.

13.5 Case study

The case study for this section comes from The Netherlands: Bots, P.W. and Hulshof, J.A., 2000. Designing multi-criteria decision analysis processes for priority setting in health policy. *Journal of Multicriteria Decision Analysis, 9*(1–3):56. The authors use MCDA to provide insight into the potential application of this approach to real life policy-making. It is particularly relevant because it looks at the application of MCDA in the context of public health policy-making. The authors proceed by assessing (i) the most important health problems in The Netherlands and (ii) efficiency gains in the health sector. A rational model of policy-making is presented whereby the policy-making process is made up of the five distinct activities of 'intelligence gathering–design–choice–implementation–review'. The rationality of the model comes through the assumption that policy development is based on sound information and that the chosen policy is consistent with this information. It is argued that MCDA is especially apt in this case because the focus on operational objectives gives the analyst well-defined criteria that can be used to compare a set of alternative policy instruments. In order to choose which MCDA technique to use, techniques were rated in terms of transparency, simplicity of the analysis, sensitivity to different ways of standardization, ability to deal with quantitative and/or qualitative data and the eventual ranking result' (Bots and Hulshof, 2000, p. 59).

It was decided to base the analysis around the simple multi-attribute rating technique (SMART) because quantitative data were available, the alternatives were to be ranked on a linear scale (Von Winterfeldt and Edwards, 1993. The SMART is based on the linear additive approach mentioned in section 13.2.1. They identify the main roles within the MCDA as an expert role and a decision-maker role. These people would then meet in an electronic meeting system to take part in four group activities, as follows:

1. Consensus building on impact matrix and impact scores
   The impact matrix is directly comparable with the performance matrix discussed in section 13.2.1. Its rows consist of policy options and its columns the criteria by which these are judged.
2. Prioritizing criteria
   It is possible to prioritize criteria according to pairwise comparison, ranking, scoring, weight allocation, etc. These methods are supported by electronic meeting systems such as Ventana's *Group Systems* (Dennis et al., 1988).
3. Ranking options
   Here, the ranking of options is based on the weighted sum of scores. This can be achieved using the Microsoft™ Excel package. By sorting the rank order of different weight sets it is possible to conduct the next activity of identifying robust options.
4. Identifying robust options
   An option is 'robust' if it maximizes all or most of the weight sets.

   This study aimed to assess (i) the most important health problems in The Netherlands and (ii) potential efficiency gains in the health sector. This case was developed by initially clustering the diseases that needed to be taken into account. The authors then determined the criteria to be used to rate these clusters by importance. These criteria were prevalence, potential years of life lost, and cost of health care. The next step was to find data on all the criteria for all the disease clusters and using these data, the three criteria scores were aggregated in order to determine the rank order. This was the basic structure of the MCDA in this case. The rest of the process involved policy design where MCDA can be used to rank diseases in order of importance which can then be used to inform policy goals and instruments. These policy instruments were categorized as relating to 'cure', 'care', and 'prevention', and were defined for the 15 most 'important' disease clusters, resulting in 42 distinct policy instruments. The disease clusters were: coronary heart disease, stroke, accidents, chronic obstructive lung disease, diabetes mellitus, dementia, lung cancer, breast cancer, colon/rectum cancer, arthrosis, pneumonia/acute bronchitis, learning difficulties, neonatal complications, rheumatoid arthritis, and depression.

Summary of Chapter 13

In this chapter we have outlined the main characteristics and processes associated with conducting MCDA. Increasingly, within the health economics community, there are calls for a wider approach to guide resource allocation decisions in public health that look beyond cost-effectiveness alone. For example, some commentators have suggested that budget impact should be another criterion to be considered when making resource allocation decisions (Cohen et al., 2008; Niezen et al., 2009). Further, it is recognized that the QALY approach (presented here in Chapter 8), whilst able to show QALY gains well below the NICE threshold of £20,000–£30,000 per QALY for many PHIs, fails to reflect the full range of benefits that may be important to society. These include benefits such as improved educational attainment in school children, productivity, improvement in subjective well-being, 'process of care' utility, and reduction in health inequalities. In the United Kingdom, NICE is moving in the direction of the more explicit treatment of other criteria and this is where MCDA could be particularly useful.

MCDA does not decide which criteria to include; this is a matter for judgment. Neither does it decide what weight to place on each criterion. This can be seen as a limitation of MCDA as it currently exists, however an additional exercise using trade-off methods such as discrete choice experiments are feasible. Once this preference-based valuation of final criteria has been conducted, MCDA can potentially support complex decision-making in a transparent way necessary in public health where there is likely to be more than one policy goal of equal importance. Decisions do not have to be based on heuristic judgement alone by formalizing the process, and while these techniques do not replace decision-making, they can facilitate the process of deciding how to allocate scarce resources in health care.

References

Abbas, A.E. and Sun, Z., 2015. Multiattribute utility functions satisfying mutual preferential independence. *Operations Research*, 63(2): 378–93.

Baltussen, R. and Niessen, L., 2006. Priority setting of health interventions: the need for multi-criteria decision analysis. *Cost Effectiveness and Resource Allocation*, 4(1): 14.

Bots, P.W. and Hulshof, J.A., 2000. Designing multi-criteria decision analysis processes for priority setting in health policy. *Journal of Multicriteria Decision Analysis*, 9(1–3): 56.

Ciomek, K., Kadziński, M., and Tervonen, T., 2017. Heuristics for prioritizing pair-wise elicitation questions with additive multi-attribute value models. *Omega*, 71: 27–45.

Cohen, J.P., Stolk, E., and Niezen, M., 2008. Role of budget impact in drug reimbursement decisions. *Journal of Health Politics, Policy and Law*, 33(2): 225–47.

Department for Communities and Local Government, 2009. Multi-Criteria Analysis: A manual. London: Department for Communities and Local Government. Available at: <https://www.gov.uk/government/uploads/system/uploads/attachment_data/file/7612/1132618.pdf> (Accessed 16 October 2018).

Dennis, A.R., George, J.F., Jessup, L.M., Nunamaker Jr, J.F., and Vogel, D.R., 1988. Information technology to support electronic meetings. *MIS Quarterly*, 591–624.

Devlin, N. and Sussex, J., 2011. *Incorporating Multiple Criteria in HTA. Methods and Processes*. London: Office of Health Economics.

Edgeworth, F.Y., 1881. *Mathematical Psychics: An Essay on the Application of Mathematics to the Moral Sciences*. London: Kegan Paul.

Edwards, R.T., Charles, J.M., Thomas, S., Bishop, J., Cohen, D., Groves, S., Humphreys, C., et al., 2014. A national Programme Budgeting and Marginal Analysis (PBMA) of health improvement spending across Wales: disinvestment and reinvestment across the life course. *BMC Public Health*, 14(1): 837

Figueira, J., Mousseau, V., and Roy, B., 2005. ELECTRE methods. In: J. Bloggs and T. Moggs (eds), *Multiple Criteria Decision Analysis: State of the Art Surveys*. Springer New York, NY: Springer, pp. 133–53.

Howard, R.A., Matheson, J.E., and **Miller, K.L.** (eds), 1977. *Readings in Decision Analysis.* Stanford, CA: Decision Analysis Group, Stanford Research Institute.

Keeney, R.L. and **Raiffa, H.,** 1993. *Decisions with Multiple Objectives: Preferences and Value Trade-Offs.* Cambridge: Cambridge University Press.

Köksalan, M., **Wallenius, J.,** and **Zionts, S.,** 2013. An early history of multiple criteria decision making. *Journal of Multi-Criteria Decision Analysis, 20*(1–2): 87–94.

Kujawski, E. 2003. Multi-criteria decision analysis: Limitations, pitfalls, and practical difficulties. *INCOSE International Symposium, 13*(1): 1169–76.

Marsh, K., **Lanitis, T., Neasham, D., Orfanos, P.,** and **Caro, J.,** 2014. Assessing the value of health care interventions using multi-criteria decision analysis: A review of the literature. *Pharmacoeconomics, 32*(4): 345–65.

National Institute for Health and Care Excellence, 2014, Guide to the process of technology appraisal. Available at: <https://www.nice.org.uk/article/pmg19/chapter/3-The-appraisal-process> (Accessed 16 October 2018).

Niezen, M.G., **de Bont, A., Busschbach, J.J., Cohen, J.P.,** and **Stolk, E.A.,** 2009. Finding legitimacy for the role of budget impact in drug reimbursement decisions. *International Journal of Technology Assessment in Health Care, 25*(1): 49–55.

Parliamentary Office of Science and Technology, 2015. Value Based Assessment of Drugs, Postnote No. 487. Available from: <https://researchbriefings.parliament.uk/ResearchBriefing/Summary/POST-PN-487> (Accessed 1 November 2018).

Raiffa, H. and **Schlaifer, R.,** 1961. Applied Statistical Decision Theory. Boston: Clinton Press

Ramsey, F.P., 1928. A mathematical theory of saving. *The Economic Journal, 38*(152):543–59. Available at: <http://doi.org/10.2307/2224098> (Accessed 16 October 2018).

Thokala, P. and **Duenas, A.,** 2012. Multiple criteria decision analysis for health technology assessment. *Value in Health, 15*(8):1172–81.

Thokala, P., **Devlin, N., Marsh, K., Baltussen, R., Boysen, M., Kalo, Z., Longrenn, T., Mussen, F.,** et al., 2016. Multiple criteria decision analysis for health care decision making—an introduction: report 1 of the ISPOR MCDA Emerging Good Practices Task Force. *Value in Health, 19*(1): 1–13.

Von Winterfeldt, D. and **Edwards, W.,** 1993. *Decision Analysis and Behavioral Research.* New York, NY: Cambridge University Press.

Von Neumann, J. and **Morgenstern, O.,** 1947. *Theory of Games and Economic Behavior.* Princeton, NJ: Princeton University Press.

Chapter 14

To disinvest or invest? The role of programme budgeting and marginal analysis (PBMA) for economic evaluation and prioritization between public health interventions

Joanna M. Charles and Rhiannon T. Edwards

14.1 Introduction to programme budgeting and marginal analysis (PBMA)

Programme budgeting is a way of tracking expenditure in different programme categories. This evidence-based decision-making process can help decision-makers to maximize the impact of health care resources on the health needs of a local population.

Programme budgeting refers to reviewing the resources allocated to specified programmes. Marginal analysis refers to the assessment of the added benefits and added costs of a proposed investment or the foregone benefits and lower costs of a proposed disinvestment in those specified programmes, or in some cases the costs and benefits of proposed alternative programmes (Brambleby and Fordham, 2003). Decisions do not necessarily need to be a dichotomous choice between investment or disinvestment; some programmes can absorb a degree of contraction whilst still continuing, for example through better targeting. It is important to be aware of opportunity costs and how changes in expenditure on one programme may impact on others (Brambleby and Fordham, 2003). Brambleby and Fordham describe programme budgeting and marginal analysis (PBMA) in eight stages, detailed in Box 14.1 (Brambleby and Fordham, 2003).

14.2 Step 1—Choose a set of meaningful programmes

PBMA is a framework used to identify activity in a specific budget. PBMA could be applied to assess a specific care pathway or a specific set of prevention programmes/interventions in a public health setting. The activity the PBMA framework is applied to could be defined by yourself, by a specific research question, or by a service

Box 14.1 Stages of PBMA

1. Choose a set of meaningful programmes
2. Identify current activity and expenditure in those programmes
3. Think of improvements
4. Weigh up incremental costs and incremental benefits and prioritize a list
5. Consult widely
6. Decide on changes
7. Effect the changes
8. Evaluate progress

Source: data from Brambleby, P. and Fordham, R. 2003. What is PBMA. What is?... bulletins, 4(2). Copyright © PBMA.

commissioner wishing to undertake an audit. A PBMA panel is typically established during this first stage. This PBMA panel will be responsible for making the resource reallocation decisions. It is recommended that this panel has membership from experts in the field of the activity under scrutiny and representation from relevant stakeholder groups. A further consideration is to include membership or representation from heads of departments, service managers, and finance managers who are in a position of power to effect changes resulting from the PBMA exercise.

In order to make resource reallocation decisions, an element of discussion and debate is likely to occur amongst the panel. The appointment of a chairperson within the panel could help to facilitate this discussion, and summarize the key points to help the panel make its decisions.

14.3 Step 2—Identify current activity and expenditure in those programmes

Once the budget has been identified, the next stage is to establish the activity and expenditure in this budget. This could be done by establishing a group that will operationalize the PBMA exercise. There is a distinction between this operational group who would be tasked with running the PBMA exercise and the PBMA panel who will be tasked with making the resource reallocation decisions. It is advisable that the operational group contains experience and expertise of the programme, service, or intervention under scrutiny. Relevant finance staff expertise is essential to establish the proportional spend for each activity and calculate potential cost savings based on alternative scenarios of resource allocation. Health economics expertise in this group is also advisable to guide the PBMA exercise and to explain the two most important notions of this priority-setting framework: opportunity cost and the principle of the margin, discussed in Chapter 2 of this book. Opportunity cost refers to the concept of the benefits foregone from the use of resources in their next best use. With regards to PBMA, the panel must weigh up the potential loss of benefits from releasing resources from one activity and the potential gains from reinvesting these resources into another activity or activities. The principle of the margin refers to altering the current pattern of resource use to achieve the most efficient use of resources. For example, in the case of funding cuts, a panel may wish to take resources from activities that show limited or no benefit so as to reduce the impact of the cuts on the population the activity serves. The best use of resources is established by examining the costs and benefits of the activity and its alternatives at the margin (Mitton and Donaldson, 2004).

14.4 **Step 3—Think of improvements**

Once the activities contained in the budget have been identified, the next step is to think of improvements to the current resource allocation structure. This could be done through liaising with stakeholders and experts to ascertain what they would do differently; for example, increasing activity in one area or investing in a completely new area. Platforms such as online surveys, engagement events, focus groups, one-to-one interviews, and previous audits or reviews undertaken by the service could be used to gain suggestions for improvements. Seeking expert opinion in this manner could provide the panel with candidates for expansion or contraction (i.e. reallocation), whilst also providing an audit trail with justification of why these candidates were suggested to the panel.

14.5 **Step 4—Weigh up incremental costs and incremental benefits and prioritize a list**

Before a list of candidates for resource reallocation can be weighed up and prioritized, it is recommended that the panel creates a list of criteria that will be used to appraise the candidates. These criteria could range from population need, equity concerns to value for money, and service quality. The panel should also assign rankings to the chosen criteria or state weightings that are assigned to each criteria (e.g. criteria X is worth 1 point, criteria Y is worth 2 points, and criteria Z is worth 3 points) so it is clear how the candidates were appraised. It is recommended that evidence be presented for each candidate for resource reallocation. As budgets can contain multiple activities, those conducting PBMA exercises should consider the importance of keeping evidence consistent across the multiple candidates to allow for cross-comparisons. Evidence could be gathered for each activity using a range of methods; for example, systematic reviewing, collaboration with librarians (e.g. Public Health Wales Library in the case study reproduced in the following), collaboration with finance staff, and, in some cases, conducting focus groups. Economic evidence, for example, cost per quality adjusted life years (QALYs), could also be appraised using thresholds such as the £20,000–£30,000 per QALY threshold used by the National Institute for Health and Care Excellence (NICE) (National Institute for Health and Care Excellence, 2013). Individuals conducting PBMA exercises should consider how evidence is presented to their PBMA panel such as accessibility of information, by explaining terminology that may be unfamiliar such as QALYs.

14.6 **Step 5—Consult widely**

It is recommended that the PBMA panel has plenty of opportunity and time to discuss the budget, activity and review the related evidence. Making the evidence gathered on candidates available prior to discussion allows panel members time to digest the evidence and come prepared to discussion sessions. Discussion (facilitated by a chairperson) is encouraged to assist the panel to reach disinvestment and reinvestment recommendations; therefore, face-to-face meetings may provide an ideal platform for these discussions. Where a PBMA exercise includes a crossover between prevention and clinical treatment services, in our experience it has proved essential that clinicians, for example, hospital consultants, commit to the PBMA process. It may also be beneficial to have representation from finance staff and those who gathered the evidence at these meetings to answer specific questions during the discussion.

14.7 **Step 6—Decide on changes**

Based on the discussions undertaken by the panel, keeping in mind the criteria and aims of the PBMA exercise, recommendations should be presented. These recommendations could take the form of dichotomous 'disinvest' or 'invest' choices for each candidate/activity. Conversely, the panel could decide which of the candidates/activities contained in the budget are of high or low priority, then progress to decisions such as disinvesting in low priorities and reinvesting in high priorities. Once the panel has made their recommendations, it should move on to state how much in monetary terms it wishes to disinvest and reinvest. How the panel makes these recommendations could be achieved by holding a vote, conducting a ranking exercise, or group consensus as decided by the chairperson in their independent role (based upon the tone of the discussion). If the panel was to make its recommendations by holding a vote there are a number of options available such as an open vote, where each member of the panel is aware of the co-members' decision, or anonymous voting where each panel member is unaware of their co-members' decisions. Electronic systems could be used to conduct the voting which have the advantage of displaying the results quickly in graphical format. Displaying the results immediately after voting could facilitate a follow-up discussion and reflection, with a chance to vote again if the panel feels this would be appropriate.

14.8 **Step 7—Effect the changes**

Once the panel has considered all activities and made its recommendations, these recommendations should be presented to the appropriate managers and directors who have the power to implement them. The format of the presentation could be a report or verbal presentation. If representation from managers and directors has been incorporated into the PBMA panel membership, this could provide a wealth of background information during this stage. The manager or director who took part in the discussions would have an understanding of the context and discussions that led to the recommendations. In cases where is it deemed inappropriate to have manager or director representation during the exercise, individuals are encouraged to bear in mind the importance of providing the audit trail to candidate generation and a summation of the key points raised in the discussions, in order to provide a transparent account of the PBMA exercise undertaken.

14.9 **Step 8—Evaluate progress**

It is advised that PBMA be viewed as a form of iterative audit. Once the recommendations from the current PBMA exercise have been implemented, the programme should be re-evaluated in the future to ensure that the most effective and beneficial resource allocation with respect to defined policy or service goals has taken place. This is of particular importance as new programmes, initiatives, and technologies may become available in the future which could be considered a better use of resources than previous activity considered in an earlier PBMA exercise. There is no guideline to state when to re-evaluate a PBMA exercise. Individuals should be guided by factors that could affect the previous recommendations, for example, the availability of new programmes, initiatives, and technologies, relevant guidelines, new polices, change in directorship, and further restrictions on budgets.

14.10 **Potential for use of PBMA in public health settings**

PBMA is an example of a type of multi-criteria decision analysis (MCDA) discussed in Chapter 13. PBMA's origins lie in US Defence Budgeting in the 1960s. It was developed as a way of defining costs and outcomes in order to rationalize defence budget spending (Brambleby and Fordham, 2003). Ruta and colleagues debated why PBMA had not been used further in the National Health Service (NHS) given the suitability of the method and its wide applications in health care outside of the United Kingdom (Ruta et al., 2005). Early applications of the framework in a UK health setting occurred in the 1990s (Cohen, 1994; Craig et al., 1995). Since then, the use of PBMA in health care has increased, with health care commissioners applying this framework to assist resource reallocation decisions or as part of their planning strategies. In the United Kingdom, PBMA has been employed in maternity services (Ratcliffe et al., 1996), gynaecology services (Twaddle and Walker, 1995), GP-led community hospital care for stroke patients (Henderson and Scott, 2001), and respiratory care (Charles et al., 2016). Outside the United Kingdom, PBMA has been used in health organizations in Australia (Crockett et al., 1999; Haas et al., 2001), Canada (Mitton et al., 2003) and New Zealand (Bohmer et al., 2001; Grocott, 2009). Economic recession has led to PBMA being used as a method for evidence-based disinvestment (Donaldson et al., 2010), which is discussed further in our case study, reviewing a ministerial health improvement budget in Wales (Edwards et al., 2014). In the case study in section 14.11, we show that the use of PBMA is particularly pertinent in constrained budgets of NHS-based public health, where new money is rarely introduced into services; therefore, the best use of current resources must be made.

Table 14.1 Summary of key activities and considerations for each PBMA stage

PBMA Stage	Activities	Considerations
1. Choose a set of meaningful programmes	Identify activity in a specific budget or spend Establish a PBMA panel	An awareness of boundaries is essential to consider at this stage. If activity occurs across boundaries it can be difficult to attribute spending and outcomes to specific activities. It is recommended that a PBMA panel comprise of experts in the field of the activity under scrutiny and have representation from relevant stakeholder groups. A further consideration is to include membership or representation from heads of departments, service managers, and finance managers who are able to effect changes resulting from the PBMA exercise. A chairperson may also be appointed to facilitate panel discussion and summarize the key points to help the panel make its decisions.
2. Identify current activity and expenditure in those programmes	Identify current activity Identify expenditure of that activity Establish an operationalization group	Relevant finance staff expertise could be beneficial to establish the proportional spend for each activity and calculate potential cost savings based on alternative scenarios of resource allocation. It is advised the operationalization group contains expertise of the programme, service, or intervention under scrutiny and health economists.
3. Think of improvements	Liaise with experts and stakeholders	Use of platforms such as online surveys, engagement events, focus groups, one-to-one interviews, and previous audits or reviews undertaken by the service can be utilized to gain suggestions of improvements. Seeking expert opinion in this manner provides justification of why these candidates were suggested to the panel.
4. Weigh up incremental costs and incremental benefits and prioritize a list	Create a list of criteria to appraise resource reallocation candidates Rank or assign weightings to these criteria Create a list of candidates and gather evidence for each one	The panel should create a list of criteria that will be used to appraise the resource reallocation candidates. The panel should also assign rankings to their chosen criteria, or state weightings that are assigned to each criteria so it is clear how the candidates were appraised. The aims of the PBMA exercise should also be considered and decided upon by the panel. This is particularly relevant if there is a target amount of cost savings the PBMA exercise needs to achieve due to shrinking budgets. The aim provides a steer for discussions and outcome for the exercise. Evidence should be presented consistently for all candidates to allow for cross-comparisons. Evidence should be presented in an accessible format and explain any terminology that may be unfamiliar (e.g. QALYs).

(continued)

Table 14.1 Continued

PBMA Stage	Activities	Considerations
5. Consult widely	Allow the PBMA panel to review the evidence and discuss the candidates for resource reallocation	The PBMA panel should have plenty of opportunity and time to discuss the budget, activity, and review the related evidence. Making the evidence gathered on candidates available prior to discussion allows panel members time to digest the evidence and come prepared to discussion sessions. Discussion (facilitated by a chairperson) to assist the panel to reach disinvestment and reinvestment recommendations. Presence of those who gathered evidence and prepared finance information is recommended so the panel may ask questions.
6. Decide on changes	Recommendations for disinvestment and investment State the monetary value of the disinvestment and investment recommended	Based on the discussions undertaken by the panel (keeping in mind the criteria and aims of the PBMA exercise) recommendations should be presented. These recommendations could take the form of dichotomous 'disinvest' or 'invest' choices for each candidate/activity, or which candidates/activities are high or low priority. The panel should progress to state how much in monetary terms it wishes to disinvest and reinvest. Recommendations could be achieved by; ♦ holding a vote (using open or closed/electronic techniques) ♦ conducting a ranking exercise ♦ chairperson judgement of the consensus in the room
7. Effect the changes	Present recommendations for disinvestment and investment to managers and directors who have the power to implement them	The format of the presentation could be in the form of a report or verbal presentation. Representation from managers and directors during the PBMA exercise would provide an understanding of the context and discussions that led to the recommendations. In the absence of this, individuals are encouraged to bear in mind the importance of providing the audit trail to candidate generation and a summation of the key points raised in the discussions.
8. Evaluate progress	Re-evaluate recommendations in the future	PBMA should be viewed as a form of iterative audit. The recommendations from the current PBMA exercise should be re-evaluated in the future. Individuals should be guided by factors that could affect the previous recommendations; for example, the availability of new programmes, initiatives, and technologies, relevant guidelines, new polices, change in directorship, and further restrictions on budgets to decide when to undertake this re-evaluation.

14.11 Case study: PBMA of health improvement budget of the Welsh Minister for Health and Social Care

This case study has been reproduced from Edwards, R.T., Charles, J.M., Thomas, S., Bishop, J., Cohen, D., Groves, S., Humphreys, C., Howson, H. and Bradley, P., 2014. A national Programme Budgeting and Marginal Analysis (PBMA) of health improvement spending across Wales: disinvestment and reinvestment across the life course. *BMC Public Health, 14*(1): 837. doi:10.1186/1471-2458-14-837.

14.11.1 Background

14.11.1.1 Public health challenges in Wales

Despite an increase in healthy life expectancy in Wales in recent years, local authorities continue to experience among the worst life expectancies in the United Kingdom, and the gap between the most and least deprived remains wide. Smoking causes about one in five deaths in Wales (Public Health Wales Observatory, 2012). Prevalence is currently 23 per cent and is highest in young males aged 25–34 at 38 per cent (Public Health Wales Observatory, 2012). About 45 per cent of the population drink above guideline amounts of alcohol, over 1000 people a year die from alcohol in Wales, and there are over 55,000 hospital admissions due to alcohol in Wales per year (Public Health Wales Observatory, 2010). Only about a third of adults eat five portions of fruit and vegetables a day, under a third meet physical activity guidelines, with about 30 per cent of the adult population taking no exercise in a typical week (Public Health Wales Observatory, 2010). As a consequence of unhealthy eating and low physical activity, 57 per cent of the Welsh adult population is overweight or obese (Public Health Wales Observatory, 2010). There is a growing call from policy-makers for interventions that address these challenges, and interventions that are also considered a good use of public resources. The cost-effectiveness evidence base for PHIs is beginning to grow.

14.11.2 Growing evidence of the cost-effectiveness of public health interventions (PHIs)

Owen and colleagues have synthesized the evidence of the cost-effectiveness of PHIs underpinning NICE Public Health Guidance from 2006 to 2010 (The paper by Owen and colleagues paper is reproduced in full in Chapter 8). They analysed 200 base-case cost-effectiveness estimates. Findings showed the majority of PHIs assessed were highly cost-effective, 85 per cent of which had an incremental cost-effectiveness ratio less than £20,000 per QALY and 89 per cent at the higher threshold of £30,000 per QALY (Owen et al., 2012). The authors conclude that the next step would be to develop a framework that allows the combination of economic analysis and other criteria to support local decision-makers to make better investments. Although there is a need for quality evidence from randomized controlled trials (RCTs) that pay particular attention to the challenges of conducting economic evaluations of complex (as defined by the Medical Research Council (MRC)) (Craig et al., 2008), public health interventions as recommended by Kelly and colleagues (2005), McDaid and Needle (2009), and Weatherly and co-workers (2009), there is also a need for expert opinion and common sense. PBMA can be employed as a means of using expert opinion as a part of evidence-based decision-making.

14.11.3 **PBMA**

PBMA is a process that helps decision-makers maximize the impact of health care resources on the health needs of a local population or meet other specified goals such as equity considerations. Programme budgeting is an appraisal of past resource allocation in specified programmes, with a view to tracking future resource allocation in those same programmes. Marginal analysis is the appraisal of the added benefits and added costs of a proposed investment or the lost benefits and lower costs of a proposed disinvestment (Brambleby and Fordham, 2003). Some programmes can absorb a degree of contraction, whilst still continuing e.g. through better targeting. It is important to be aware of the links across programmes and, therefore, how changes in expenditure on one programme may impact on others. The PBMA process requires information on expenditure by programme; for example, by an annual budget and/ or numbers of full-time equivalent posts (FTE). The stages of a PBMA exercise are shown in Table 14.2.

A published literature review considered factors that may explain the success or otherwise of PBMA exercises (Tsourapas and Frew, 2011). Tsourapas and Frew found 28 applications of PBMA spread across the United Kingdom, Australia, New Zealand, and Canada. Findings showed PBMA was successful in 52 per cent of cases where success was defined in terms of the participants gaining a better understanding of the area under scrutiny. PBMA was successful in 65 per cent of cases where success was defined as 'implementation of all or some of the PBMA panel's recommendations'. Forty-eight per cent of the studies were successful where success was defined in terms of disinvesting or resource reallocation, and in 22 per cent where success was defined in terms of adopting the framework for future use. The authors concluded that the definition of success influenced the rate of successful PBMA applications. They argue for

Table 14.2. The eight stages of PBMA by Brambleby and Fordham (2003)

Stage	Description
1	Choose a set of meaningful programmes/initiatives.
2	Identify current activity and expenditure in those programmes/initiatives.
3	Think of improvements.
4	Weigh up incremental costs and incremental benefits and prioritize a list.
5	Consult widely
6	Decide on changes
7	Effect the changes
8	Evaluate progress

Source: data from Brambleby, P. and Fordham, R. 2003. What is PBMA. What is?... bulletins, 4(2). Copyright © PBMA.

a broadly accepted definition of success to allow greater comparability within the field (Tsourapas and Frew, 2011).

There has also been more recent use of PBMA as a framework for disinvestment (Donaldson et al., 2010). When conducting a rapid review of applied PBMA framework, we found papers describing PBMA exercises of maternity services (Ratcliffe et al., 1996), surgical department (Mitton et al., 2003), gynaecology services (Twaddle and Walker, 1995), and GP-led community hospital care for stroke patients (Henderson and Scott, 2001). This case study describes a national PBMA exercise of the annual health improvement budget of the Welsh Minister for Health and Social Care. We believe this to be the first published description of a PBMA exercise at a national level (Edwards et al., 2014).

14.11.4 Methods

We describe the process of conducting the PBMA exercise, with particular reference to the perspective, development of the panel, gathering of evidence, and the marginal analysis task.

14.11.5 Perspective of the health improvement review

This PBMA exercise was completed on behalf of Public Health Wales and considered PHIs at a national level, taking into account NHS services and those provided by public and private partners. This PBMA exercise assessed the health improvement budget of the Minister for Health and Social Care. At the beginning of the process, health improvement was defined under the Ottawa Charter (1986). This definition of health improvement highlights the importance of reorienting health services, creating supportive environments, improving personal skills, community action, and the role of healthy public policy. Once the perspective was defined, a panel was established to review the evidence gathered and reach the disinvestment/investment decisions.

14.11.6 Development of a PBMA panel

An expert panel list of 30 potential members was established with representatives from Public Health Wales, Welsh government, NHS Health Boards, third sector, local government, and primary care. Each member of the suggested panel was sent an invitation to participate in the PBMA exercise by e-mail. The e-mail described the purpose of the exercise, the invited member's role in the panel, the commitment required, and the dates and times of the proposed meetings. The invited members were able to decline to participate, and panel members who agreed to participate were able to withdraw their membership at any time. As this was a government-initiated, evidence-based, decision-making exercise, ethical approval was not required.

Once the budget was defined, the researchers were informed that the budget contained 25 initiatives, accounting for the total £15.1 million of the Minister's expenditure on health improvement across Wales. The panel drew upon evidence collated for each initiative from the review subgroups, stakeholder consultation, and an NHS/primary care subgroup to explore potential alternative modes of health improvement delivery across Wales. The PBMA panel met three times and the sessions were facilitated by a session leader. The sessions started with an explanation of the exercise and the review of evidence undertaken. A discussion of the criteria to appraise the evidence was also conducted with a list of six final criteria agreed by the panel. These criteria were as follows: considered a priority health issue for Welsh government, opinions of experts, stakeholder views, presence and robustness of evidence of effectiveness, presence and robustness of evidence of cost-effectiveness, and impact or potential impact on reducing inequalities in health. The options above were used as part of the electronic voting exercise. The panel were then asked to vote electronically on the preferred objective of the Health Improvement Review, the top four criteria for the health improvement review from 12 PBMA panel members, and to agree the most relevant time horizon for this PBMA exercise. The vote was conducted and then the results were displayed electronically using graphics and discussed, with an opportunity to repeat the voting if required. The panel were given the evidence underpinning each of the initiatives to read between the second and third session. At the third session, the panel were asked to vote for candidates for investment and disinvestment. The vote was conducted, the results were displayed and discussed, with an opportunity to vote again if required.

14.11.7 **Boundaries of the programme budget**

This programme was a historically determined programme budget of Ministerial resources currently devoted specifically to health improvement at an All-Wales level. There are other resources known to be used for health improvement purposes, sometimes matched with local government or voluntary sector spending. However, these were considered outside the remit of this analysis.

The review established five operational subgroups to support the review, as outlined in the following. Information from each of these groups was summarized and then combined and collated into summary booklets for each initiative. During this summary process, the review teams decided that a scoring system was required to help guide the panel. A traffic-light system was agreed as the most appropriate and visually effective structure. Each of the evidence review sub-teams applied a traffic-light rating system to their particular stream of evidence and then an overall traffic-light grading was assigned to each initiative based upon all the available evidence gathered by the subgroups. The overall traffic-light grading was as follows:

Red—based on published evidence and consultation, this intervention is unlikely to bring a population health benefit and alternatives should be explored to achieve these health goals.

Amber—greater evidence needs to be found for the impact of this initiative at a population level and/or there are elements of the programme that need substantial revision or there is insufficient evidence available to make a judgment.

Green—this is a sound programme with a reasonable evidence base; however, we need to ensure that reach is maximized and it is cost-effective.

See Edwards et al., 2014 for a description of the evidence booklet methodology. These booklets were distributed to the PBMA panel members for their consideration before the sessions.

14.11.8 **Protocol for review of effectiveness evidence**

A pragmatic search strategy was designed using specified health databases (NHS Evidence, Cochrane Collaboration, Campbell Collaboration, Health Evidence Canada) and the search engines (PubMEd and Google Scholar). For initiatives where recent high-quality secondary analyses of the primary literature were found, searches were narrower and terminated at an earlier stage. Searches for questions that yielded little high-quality data initially were broadened by date or by search terms in an attempt to capture related work. Retrieved articles were screened for inclusion by two independent reviewers (disagreements resolved by discussion) on the basis of direct relevance to the initiative or component interventions and type of article, thus single studies were not included if higher-level evidence was available. Evaluations of interventions in practice were also sought and interventions were assigned an overall evidence rating taking into account potential and actual evidence of effectiveness.

14.11.9 **Protocol for review of cost-effectiveness evidence**

Relevant articles identified from an evidence search (2002–2012) of the NICE, PubMed, and the Centre for Reviews and Dissemination (CRD) databases using key terms from each of the 25 initiatives were sourced and then appraised. Evidence was defined as; *directly* relevant (i.e. an economic evaluation of a specific intervention delivered through the programme/initiative stated in the list of included programmes); or *indirectly* relevant (where directly relevant evidence is unavailable); that is, evaluation of related intervention similar to the one delivered through the programme/initiative or as part of the intended aims of the programme/initiative stated in the list of included programmes by either method of delivery (school-based smoking cessation) or target population (pregnant women). The checklist developed by Drummond and colleagues for a sound economic evaluation was used to appraise evidence found in the electronic searches (Drummond et al., 2015). A subjective judgement of the overall balance of economic evidence was made by the economic evidence subgroup and a traffic-light system of grading was used.

14.11.10 **Stakeholder consultation process**

The review involved wide consultation to gain opinions of stakeholders such as practitioners delivering the initiatives and the public who may have come into contact with particular initiatives. These were used in the evidence booklets to give the panel an indication of stakeholder views. This was undertaken as part of a wider 'change management' strategy to ensure the public had opportunity to discuss any possible changes to services and relay their concerns so policy-makers could understand the potential impacts. The consultation process involved a range of engagement events including visits to local public health teams across the seven health boards,(these teams were often involved with the delivery of health improvement programmes) and visits with Public Health Wales staff. Beaufort Research was commissioned to undertake a public survey and to conduct six focus groups and six in-depth family interviews. Eight consultation events were held across Wales addressing the initiatives with regards to different stages of the life course. An open online feedback form was hosted on the bilingual review web pages on the Public Health Wales website to engage the public and staff further. Responses were assigned a traffic-light system based upon the overall majority of positive, negative, and mixed feedback from each of the groups.

14.11.11 Equity review

The extent to which each of the initiatives addressed equity concerns was also supplied in the evidence booklets. A traffic-light categorization system was developed to grade the degree of equality/equity focus of each initiative under review. Some of these initiatives have a degree of complexity which required explanation in addition to the traffic-light grading. These include some where there has been a change of focus since inception and others where programme employees act as intermediaries and local areas are largely autonomous in the way initiatives are delivered. It should be noted that the categories apply to the intention of the programme rather than the supporting evidence, effectiveness, or cost-effectiveness, which have been reviewed separately.

14.11.12 NHS/primary care consideration

The evidence booklets also detailed options for alternative modes of delivery through existing mainstream services. The mechanism of delivery was summarized with consideration given to alternatives where appropriate.

Those directly involved in the intervention delivery or commissioning of services were invited to correct matters of accuracy and supply additional evidence for consideration. This was reviewed and a final assessment agreed by the panel.

We went on to undertake a pragmatic, high-level marginal analysis task as part of the PBMA process.

14.11.13 Marginal analysis

Three months following the PBMA sessions all members of the PBMA panel and Health Improvement Advisory Board (HIAG), which oversaw the PBMA exercise, received a high-level pragmatic marginal analysis electronic task and supporting document. The supporting document provided the recipients with a refresher of the PBMA sessions, including grading of evidence and the outcomes of electronic voting for criteria and investment/disinvestment decisions. As the panel did not wish to continue investing in any of the current programmes, based on available evidence, a high-level task was developed in which the recipients were asked to consider what Public Health Wales should do with a hypothetical £5 million. This sum of money was chosen based upon the median amount of monies released from the recommended disinvestment and partial disinvestment decisions made by the panel. The panel and HIAG members were asked to rank, in order of importance, their top 3 priority areas (out of a choice of 11) and their top 3 life-course stages (out of a choice of 6), in which new approaches to health improvement should be developed with this hypothetical £5 million. They were also asked to state how much of the £5 million they would allocate to each of their top three choices and to give a brief rationale for their choices.

14.11.14 **Results**

14.11.14.1 The programme budget

We identified 25 specific health improvement initiatives within the programme budget (see Table 14.3). See Edwards et al., 2014 for a brief description of each of the initiatives. There were a number of initiatives where no or little evidence was available. Economic evidence was sparse, with 11 of the 25 initiatives having no available evidence of cost-effectiveness, cost utility, or cost benefit. A total of 12 panel members attended each of the 3 PBMA sessions.

The 25 initiatives identified in the PBMA exercise with an overall traffic-light grading and summary statement from the five evidence subgroup categories (total of £15 million expenditure).

Nineteen of the 25 initiatives included in the PBMA exercise received an overall evidence traffic-light grading of red or amber, stating alternatives should be explored to achieve the health improvement goals outlined by the initiative or required further evidence. Fifteen of the 25 initiatives had no economic evidence.

14.11.15 **Spending by life-course stage**

Figure 14.1 illustrates the prevailing spending per life-course stage of the £15 million of the identified programme budget.

14.11.16 **Establishing criteria for evaluating the programme and candidate interventions for investment and disinvestment**

The 12 PBMA panel members were asked, using electronic voting, to identify criteria with which to judge the relative merit of candidate interventions for investment and disinvestment (see Tables 14.4, 14.5, and 14.6).

14.11.17 **Generating candidate initiatives for investment and disinvestment**

Figure 14.2 illustrates that the PBMA panel was able to reach a majority vote to recommend disinvestment in 7 out of 25 initiatives, releasing £1.5 million per annum (The Cooking Bus, Smoke Bugs, Skin Cancer Awareness, Health Challenge Wales Website, Mind, Exercise, Nutrition ... Do it! (MEND), Mental Health First Aid and Smokers Helpline). Although the overall health improvement goals were rational, it was stressed that this was on the basis of a lack of evidence of effectiveness, cost-effectiveness, or support from local public health teams, or any evidence of impact on inequality.

These results did not mean that the target stages of the life course (e.g. primary school children), or the goal of limiting health-harming behaviours were less important than other goals, rather that such goals should be addressed in other, evidence-based ways (e.g. environmental change). The PBMA panel also recommended partial disinvestment in a further three interventions, releasing £7.3 million of resources, including some big spend areas such as Designed to Smile and National Exercise Referral Scheme. Because of a lack of published evidence at the time on effectiveness,

Table 14.3 The 25 initiatives identified in the PBMA exercise

Initiative	Approx. spend 2012/13	Assessment category
Cooking Bus	£655,000	Red—Based on published evidence and consultation, this intervention is unlikely to bring a population health benefit and alternatives should be explored to achieve these health goals.
MEND	£480,000	
Mental Health First Aid	£143,000	
Smokebugs	£131,000	
National Breastfeeding Programme—Breastfeeding Peer Support Programme (BPSP)	£31,000	
National Breastfeeding Programme—Breastfeeding Welcome Scheme (BFWS)	£11,000	
Health Challenge Wales website Cost	£38,000	
Smokers Helpline	£30,000	
Smoking Resources	£30,000	
Skin Cancer Awareness	£15,000	
Designed to Smile	£3.75 million	Amber—Greater evidence needs to be found for the impact of this initiative at a population level; and/or there are elements of the programme that need substantial revision; or there is insufficient evidence available to make a judgment
Welsh Network of Healthy Schools Schemes (WNHSS)	£2.3 million	
Stop Smoking Wales—Pre Surgery	£2.2 million (N.B. total spend on SSW over five programmes as it was not possible to break spend down to individual programmes)	
Stop Smoking Wales (SSW)—Pregnancy		
Stop Smoking Wales—Vulnerable Groups		

Table 14.3 Continued

Initiative	Approx. spend 2012/13	Assessment category
Stop Smoking Wales—Brief Intervention Training		
Fresh Start Wales	£700,000	
Alcohol Brief Interventions in Primary Care Training	£100,000	
HIV Prevention	£56,000	
National Exercise Referral Scheme	£3.5 million	Green—This is a sound programme with a reasonable evidence base; however, we need to ensure that reach is maximized and it is cost-effective.
Stop Smoking Wales—Adults	£2.2 million (N.B. spend over five programmes as it was not possible to break spend down to individual programmes)	
ASSIST	£300,000	
National Breastfeeding Programme—Baby-Friendly initiative (BFI)	£110,000	
No Smoking Day	£27,000	
Teenage Pregnancy Pilot	£150,000	White—a Pilot
Steroids and Image-Enhancing Drugs	£50,000	White—insufficient information to make an assessment.
Champions for Health	£30,000	White—It is not clear what theoretical or evidence base has been used in planning this intervention. Without an evaluation (which specifies and measures primary outcomes) wider implementation cannot be recommended.

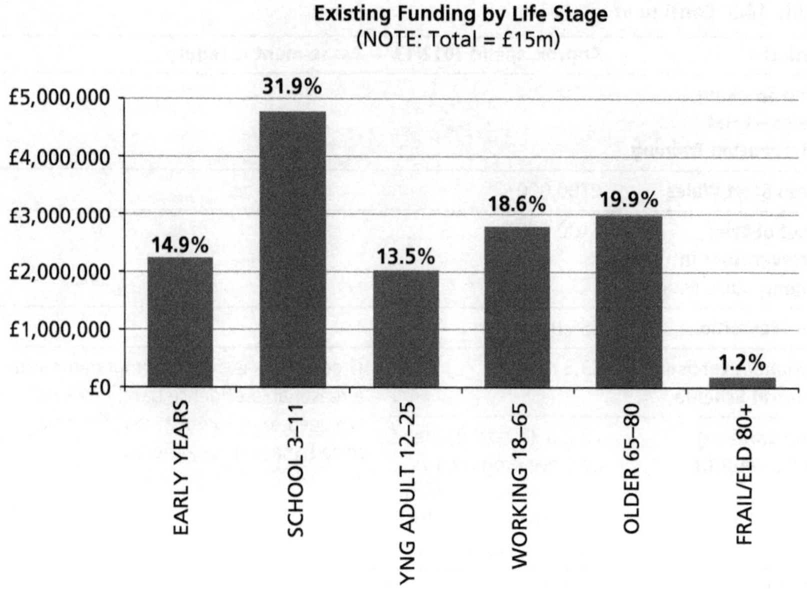

Existing Funding by Life Stage
(NOTE: Total = £15m)

Figure 14.1 Spending by life-course stage of the 25 health improvement initiatives. Spending on the 25 health improvement initiatives by each life-course stage.

cost-effectiveness, and impact on inequalities, the panel did not vote in any majority fashion to invest further in any of the 25 interventions under review. Following this, a high-level marginal analysis task was developed to assess which priority areas and life-course stages the PBMA group would like to invest in. Priority areas were defined by the Welsh government's 'Our Healthy Future' report (Public Health Wales, 2013).

14.11.18 **Results of the marginal analysis task**

We received 9 completed marginal analysis tasks from the panel and HIAG members out of a possible 30 responses. Though disappointing, the nine respondents

Table 14.4 Preferred objective of the health improvement review electronic vote results

Objective	Percentage vote	n
A housekeeping exercise of current patterns of spending	8%	1
A means of bringing a culture of evidence-based decision- making into routine policy	42%	5
An academic exercise to explore the degree of success achieved in applying PBMA	8%	1
A means of bringing evidence of cost-effectiveness into resource planning	42%	5

Table 14.5 The top four criteria for the health improvement review electronic vote results.

Criteria	Percentage vote	*n*
Stakeholder views	20%	2
Presence and robustness of evidence of effectiveness	34%	4
Presence and robustness of evidence of cost-effectiveness	27%	3
Impact or potential impact on reducing inequalities in health	19%	2

were representative of the wider panel with regards to their role and expertise spanning Public Health Wales, Welsh government, Health Boards, local government, and primary care.

As shown in Table 14.7, respondents allocated the largest proportion of the hypothetical £5 million to their first-choice priority area and the smallest proportion to their third-choice priority area. Only one respondent gave an equal division of the £5 million to each of the three rankings. Obesity was given the largest proportion of the £5 million, followed by: mental health and well-being, tobacco control, nutrition, substance misuse, physical activity, injuries, and finally oral health. The rationale for respondents' choices were mainly based upon the large adverse costs and impacts on the population of poor population health in these priority areas, with the potential for large benefit if these areas were given funding and priority. One respondent stated that their decisions were based upon key local priorities. Another respondent stated that their decisions were based on their view that two priority areas were generally underfunded, though could have wide-ranging benefits.

As shown in Table 14.8 and Figure 14.3, the majority of respondents allocated the largest proportion of the hypothetical £5 million to their first-choice life-course stage and the smallest proportion to their third-choice life-course stage. However, one respondent allocated the largest proportion to their third ranking as they felt this life area was often neglected and underfunded. The rationale for respondents' choices

Table 14.6 The most relevant time horizon to assess outcomes of the health improvement programmes under review

Time horizon	Percentage vote	*n*
1 year	8%	1
5 years	50%	6
10 years	17%	2
15 years	8%	1
20 years	17%	2
Other	0%	0

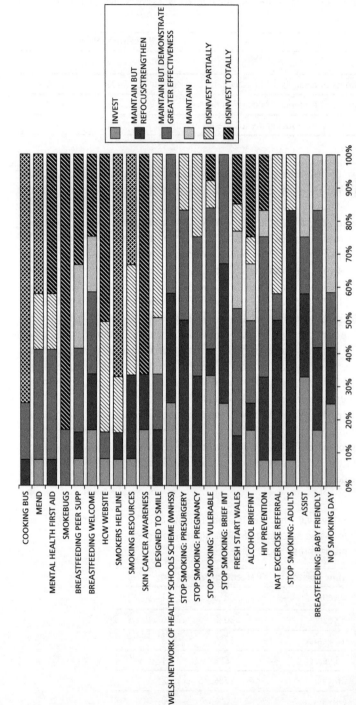

Figure 14.2 Investment and disinvestment decisions made by the panel for each of the 25 initiatives. Candidates for investment and disinvestment recommendations from votes made by the PBMA panel (*n*=12) for the 25 initiatives under review. Please note the initiatives considered as pilots (Teenage Pregnancy Pilot, Steroids and Image-Enhancing Drugs, and Champions for Health) were not included in the voting.

Table 14.7 Results of the marginal analysis ranking exercise for the eleven priority areas from the nine respondents

Priority area	Total number of times the area was assigned first ranking	Total number of times the area was assigned second ranking	Total number of times the area was assigned third ranking
Tobacco control	1	2	2
Physical activity	1	0	0
Nutrition	0	0	2
Oral health	0	0	1
Obesity	3	3	1
Substance misuse	0	1	1
Sexual health	0	0	0
Injuries	1	0	0
Mental health and well-being	3	2	1
Public health education	0	0	0
Work and health	0	1	1

was mainly based upon the view that focusing on early intervention could provide the greatest potential to gain in the long term. The early years' life-course stage received the highest number of first rankings. Respondents also stated that keeping older people healthy for as long as possible could have huge potential public health gains and savings to the NHS and social care sectors.

Table 14.8 Results of the marginal analysis ranking exercise for the six life-course stages from the nine respondents

Life-course stage	Total number of times the stage was assigned first ranking	Total number of times the stage was assigned second ranking	Total number of times the stage was assigned third ranking
Early years (including prenatal and maternal health)	4	2	2
School aged children (3–11 years)	1	2	0
Children and young adults (12–17 years)	2	2	2
Working aged adults (18–65 years)	2	1	2
Older people (66–80 years)	1	0	2
(Frail) elderly (80+years)	0	1	1

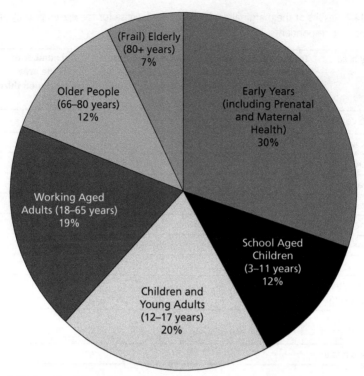

Figure 14.3 Results of the marginal analysis exercise—proportion of the total allocation of the hypothetical £5 million for the six life-course stages from the nine respondents.

14.11.19 Which of UK's NICE recommendations are not being implemented in Wales?

As part of the next steps of the PBMA exercise and recommendations, it was stated that the evidence-gathering exercise identified areas where Wales was not implementing existing NICE public health recommendations. Unlike NICE clinical guidelines, NICE public health guidance is not commissioned by the Welsh government. Nonetheless, the recommendations of NICE are evidence-based and would have similar value in Wales as in England. There is limited information on the extent of implementation of NICE public health guidance in Wales. There is potential for the introduction of systematic implementation and monitoring of NICE recommendations in Wales. There are a number of existing programmes where greater impact could be achieved through more systematic targeting and implementation, more robust monitoring, and greater reach. There are a number of interventions with evidence of effectiveness not currently being implemented in Wales (see Edwards et al., 2014).

14.11.20 Case study discussion

This PBMA exercise has generated practical policy lessons for the Welsh Government, Public Health Wales, and their partner agencies. Although PBMA has been applied in a range of clinical settings in the United Kingdom and internationally such as maternity services, it has not to our knowledge been used at a national level to review a whole programme of public health spending. The results from this PBMA exercise were used to inform the Public Health Wales report, 'Transforming Health Improvement in Wales', which makes recommendations for reinvestment and disinvestment decisions and detailed actions for the future for health improvement in Wales (Public Health Wales, 2013). The budget presented for this PBMA exercise was historically within the behest of the Minister for Health and Social Care for Wales. It was split; 70 per cent allocated via Public Health Wales and 30 per cent directly allocated by Welsh government. What became clear through the PBMA process was the importance of a programme having a logical and comprehensive boundary. The £15.1 million did not represent the total spending on health improvement across Wales and it is likely that many examples might be found of matched funds, through arrangements between Welsh government, local government, the voluntary sector, and other agencies. It became difficult for the members of the PBMA group to undertake the task of reallocating the £15.1 million without full knowledge of what resources, and what interventions, were being devoted to tackling health improvement issues outside the programme budget under review. The same argument could be made for previous published PBMA exercises. For example, Twaddle and Walker reviewed gynaecological services in Glasgow (Twaddle and Walker, 1995). In hindsight, they may have benefited from consideration of a wider context of spending, for example across primary care, other hospitals, and other related agencies.

14.11.21 QALYs in public health

Despite a growing view that QALYs may be an insufficient outcome measure to capture the benefits of public health interventions in full (Kelly et al., 2005; McDaid and Needle, 2009; Weatherly et al., 2009; Payne et al., 2013), 85 per cent of 200 cost per QALY estimates relating to NICE Public Health Guidance produced a cost per QALY of under the NICE threshold of £20,000 per QALY (Owen et al., 2012). We found that in reviewing evidence of cost-effectiveness it was necessary to try to find common units of benefit with which to compare across a whole range of health improvement interventions. QALYs, Disability-adjusted life years (DALYs), and life years gained were most useful. What proved to be more difficult was the ability to use information on cost-effectiveness studies which used natural units of effect directly relevant to the public health intervention concerned (e.g. point change on a child behaviour index, minutes of exercise per week, number of smokers quitting). This PBMA exercise reinforced the argument for common units of benefit for the purpose of comparing across a whole programme of interventions, even in a public health setting.

We found few return on investment studies, or cost–benefit studies of public health improvement interventions. Placing monetary values on health outcomes, whether clinical or public health, remains difficult, though cost–benefit analysis and cost–consequence analysis are recommended by NICE (National Institute for Health and Care Excellence, 2012).

14.11.22 **Public health: Invest to save**

There is a growing interest amongst health care commissioners and local government for the concept of 'invest to save' to be applied to PHIs. This was also demonstrated by the PBMA panel in the marginal analysis task. The early years' life-course stage received the highest number of first rankings. The early years of the life-course stages also received a higher proportion of the £5 million that later stages of life with reasons highlighted that focusing on early intervention could provide the greatest potential to gain in the long term. It is worth noting there is no similar pressure for clinical services to be assessed in this way. From an economic perspective, clinical and PHIs can both be seen as having a common objective—to produce health benefits—and the key issue should therefore be to identify which types of intervention produce the most health benefits and wider social benefits per pound (£) on the margin. It is thus arguably disingenuous to demand that PHIs demonstrate an 'invest to save' benefit when we do not expect this of new drugs and surgical interventions in the NHS (Woolf et al., 2009).

14.11.24 **Limitations of the PBMA exercise**

This PBMA exercise was the result of a direct request from the Minister for Health and Social Care in Wales to review the specific health improvement budget of £15.1 million. This gave the exercise momentum; however, beyond these contexts where high level of political support does not exist, the generalizability of this PBMA exercise may be limited. It was recognized that across Welsh government there were other budgets that could be linked with health improvement activities, such as through matched funding with local government and the voluntary sector. This meant that we were, at best, undertaking a 'partial analysis', and needed to keep in mind wider patterns of spending, as far as these could be identified in the time allowed. Common themes and concerns highlighted by the authors that emerged from the three PBMA sessions are summarized in Table 14.9.

Another limitation of the PBMA exercise was the marginal analysis task. Due to time constraints, the panel were unable to complete the task as part of the face-to-face group discussion sessions. Rather than omit this step, a pragmatic, high-level e-mail-based task was devised. This task was used to indicate the direction of travel and provide further recommendations for next steps; it is also worth noting a strength of this task was that it made the panel consider opportunity cost. However, only nine PBMA panel members completed the marginal analysis task. Although these members were representative of the wider group with regards to role and expertise, the lack of response limits the potential wider applications of the recommendations given in this task. As the panel included front line clinical staff, we had three sessions to make participation in this PBMA exercise as manageable as possible given the work commitments of the members. As many PBMA exercises are shown to be unsuccessful (Tsouparas and Frew, 2011), it was important that the panel completed all stages of the process, including a marginal analysis task though the limitations of the pragmatic task chosen here are noted above. The smaller response rate may be attributed to the fact that this task was conducted via e-mail rather than in person.

Table 14.9 Key themes and concerns emerging from the PBMA process and sessions as noted by the authors

Number	Key themes and concerns
1	There is no readily available source of information on wider spending in Welsh government and Public Health Wales on health improvement to provide the 'big-picture' context to the exercise.
2	It is very difficult to find evidence of effectiveness and cost-effectiveness relating specifically to different time horizons or national versus local provision.
3	The panel may need information about the proportion of the population who may take up a service when thinking about budget share (i.e. population affected).
4	What is the (purpose/function) role of the 'budget' (i.e. the pot of money under consideration)? What makes it different from other budgets/pots of money?
5	How we might best assess the effect of combined interventions and integrated approaches?
6	How we might best assess the effect of combined interventions and integrated approaches?
7	Government priorities can sometimes be based upon serial decision making rather than parallel decision-making.

14.11.23 Strengths of the PBMA exercise

This Health Improvement Review and the PBMA exercise offered the first transparent detailed breakdown of spending on 25 health improvement initiatives within a ministerial budget. This provided a starting point for the Welsh government and Public Health Wales to expand the scope, if required, and to gain a greater understanding of what is spent on health improvement in Wales. The review of initiatives allowed the panel to see what programmes are currently operating in Wales and suggest further improvements for initiatives (e.g. targeting), alternate delivery systems, or new initiatives based upon NICE guidance. The PBMA exercise also generated a list of interventions recommended by NICE that are not currently being delivered in Wales as part of potential next steps and further research. A next step would be to generate evidence booklets for these, estimating what could be achieved with, for example, £1 million invested in any one of these new interventions. There would be a need to see how they would dovetail with existing interventions and goals. Using the definitions of success categorized by Tsouparas and Frew (2011) in their review, we argue our PBMA exercise would be considered successful in terms of the participants gaining a better understanding of the area under interest. It would also be considered successful as the recommendations were taken further in a report to the Minister, with changes to resource allocation made, and the promotion of an evidence-based culture in order to aid future resource allocation decisions.

14.11.24 **Case study: Conclusions**

The PBMA exercise provided a useful platform to discuss and prioritize public health initiatives in Wales, taking account of the budget, their evidence base (including clinical effectiveness, cost-effectiveness, and equity considerations), stakeholder views on and alternative options for delivery. The electronic voting on candidates for investment and disinvestment showed a clear recommendation for total disinvestment in four initiatives and a recommendation for partial disinvestment in six further initiatives due to lack of evidence for their effectiveness and cost-effectiveness at the time. The marginal analysis exercise indicated the direction of travel, the PBMA panel and HIAG group members advocated shifting funding to prioritize areas associated with large adverse health- and social care costs. Priority was given to interventions that impact on sections of the population with the poorest health (e.g. obesity and tobacco control). The panel also advocated focusing on early intervention, as this has the potential to result in large gain in the long term. The evidence sub groups were able to suggest which interventions Wales could be prioritizing based upon NICE guidance. Wales spends a very small proportion of its NHS budget on health improvement. This exercise helped demonstrate the activity currently undertaken in the budget and its impact on the population, which was currently unknown. This was a necessary process to promote an evidence-based culture to help resource allocation decisions, which has been promoted further since the completion of the exercise. Within the current climate of 'prudent health care', we have demonstrated that, at a national level, the PBMA process can reach decisions about potential candidates for disinvestment and potential investment in priority areas and life-course stages. The next steps are to estimate the financial and health gain returns from reallocating resources released in this process.

14.12 **Challenges of conducting PBMA exercises**

As with any approach, there are certain challenges that can occur when conducting a PBMA exercise. First, PBMA can take time, usually requiring more than six months from inception to completion. The largest proportion of this time is spent establishing the operational group, PBMA panel, and gathering the evidence relating to the costs and outcomes of current activity and any additional proposals for disinvestment or investment. As this framework can take time to apply, it is recommended there is buy-in and sponsorship from the highest level of an organization in order to facilitate the process to conclusion. As mentioned earlier, collaboration with finance and clinical staff can be valuable during evidence gathering. However, in the absence of availability of this expertise individuals conducting the PBMA exercise may need to undertake detailed literature searches or contact other staff for this information, all of which could increase the time required to undertake the PBMA exercise. It is recommended to define the boundary of the budget and scope of the exercise as early as possible. Challenges can occur when activities span multiple boundaries, as this can make it very difficult to calculate proportional costs and attribute specific outcomes. There is a need for awareness of the culture and context of 'the budget' outside of the exercise. Certain budgets or activities may be ring-fenced or under a time-specific commitment, therefore it may not be possible to alter the amount of resources allocated to them. The panel should be informed of what is possible and what is not, before beginning its recommendation process and initiating discussion. This does not mean that the panel cannot make suggestions as part of a wider set of recommendations resulting from the exercise. However, these wider recommendations should be perhaps viewed as longer-term proposals or ideas for future exploration, and would not be included in any vote, due to current context and challenges to eventual implementation. Use of voting during discussions also has wider considerations. When using open voting, members could be susceptible to 'herd mentality' voting. Individuals may go along with the consensus rather than air their real opinions and views, especially if they contradict the current thinking in the room. This bias could be alleviated by using anonymous voting techniques and conducting one-to-one meetings instead. Another challenge is obtaining relevant evidence of the outcomes and benefits of services that have not previously been evaluated, and therefore have no established evidence base. In this situation, engagement events with the staff delivering the service/s and events with members of the public who are service users could provide a form of feedback to be used in evidence presented to the panel.

14.13 Summary - Some reflections on the case study

In retrospect, we might offer the following reflections:

- As health economists we were asked, with a blank canvas, to review health improvement spending across Wales and chose to adopt a PBMA approach. What we did not start with was any maximand or societal goal. We did not start with an allocative efficiency question about what public health prevention services should be produced and then go on to talk about 'how' these services might best be delivered—a technical efficiency question. We ended up being lost somewhere between the allocative efficiency question and the technical efficiency question. In future we would suggest that we, as health economists, should ask policy-makers to define their goal (e.g. improving child nutrition and education), and then, as 'dispassionate analysts', health economists are well-placed to present evidence on the relative cost-effectiveness of alternative strategies to achieve this policy goal.

- The most salient lesson we learnt from our experience in Wales was that even with a Ministerial health improvement budget of over £15 million, we were only in a position to undertake a 'partial' analysis in our PBMA exercise. What we lacked (and in the timescale available were unable to gather) was a complete picture of spending on prevention services across the whole of Welsh government. If spending on school-based interventions looked under-represented in our programme budget, we did not know whether this was the case or whether spending on prevention through schools was actually occurring from other budgets held by other government departments and local authorities.

- We made a fairly comprehensive effort of reviewing evidence of effectiveness and cost-effectiveness—this is the technical efficiency question.

- Out of the review came a reinforcement of a need to monitor uptake of public health programmes, potential barriers to uptake (equity concern), and a need to link with routine data collection systems (government, schools, primary care).

Summary of Chapter 14

This chapter:

♦ Presented an overview of PBMA, and described the potential application of this method as an evidence-based framework to make resource allocation decisions.

♦ Outlined methods for conducting each of the eight stages of PBMA, including wider considerations such as; the perspective of the PBMA exercise, objective of the PBMA exercise, criteria for appraising evidence and alternatives and time horizon.

♦ Presented a case study of PBMA to appraise a national health improvement budget, detailing the methods used to undertake the exercise.

♦ Offered reflections from this case study and lessons learnt, which may assist others wishing to use PBMA in the future.

References

Bohmer, P., Pain, C., Watt, A., Abernethy, P., and Sceats, J., 2001. Maximising health gain within available resources in the New Zealand public health system. *Health Policy,* 55(1): 37–50.

Brambleby, P. and Fordham, R., 2003. What is PBMA. *What is?... series. EPRINTS-JOURNAL,* 4(2).

Charles, J.M., Brown, G., Thomas, K., Johnstone, F., Vandenblink, V., Pethers, B., Jones, A. et al., 2016. Use of programme budgeting and marginal analysis as a framework for resource reallocation in respiratory care in North Wales, UK. *Journal of Public Health,* 38(3): e352–e361.

Cohen, D., 1994. Marginal analysis in practice: an alternative to needs assessment for contracting health care. *British Medical Journal,* 309(6957): 781.

Craig, N., Parkin, D., and Gerard, K., 1995. Clearing the fog on the Tyne: programme budgeting in Newcastle and North Tyneside Health Authority. *Health Policy,* 33(2): 107–25.

Craig, P., Dieppe, P., Macintyre, S., Michie, S., Nazareth, I., and Petticrew, M. 2008. Guidance on the development, evaluation and implementation of complex interventions to improve health. Available at: <http://www.mrc.ac.uk/documents/pdf/complex-interventions-guidance/> (Accessed 16 October 2018).

Crockett, A., Cranston, J., Moss, J., Scown, P., Mooney, G., and Alpers, J., 1999. Program budgeting and marginal analysis: A case study in chronic airflow limitation. *Australian Health Review,* 22(3): 65–77.

Donaldson, C., Bate, A., Mitton, C., Dionne, F., and Ruta, D., 2010. Rational disinvestment. *Quarterly Journal of Medicine,* 103(10): 801–7.

Drummond, M.F., Sculpher, M.J., Torrance, G.W., O'Brien, B.J., and Stoddart, G.L., 2015. *Methods for the Economic Evaluation of Health Care Programmes.* Oxford: Oxford University Press.

Edwards, R.T., Charles, J.M., Thomas, S., Bishop, J., Cohen, D., Groves, S., Humphreys, C., et al., 2014. A national Programme Budgeting and Marginal Analysis (PBMA) of health improvement spending across Wales: disinvestment and reinvestment across the life course. *BMC Public Health,* 14(1): 837.

Grocott, R., 2009. Applying Programme Budgeting Marginal Analysis in the health sector: 12 years of experience. *Expert Review of Pharmacoeconomics & Outcomes Research, 9*(2): 181–7.

Haas, M., Viney, R., Kristensen, E., Pain, C., and Foulds, K., 2001. Using programme budgeting and marginal analysis to assist population based strategic planning for coronary heart disease. *Health Policy, 55*(3): 173–86.

Henderson, L.R. and Scott, A., 2001. The costs of caring for stroke patients in a GP-led community hospital: an application of programme budgeting and marginal analysis. *Health & Social Care in the Community, 9*(4): 244–54.

Kelly, M.P., McDaid, D., Ludbrook, A., and Powell, J., 2005. *Economic Appraisal of Public Health Interventions.* London: Health Development Agency. Available at: <http://citeseerx.ist.psu.edu/viewdoc/download?doi=10.1.1.476.3820&rep=rep1&type=pdf> (Accessed 1 November 2018).

McDaid, D. and Needle, J., 2009. What use has been made of economic evaluation in public health? A systematic review of the literature. In: S. Dawson and S. Morris (eds), *Future Public Health* (pp. 248–264). Basingstoke, Palgrave Macmillan, pp. 248–64.

Mitton, C. and Donaldson, C., 2004. Health care priority setting: principles, practice and challenges. *Cost Effectiveness and Resource Allocation, 2*(1): 3.

Mitton, C., Donaldson, C., Shellian, B., and Pagenkopf, C., 2003. Priority setting in a Canadian surgical department: a case study using program budgeting and marginal analysis. *Canadian Journal of Surgery, 46*(1): 23–29.

National Institute for Health and Care Excellence (NICE). 2012. Methods for the development of NICE public health guidance. Available at: <http://www.nice.org.uk/guidance/ph1/resources/methods-for-development-of-nice-public-health-guidance2> (Accessed 16 October 2018).

National Institute for Health and Care Excellence (NICE). 2013. *Guide to the methods of technology appraisal.* London: National Institute for Health and Clinical Excellence.

Owen, L., Morgan, A., Fischer, A., Ellis, S., Hoy, A., and Kelly, M.P., 2012. The cost-effectiveness of public health interventions. *Journal of Public Health, 34*(1): 37–45.

Payne, K., McAllister, M., and Davies, L.M., 2013. Valuing the economic benefits of complex interventions: when maximising health is not sufficient. *Health Economics, 22*(3): 258–71.

Public Health Wales: Transforming Health Improvement in Wales. 2013. Available at: <http://www.wales.nhs.uk/sitesplus/documents/986/PHW%20Health%20Improvement%20Review%20Final%20Report%20-%20260913.pdf> (Accessed 1 November 2018).

Public Health Wales Observatory: Tobacco and Health in Wales. 2012. Available at: <http://www2.nphs.wales.nhs.uk:8080/PubHObservatoryProjDocs.nsf/85c50756737f79ac80256f2700534ea3/509486bfd300fdef80257a29003c3c67/$FILE/Eng%20Smoking%20Report%20LowRes.pdf> (Accessed 1 November 2018).

Public Health Wales Observatory: Lifestyle and health: Wales and its health boards. 2010. Available at: <http://www2.nphs.wales.nhs.uk:8080/PubHObservatoryProjDocs.nsf/public/A1E8A36C3D05AB5C802576F5005054EB/$file/Lifestyle_Wales_Final_E.pdf> (Accessed 1 November 2018).

Ratcliffe, J., Donaldson, C., and Macphee, S., 1996. Programme budgeting and marginal analysis: a case study of maternity services. *Journal of Public Health, 18*(2): 175–82.

Ruta, D., Mitton, C., Bate, A., and Donaldson, C., 2005. Programme budgeting and marginal analysis: bridging the divide between doctors and managers. *British Medical Journal, 330*(7506): 1501–3.

The Ottawa Charter for Health Promotion. Available at: <http://www.who.int/healthpromotion/conferences/previous/ottawa/en/index.html> (Accessed 16 October 2018).

Tsourapas, A. and Frew, E., 2011. Evaluating 'success' in programme budgeting and marginal analysis: a literature review. *Journal of Health Services Research & Policy*, *16*(3): 177–83.

Twaddle, S. and Walker, A., 1995. Programme budgeting and marginal analysis: application within programmes to assist purchasing in Greater Glasgow Health Board. *Health Policy*, *33*(2): 91–105.

Weatherly, H., Drummond, M., Claxton, K., Cookson, R., Ferguson, B., Godfrey, C., Rice, N., et al., 2009. Methods for assessing the cost-effectiveness of public health interventions: key challenges and recommendations. *Health Policy*, *93*(2):85–92.

Woolf, S.H., Husten, C.G., Lewin, L.S., Marks, J.S., Fielding, J.E. and Sanchez, E.J., 2009. *The Economic Argument for Disease Prevention: Distinguishing Between Value and Savings*. Washington, DC: Partnership for Prevention.

Chapter 15

International perspectives and future directions for research and policy

Rhiannon T. Edwards, Emma McIntosh, and Eira Winrow

15.1 Introduction

The three major causes of premature death in the United Kingdom—heart disease, lung cancer, and stroke—are all largely preventable. The Department of Health in England calculates that 70 per cent of total health and social care expenditure in England is for the treatment and care of people with long-term conditions such as diabetes and heart disease. Yet, many lifestyle choices, such as smoking, poor diet, alcohol misuse, and sedentary lifestyles, contribute towards developing these conditions, and all are avoidable (Department of Health, 2010; Davies et al., 2016).

Bayer and Galea identify the 'many frameworks that recognize multiple contributors to the production of population health' (Bayer and Galeo, 2015). One focus of this book was to identify and describe economic evaluation methods that handle with such multiple contributions as well as the resulting multiple outcomes. The purpose of economic evaluation with respect to public health is to inform decision-making as to how best to use society's scarce and limited public resources across all government departments, beyond the health sector/non-health sector interface, in order to achieve public health goals. These may be the goals of national or devolved governments (e.g. policies that have related to smoking bans in public places, proposed minimum alcohol pricing, and sugar taxes), local authorities, the National Health Service (NHS), and the voluntary sector.

Public health is essentially concerned with the complex business of prevention of disease and disability which often requires behavioural change, is highly sensitive to socio-economic factors, the environment in which people live, and the interactions between people and sectors. This book is concerned with the economic evaluation of public health interventions (PHIs). These multifaceted, complex interventions are typically delivered outside the health sector (i.e. education, housing, community and transport sectors) and often impact multiple sectors of society, hence making this evaluation role a challenging one, particularly with respect to measuring outcomes (as outlined in Chapter 6). Health economists assume the role of dispassionate analyst (Culyer, 2012), but we must also develop and test alternative methods of analysis in economic evaluation if we are aware that our traditional tools are likely to fail to capture the full range of relevant costs and benefits in relation to the economic evaluation of public health interventions. This book has identified a number of possible alternative frameworks and methods that may have a role to play in the economic evaluation of PHIs, including multi-criteria decision making (MCDA), social return on investment (SROI), cost–consequence analysis (CCA), and impact evaluation. Further, PHI economic evaluation will benefit from developments in research designs and other evaluative approaches such as natural experiments for evaluation of data from observational data (Deidda et al., 2018), advances in systems modelling methods such as agent-based modelling (ABM), and expansions in the outcome space such as increased use of contingent valuation approaches, capability well-being, development index approaches, and increased creativity with our interpretation of 'effectiveness' outcomes.

Public health policy often focuses heavily on reducing inequalities in health and improving the health of the most deprived in society. That means that economic evaluations of PHIs need to take account of equity implications through subgroup or sensitivity analysis. A single mean incremental cost-effectiveness ratio is probably not sufficient; it is often necessary to make such estimates context-specific (e.g. age group, geographical setting, or socio-economic circumstances). A forthcoming handbook in this series (Cookson et al., 2019) will explore equity-informed economic evaluation in more depth. Many PHIs targeting the most deprived groups can often realize substantial cost savings (Owen et al., 2011). Indeed, the toothbrushing population health economic evaluation (Anopa et al., 2015), highlighted in Chapter 1, provides a prime example of how PHI's can reduce the inequalities gradient, increase health outcomes, and produce cost savings—an economic 'win–win' scenario (see Figure 15.1).

There are efficiency and equity arguments for investing in prevention (Merkur, 2013), however the traditional toolbox of methods of economic evaluation has arguably been too limited to capture all relevant costs and benefits and conduct equity-informed economic evaluations. Within this book we have tried to suggest ways of expanding this toolbox, and means of thinking 'outside the box' whilst acknowledging that some practical gains come at the expense of theoretically preferred approaches. The National Institute for Health and Care Excellence guidance has acknowledged this sea-change by recommending an increased use of CBA and CCA (National Institute for Health and Care Excellence, 2012. This book, the fifth in the series of handbooks in health economics evaluation, emphasizes that 'no one size fits all', and that there is a need for creativity in design, conduct, and analysis of economic evaluation of PHIs. The next book in the series provides readers with a guide to equity informed economic evaluation (Cookson et al., 2019).

15.2 **International perspective**

In researching this book, it became apparent that many countries, including Finland, Australia, Norway, Canada, and the United Kingdom, all use a broad range of economic evaluation methods and research designs to explore the relative cost-effectiveness of investing in prevention. We include some illustrative examples in the sections to follow.

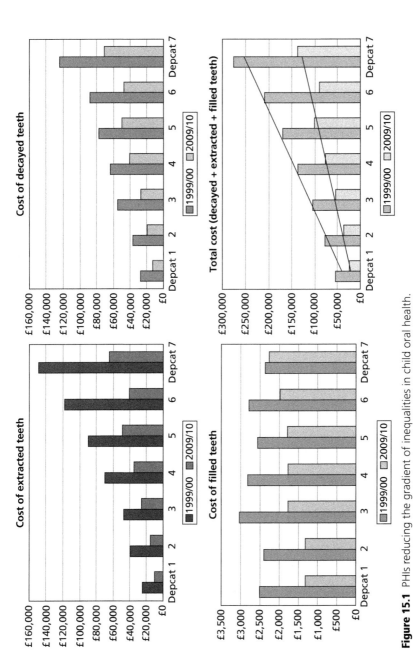

Figure 15.1 PHIs reducing the gradient of inequalities in child oral health.

15.2.1 **Finland**

Finland had the highest cardiovascular disease (CVD) mortality rate in the world at the beginning of the 1970s. As a consequence, a cross-sectorial, community-based approach to educate the population and reduce the risk factors (smoking, cholesterol, and hypertension) was initiated in the form of the North Karelia Project in 1972. Evaluation of the programme highlighted that between 1970 and 1995, the heart disease-related mortality rate was reduced by 73 per cent in Finland and 65 per cent in North Karelia (Puska, 2002). The cost-effectiveness analyses of the study found the intervention to be cost-effective with the cost per quality-adjusted life year (QALY) gained of US$3612 at zero discount and $5830 at 10 per cent discount over a five-year time horizon (Nissinen et al., 1986).

15.2.2 **Australia**

One of the most comprehensive examples of modelling the potential cost-effectiveness of public health prevention initiatives, the ACE–Prevention study, was undertaken in Australia (Vos et al., 2010). ACE–Prevention made an important contribution to the evidence base for priority setting in prevention by its evaluation of prevention for non-communicable disease in Australia, using comparable methods across 150 interventions and evaluating combinations of prevention approaches for major health risks (such as alcohol, diet, and cardiovascular risks). To ensure valid comparisons between results, each intervention was modelled to apply to the relevant 2003 Australian population and the costs and health outcomes were measured for as long as they occurred, often over a lifetime. All results were expressed as a cost per disability-adjusted life year (DALY) averted. Best available evidence on effectiveness was derived from the international literature, using estimates that were pooled across all available studies. Costs and outcomes were modelled based on expectations of how interventions would be implemented under routine health service conditions in Australia. The ACE–Prevention project took an Australian government perspective (as third-party payer) and aimed to assist policy-makers and health service managers in making practical decisions about prevention services. The main aim of the indigenous component of ACE–Prevention was to estimate the difference in cost-effectiveness between preventive interventions addressing indigenous and non–indigenous Australian populations, and to advise on the appropriate distribution of resources. Costs and benefits were measured in a consistent manner in the indigenous and non-indigenous analyses; separately, the indigenous cost-effectiveness ratios were recalculated using a broader concept of benefit as developed in consultation with the representatives of the indigenous population. For the whole population, benefits were modified for equity, feasibility, and acceptability. A standard method for collecting cost information was used. Costs were discounted at 3 per cent using a reference year of 2003. Extensive sensitivity analysis was undertaken.

Using cost–utility analysis (CUA) and cost-effectiveness analysis (CEA) methods, the ACE–Prevention project advised the prioritization of government spending on taxation of tobacco, alcohol, and unhealthy foods; a mandatory limit on salt in bread, cereals, and margarine; improving the efficiency of blood pressure- and cholesterol-lowering drugs using an absolute risk approach, and choosing the most cost-effective generic drugs (or polypill that combines three blood pressure-lowering drugs and one cholesterol-lowering drug); gastric banding for severe obesity; and an intensive 'SunSmart' campaign to reduce skin cancer incidence, morbidity, and mortality through a targeted prevention and early detection program. The SunSmart return on investment (ROI) analysis showed it to be a worthwhile investment, with a AUS$2.20 return for every dollar spent. The ACE–Prevention project also acknowledged that mental health deserved special consideration in addition to providing economic arguments for the introduction of hepatitis B vaccination and HPV vaccination.

15.2.3 **Northern Ireland**

In Northern Ireland, Greenways initiative suggests that the disused railway network across the region has the potential to tackle obesity through physical inactivity by developing the railway lines into over 600 miles of walking and cycling pathways (nigreenways, 2017). Dallat undertook research involving the Connswater Community Greenway regeneration in Northern Ireland and concluded that population-based health gains were substantial and could have wider benefits beyond health (Dallat et al., 2014). If 10 per cent of the community became more active, Dallat calculated that 75 deaths could be prevented with an ICER of £4469 per DALY.

15.2.4 **Norway**

Cost–benefit analyses of walking and cycling tracks in Norway have been conducted to explore the impact of infrastructure improvement projects to promote non-motorized transport. This study took a wider approach to assessing these benefits. Alongside health benefits, the study took into consideration a reduction in 'external costs' such as reduced noise and air pollution and reduced parking costs (Sælensminde, 2004). The ROI of investing in cycle networks is suggested to be four to five times the initial investment, and because of the wide-reaching benefits, it is suggested that investing in these kinds of infrastructure projects are of great benefit to society. Sælensminde discovered that analysis of the wider benefits in the CBA uncovers 'barrier costs'; in this instance, the barriers to walking or cycling may be attributed to motorized vehicles on roads which prevent people from taking the non-motorized option due to unsafe surroundings such as passing places or a lack of safe crossings. The authors conclude that such 'barrier costs' should be considered alongside the more obvious costs in order to provide a comprehensive analysis of an intervention (Sælensminde, 2004).

15.2.5 **Canada**

In Canada, the 'Communities that Care' project is a successful example of preventing health- and life-course-harming behaviours in young people. This national programme is tailored to the specific needs of the community population by identifying the strengths and weaknesses of the community in order to strengthen the support available to help young people flourish. The results of the economic evaluation revealed that young people in the evaluation study ($n = 4407$) were 25 per cent less likely to be involved in delinquent behaviour, 32 per cent less likely to consume alcohol, 33 per cent less likely to smoke tobacco, and for every dollar invested there was a return of C$5.30 via savings to the criminal justice system, health care, and tax revenue from being active in the jobs market (Kuklinsky, 2012; 2015).

15.2.6 Mexico

In 2012, the prevalence of overweight and obesity in Mexico reached 70 per cent among adults and 30 per cent among children (Colchero et al., 2017). Although obesity and all related chronic disease are the result of many causes, evidence reveals that consumption of sugar-sweetened beverages (SSBs) is associated with weight gain, diabetes, and other chronic diseases (Malik et al., 2006, 2010). To reduce the consumption of SSBs, in January 2014 the Mexican government implemented an excise tax of one Mexican peso per litre to all non-alcoholic beverages with added sugar (including powdered SSB based on their reconstitution and flavoured/sweetened dairy products that are not milks). Colchero and colleagues show that as a result of this excise tax, in Mexico purchases of taxed beverages decreased by 8.2 per cent over the two years on average (−5.5 per cent in 2014; −9.7 per cent in 2015). Further, they show that the lowest socio-economic group had the largest decreases in taxed beverages in both years. Untaxed beverage purchases increased 2.1 per cent in the post-tax period. In Mexico, lower purchases of taxed beverages were sustained and de creased still further in the second year of the tax.

15.2.7 United Kingdom

As of 6 April 2018, the Soft Drinks Industry Levy came into effect in the United Kingdom. The aim of the levy is to encourage companies to reduce the sugar content in their soft drinks. The rates companies will need to pay are: 24p per litre of drink if it contains 8 grams of sugar per 100 millilitres; 18p per litre of drink if it contains between 5–8 grams of sugar per 100 millilitres. Commonly referred to in the United Kingdom as the 'sugar tax', this levy has already resulted in over 50 per cent of manufacturers reducing the sugar content of drinks since it was announced in March 2016— the equivalent of 45 million kilos of sugar every year. Soft drinks manufacturers who do not to reformulate their sugar content will pay the levy, which is expected to raise £240 million each year. The taxes raised will also make a contribution to the funding of programmes designed to reduce obesity. Such 'ear-marking' of taxes is relatively rare, but in the United Kingdom, the tax was introduced in the March 2016 budget with the explicit goal to 'fund a doubling of the primary schools' sports premium'. £100 million of revenue generated from the Soft Drinks Industry Levy will be used for the Healthy Pupils Capital Fund (HPCF). This fund is intended to improve children's and young people's physical and mental health by enhancing access to facilities at schools such as kitchens, dining facilities, changing rooms, playgrounds, and sports facilities (<https://www.gov.uk>). It has been agreed that even if revenue from the levy declines, funding for schools and children will stay the same.

   (Source: <https://www.gov.uk/government/news/soft-drinks-industry-levy-comes-into-effect>; <https://theconversation.com/sugar-tax-what-you-need-to-know-94520>.) Of note, a new tax on SSBs also came into effect in the US cities of Seattle and Philadelphia at the beginning of 2018.

15.3 **Research priorities for the future**

There is a burgeoning literature on public health economic evaluation. In a bid to summarise some priorities for research in this field we have set out the following suggestions, not in any particular order of priority.

15.3.1 **Increased use of behavioural economics**

Incorporation of behavioural economics (e.g. in relation to how consumers make choices) in the design of behaviour change interventions and also in the design of economic evaluation studies is an area worthy of increased routine use for public health economic evaluation. There is a wealth of evidence that many of the issues that undermine or improve our health outcomes have behavioural determinants (in addition to structural and social determinants). It is now commonly accepted that the protection and improvement of the population's health cannot be expected to rely solely on biological and medical models. There is a growing recognition that a multi-faceted approach is needed to address many of the leading public health issues, including infectious and preventable diseases, mental health, smoking, alcohol misuse, poor diet and physical inactivity. Behavioural economics comprises a key part of this approach, providing unique insights into human decision making, choices and financial incentives amongst others. The inclusion of economics within public health intervention evaluation funding bids should aim to be developing not only economic evaluation designs but behavioural economic contributions. Advances in methods of artificial intelligence and machine learning methods to complement behavioural economics in public health is an exciting and rapidly growing area of research.

15.3.2 **Ethical considerations for the use of financial incentives in achieving behaviour change**

In the exploration of whether financial incentives are cost-effective in achieving behaviour change there is a need for moral considerations reagrding the use of financial incentives. Ryan and colleagues found that financial incentives for weight loss could target at-risk groups and encourage positive behaviour change (Ryan et al., 2015. Hoddinott and co-workers found that public perception of financial incentives for stopping smoking during pregnancy and breastfeeding was mixed (Hoddinott et al., 2014). Their cross-sectional public survey revealed that agreement with incentives was mixed depending on age, gender, and type of incentive. Future research into the role of financial incentives should ensure the ethical implications are considered (see Cookson et al, 2019 for suggested methods).

15.3.3 **Valuing green space in the built environment and valuing nature**

Increasingly, health promotion activities are available in public 'green' spaces such as parks. An example of this is the Parkrun scheme, which coordinates regular 5 kilometre runs which are free and open to everyone in parks all over the world (parkrun. org, 2017). In the United Kingdom, local authorities faced with financial cuts are struggling to maintain parks. For a perspective on the value of nature, see to Juniper (2013).

The Commission on Architecture and the Built Environment (CABE) has raised concerns that local authorities list their parks and playgrounds as liabilities rather than as assets, based on their potential resale value, because they do not know or cannot operationalize the potential and actual health, environmental, and inter-generational value of such public places (CABE, 2009). The challenge for health economists is to capture, at the margin, the befits attributable to health promotion activity such as a parkrun, in some way through revealed or stated preferences; for example, to measure and value the health benefits of health promotion activities in green space (Edwards, 2017; see section 15.2.3 for an example from Northern Ireland).

The Field in Trust charity published findings of survey of a representative sample of 4000 members of the UK population. Using willingness to pay techniques conforming to the Treasury Green Book approach, they found the willingness to pay value of parks and green spaces more than doubles for lower socio-economic groups when welfare weighted, increasing from £2.00 to £4.32 per month. They found that urban residents value parks and green spaces higher than the UK average willingness to pay value at £2.89 per month, and this value increases after welfare weighting to £3.93. People who visited their park less often than once a month value the existence of parks and green spaces. However, frequent park users stated higher willingness to pay values for parks and green spaces (67 per cent higher than non-frequent users and non-users) (Fields in Trust, 2018).

Play provision provides an important context in which children can counter the effects of poverty and deprivation. A report for Public Health Wales on the economic case for investing in early years (Edwards et al., 2016) revealed that the only cost per QALY estimate for playgrounds was produced by Matrix and was high—a very expensive adventure playground! (Matrix, 2010).

15.3.4 Exploring the roll of prevention and public health in a circular economy

In the United Kingdom, the NHS was created on a principle of treatment free at the point of delivery from cradle to grave. This has proved over time to be an challenging aspiration due to an ageing population, scientific advances, and a more demanding patient population. A concept of 'cradle to cradle' (from this generation to the next generation) widens this model to start thinking about future generations within a 'circular economy' (Lacy and Rutqvist, 2016; Sundararajan, 2016).

It could be argued that a medical model of the production of health fits with a linear 'take, make, and dispose' model of a wider economy. By contrast, in a circular economy model, resources are reused through reusable design, and more effective repair, recycling, and restoration. It is useful to consider public health and prevention at the health/non-health sector interface within the context of a circular economy model. Simple examples of this are the benefits of reduced plastics and packaging used by hospitals, improved population health, and through prevention initiatives. Recent studies report that hospitals generate 33.8 pounds in weight of waste per day, per staffed bed. Multiplying this amount of waste across world hospital bed density yields a total of 100 million tons of plastics waste per year (<https://www.hprc.org/single-post/2016/06/22/HPRC-and-the-Circular-Economy>).

Policies such as the Wellbeing of Future Generations Act in Wales (Welsh Government 2016) operationalize a commitment to thinking about how current policies and future policies may affect future generations. This gives credence to using a lower discount rate for costs and outcomes in the case of PHIs, as discussed in Chapter 2. Brouwer and colleagues argued for the use of differential rates in the economic evaluation of prevention intervention (Brouwer et al., 2005), and since 2013. NICE has recommended a discount rate of 3 per cent for costs and 1.5 per cent for health outcomes (National Institute for Health and Care Excellence, 2012). A zero per cent rate, as used by the World Health Organization (WHO) sensitivity analysis, is a way of illustrating the impact of choice of discount rate on the relative cost-effectiveness of public health interventions with a long-term and sometimes intergenerational time horizon.

In the United Kingdom, it is estimated that only 4 per cent of NHS spending is on prevention (Butterfield et al., 2009). Other government sectors at the health/non-health interface such as housing, transport, education, and the environment arguably have a much greater role to play in determining population health and potentially preventing disease and disability than the NHS in the United Kingdom. This book reminds those of us focused on the technical methods of economic evaluation that first and foremost is the need to address the question of allocative efficiency. What maximands or goals is society to pursue with respect to improving population health and reducing inequalities in health? Today, one in four 5-year-old children will live to be 100. Buck and Maguire updated what is known as the Marmot curve to show that life expectancy now is determined more by where you live than your income or any other factor (Buck and Maguire, 2015). Longevity does not necessarily mean a good health-related quality of life. Up to 30 per cent of incidences of dementia could be prevented by taking action in mid-life to alter risk factors such as physical inactivity, smoking, diabetes, hypertension, obesity, depression, and mental inactivity (Public Health England, 2016).

15.3.5 Consistency in dealing with spillover costs and outcomes and the increased use of CBA methods

The case for including spillover costs and benefits to informal caregivers and family members has been made on methodological and equity grounds by Brouwer (Brouwer, 2018) amongst others. In the United Kingdom the National Institute for Health and Care xcellence (2013) provided guidance that such spillover costs and benefits should be considered where deemed relevant. All direct health effects, whether for patients or, where relevant, carers (National Institute for Health and Care Excellence, 2013). In the United States, the Second Panel on Cost-Effectiveness in Health and Medicine has proposed the use of 'impact inventories' (Sanders, 2016). McCabe has argued against the inclusion of spillover effects in Health Technology Assessment when a health service perspective is used and there is assumed to be a fixed specified budget (McCabe, 2018). This is essentially a welfarist versus extra-welfarist debate where a welfarist approach would take a societal perspective which could span many sectors and reflect spillover effects from, for example, a health intervention that was able to reduce absenteeism from work. An extra-welfarist approach would focus on the direct benefits to a patient and whether a new drug or treatment should or should not be funded by a health care system such as the NHS in the United Kingdom. What is becoming clear is that economic evaluation of PHIs requires a much wider perspective of analysis than used in Health Technology Assessment (HTA). Cost–benefit analysis represents the operationalization of such a welfarist approach. The advantages of the CBA approach for the economic evaluation of PHIs has been a recurrent theme throughout this book. Indeed, the reference to precision population health above refers to 'cross-sectoral efforts' and this really sums up the argument for a greater use of CBA and CBA-associated methodologies as it is really the only approach which can value those all-important recurrent cross-sectoral spillover costs and outcomes arising in PHIs. Economic evaluations such as 'Communities that Care' provide convincing evidence that investing at the socio-structural level is the key to improving population health and reducing inequalities and as such these 'mega projects' require broad evaluative approaches such as CBA (Korytárová and Papežíková, 2015). These CBAs for PHIs, however, are likely to benefit from being conducted using advanced modelling methods and systems approaches.

15.3.6 Standardization of ROI and SROI methods

A 2017 systematic review of ROI of PHIs identified studies that discovered that the ROI for PHIs demonstrates that PHIs at both national and local level are highly effective in terms of cost savings (Masters et al., 2017). The research suggests that cutting public health spending in wealthy countries generates a false economy and only serves to cause billions of pounds of costs to other sectors in the health service and beyond (Masters et al., 2017). The research also found that PHIs at a local level produced an average ROI of 4 (for every £1 invested, £4 is returned), but for interventions at the national level, the ROI could yield as much as £46 for every £1 of investment. ROI figures were in the main higher than Cost-benefit analysis figures, but most reports concentrate on either ROI or CBA, suggesting that methods of SROI, ROI, and CBA need to be standardized with sources of non-market or shadow prices made more easily available (Masters et al., 2017).

15.3.7 Steering research funding

The last ten years in the United Kingdom has seen a recognition of the need for dedicated research funds for public health research, including economic evaluation of PHIs, for example through the UK's National Institute for Health Research (NIHR)–Public Health Research (PHR) stream of research funding. Many topic-based funding calls have related to studies of behaviour change interventions (e.g. to promote exercise in children and adolescents), and while there has been continued priority given to studies with a randomized control design, there has been an increasing number of natural experiment and evidence synthesis studies. Figure 15.2 relates to obesity but the model can be generalized in a

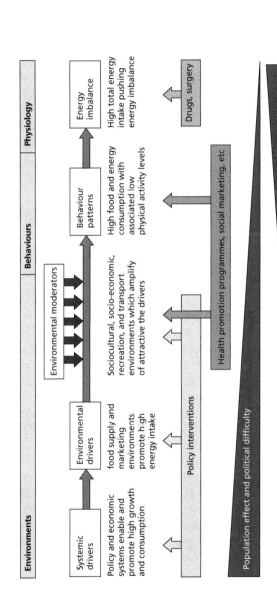

Figure 15.2 The Public Health England Economics Research landscape.

broader public health and the funding of public health research context. Most funding currently available is for studies towards the right of the diagram (i.e. behaviour patterns and behaviour change) rather than research into the effectiveness and cost-effectiveness of interventions aimed at the left-hand side of the diagram (i.e. to evaluate changes to policy and changes to environments to improve population health). The latter would probably need to have non-RCT designs. In this book we have highlighted the importance of other types of research design in public health which allow evaluation of policy interventions such as natural experiments to evaluate the reduction in drink and drive limits and the ban on smoking in public places. There is a needed for funding for the long-term follow-up of economic evaluations of PHIs, and an associated need for economic models with a long time horizons, and ways of linking short- and medium-term outcomes to longer-term economic outcomes. Figure 15.2 below is reproduced from Swinburn et al. 2011 showing the research landscape across which solutions to obesity might be tested and introduced.

15.3.8 **Precision public health**

> In sum, there is now broad consensus that health differences between groups and within groups are not driven by clinical care but by social-structural factors that shape our lives. (Bayer and Galea, 2015)

According to Vaithinathan and Asokan, precision medicine and public health share a goal (Vaithinathan and Asokan, 2017). They argue that precision medicine means 'segregating the individuals into subpopulations who vary in their disease susceptibility and response to a precise treatment' and not merely the designing of drugs or creation of medical devices. The UK's 100,000 Genomes Project is expected to sequence 100,000 genomes from 70,000 patients. Similarly, the Precision Medicine Initiative of the United States plans to increase population-based genome sequencing and link it with clinical data. A national cohort of around 1 million people is to be established in the long term to investigate the genetic and environmental determinants of health and disease and further integrated to individual's electronic health records, something that is as yet optional. Levy-Lahad and colleagues provide an example of precision medicine in a public health context with evidence that population screening was highly cost-effective compared with the current family history-based approaches (Levy-Lahad, 2015). Precision public health can be seen as administering the right intervention to a population at an appropriate time and while this may initially sound intuitive, there are a number of sceptics of such an approach. Bayer and Galea argue, in brief, that health differences between groups of people and within groups are not driven by clinical care but by social-structural factors (Bayer and Galea, 2015). Their concern is that 'an unstinting focus' on precision medicine by trusted spokespeople for health is a mistake and a distraction from the goal of producing a healthier population by investing in broad, cross-sectoral efforts to minimize the potential effect of foundational drivers of poor health.

15.3.9 **Why many public health programmes fail to demonstrate effectiveness and cost-effectiveness**

From a methodological perspective, there is a need for some forensic work on why evidence-based, large-scale government funded preventative interventions such as the Sure Start programme and Troubled Families programmes in England have failed to demonstrate effectiveness and cost-effectiveness when rolled out. We need to ask whether this was due to the implementation of the programme, or the research methods used to capture costs and benefits (Rutter, 2006).

The Sure Start programme in England aimed at 'giving children the best possible start in life' through better childcare provision, focused early education, and health and family support through community schemes. Substantial funding of over £452 million was allocated to initiate Sure Start Local Programmes (SSLPs) to target up to 150,000 children up to the age of 4 years in deprived areas across England. An economic evaluation of the programme commissioned in 2010 revealed that the programme cost was around £1300 per child, per year, from birth to age 4. By the age of 5, the SSLPs were estimated to have influenced economic benefits of between £279 and £557 per child; some of those benefits related to the parents of the children in receipt of the support of the SSLP becoming economically active through paid work, and some benefits related to behavioural aspects of the child's life which were influenced by the SSLP, such as better home learning environments and less family chaos (National Evaluation of Sure Start Team, 2010).

As the Sure Start programme was considered an investment in human capital, the evidence suggests that childhood interventions such as these generate higher returns much later in the life course (Heckman and Masterov, 2007).

The UK government claimed that £1.2 billion was saved by working with families participating in the Troubled Families programme in England, yet an evaluation of the programme revealed that it had been impossible to undertake a cost–benefit analysis of the programme due to a lack of data following the impact evaluation (Day et al., 2016). Although an estimated return of £2.11 per £1 invested was demonstrated, no comparison was made where the programme was not utilized, thus questioning the attribution of the fiscal return to the Troubled Families programme (Bate, 2017).

Complex interventions such as Sure Start and Troubled Families are often treated as simple, and the final evaluation of both programmes demonstrates that complex interventions may appear not to 'work', but it could just be that they are being judged on the wrong criteria. Linear cause and effect is (relatively) easy to look for, but that doesn't mean it is helpful to do so solely on these criteria. A whole-systems approach requires a shift from reductionist, linear, single-perspective thinking to transdisciplinary, non-linear systems thinking.

Don't forget the lessons of Geoffrey Rose: population-level prevention involves shifting the population curve in ways that may be indiscernible at the individual level (Rose, 1985; Rutter, 2006).

15.3.10 **The need for payer thresholds for changes in population health**

Health economists need to be cautious and to think about the usefulness to service commissioners of reporting economic evaluation as 'cost per unit change' on a disease-specific outcome measure, or even a percentage change in positive or negative health behaviour, for example, minutes of exercise per week (positive), number of cigarettes smoke (negative), as currently we do not have societal payer thresholds along the lines of a cost per QALY threshold used by NICE. This is why often a cost–consequences approach is useful to show a range of benefits, which might include a cost per QALY amongst them for comparison with the NICE threshold.

Related to this is the meaningfulness of cost-effectiveness thresholds for outcomes and the extent to which they are relevant for multifaceted public health outcomes. The relevance of this phenomenon for outcomes assessment is that the value of an intervention that changes the dynamic of a complex system is likely to be a function of the intervention, that is, where people may value the intervention more after implementation than before it. Preferences are no longer stable, and this undermines the validity of the methods economists use to ascertain value. Co-funding insights by Remme and colleagues add a new insight to this discussion (Remme et al., 2017). As such, economic evaluation of population health interventions will benefit from using evidence from the field of social care economic evaluation.

15.3.11 Publication of economic evaluation of PHIs

Many journals require health economics to adhere to the CHEERS checklist for publishing the results of economic evaluation studies (Husereau et al., 2013). In the case of economic evaluation of PHIs where CBAs or CCA may be the most appropriate form of analysis, this checklist may not be sufficient, and an alternative checklist is being developed. (Sanghera et al., 2015)

15.4 A review of the contents of this book

Benjamin Franklin said that an ounce of prevention is worth a pound of cure (Masters et al., 2017), and Professor Sir Michael Marmot wrote that medicine is failed prevention (Marmot, 2011). We know a growing amount about the relative cost-effectiveness of medical technologies but very little about the cost-effectiveness of prevention. This book places a marker in the sand in the emerging and challenging sub-discipline of public health economics. We have not grappled with whether to call this book applied health economics of 'population health' or 'public health'; either are equally appropriate and relevant. The book has been intended for health economists finding themselves faced with the distinct challenges posed by applying tools of economic evaluation in a public health setting, and equally for public health practitioners finding themselves faced with having to make an economic case for prevention. The book has deliberately focused on outlining methodology and presenting applied case studies.

In the United Kingdom, HM Treasury has a particular role to play in leading the way in the standardization of key factors such as discount rates and time horizons (HM Treasury). In health economics, our toolbox needs to be expanded—thinking outside the toolbox so that PHIs can be assessed on a level playing field. In this book however, we are not prescriptive about which of the methods of economic evaluation are appropriate in different settings.

In Chapter 1 of this book, we introduced readers to the work of Geoffrey Rose and his seminal article, 'Sick individuals and sick populations', in which he argued the need to distinguish between prevention for populations and prevention for high-risk individuals (Rose, 1985).

We began Chapter 1 with the three key economic questions:

1. What preventive goods and services is society to produce?

2. What technical methods of production (legislation, fiscal, i.e. taxation; shaping social norms; creating and using the built and natural environment to promote health; modifying individual behaviour directly through education and support) are in use?

3. How should access to these preventative goods and services be distributed between members of society?

If, as Professor Sir Michael Marmot has argued, we in society should do nothing that harms the current and future health of our children, then the health economist first has a role in showing the net present value to society as a whole of pursuing this overarching goal, and second has an important role in producing evidence of the technical efficiency or cost-effectiveness of achieving this goal at minimum opportunity cost—(i.e. the relative cost-effectiveness of strategies for improving the health of the population through focusing on child and adolescent health in different ways).

This book introduces the public health practitioner to the way that economists, and health economists, view the world. This is first and foremost from a neoclassical welfare economics theoretical paradigm. The concept of Pareto optimality and Pareto paralysis (an inability to judge or choose between various states of the world where no-one can be made better off without making someone else worse off), and the reason why health economists have explored a normative framework of extra-welfarism (naming 'health' as a specific goal within a social welfare function) operationalized by concepts such as the QALY and capabilities (Culyer, 1989).

In Chapter 2 we introduced the public health and health economist reader to the concept of the demand for prevention goods. Positive time preference and inaccurate knowledge about relative risks means that the markets for prevention goods (goods and services that improve our health today and prevent ill health in the future) spectacularly fail. There is, hence, a role for government to protect and improve the health of the population; many prevention goods and services are public goods. Maintenance of a cost pathway that promotes exercise and generates positive externality benefits through bringing tourism to rural areas provides an excellent example of such a public good. In the same chapter, we describe the key concepts of scarcity, choice, opportunity cost, and the margin. These concepts underpin economic evaluation. Chapter 2 illustrates how health economists deal with uncertainty: producing in a parametric and non-parametric analysis, confidence intervals around ICER point estimates relating these to probabilty that an intervention is cost-effective at different payer thresholds, and measurements of net monetary benefit.

The book shows readers how to think about investment in prevention as a one-off up-front cost with a profile over many years. For the first few years, the opportunity cost of foregone health for other patients outweighs the benefits from prevention, and at some point a break-even point is reached and from then on the benefits from prevention in terms of improved life expectancy and/or improved health related quality of life are delivered.

Chapter 3 of this book discusses the added challenges of applying the well-established toolbox of methods of economic evaluation to the evaluation of public health interventions. These interventions are often delivered in a non-health setting and more likely to be about changing environments and social norms rather than simply attempting to change individual behaviour. Probably the greatest challenge to making a pragmatic business case for investment in prevention is that benefits in the future may not accrue to the sector or stakeholder making the initial investment (Weatherly, 2009).

In Chapter 4 we discuss the importance of evidence synthesis/realist synthesis for health economists to understand the mechanisms and contexts that influence the potential effectiveness and cost-effectiveness of PHIs. This is often a case of what works for whom in what setting. We promote the use of logic models to map out processes, particularly for interventions that are often 'complex' in nature.

Chapter 5 of this book deals with the fact that economic evaluation of PHIs often requires the collection of service use and unit cost information from several different sectors. We presented a micro-costing of a toddler parenting programme to illustrate this.

Chapter 6 introduced readers to the specific challenges of measuring a much broader range of outcomes in the context of the evaluation of PHIs than is traditionally necessary in a health sector context. Chapters 7–10 discuss and present case studies for the various methods of economic evaluation. Although NICE in the United Kingdom has encouraged the increased use of cost–benefit and cost–consequence analysis methods, we recognize the continued interest and need for all methods of economic evaluation in a public health setting. We therefore provide case studies of the application of all methods, barring cost-minimization analysis, rarely applicable to the economic evaluation of PHIs in our view as editors. This is because cost minimization analysis requires confidence that outcomes of two or more interventions being compared are exactly the same, and this is rarely the case in a public health context. Of note is our argument that even if QALYs do not capture the whole range of outcomes relevant to PHIs, perhaps across health and non-health sectors, they do provide a common denominator for argument for investment in prevention when the cost per QALY is directly comparable with, and often less, than the cost per QALY of curative medical interventions as shown in Chapter 8 (Owen et al., 2011). In that chapter, we reproduce an important paper by Lesley Owen and colleagues at NICE. It illustrates that there is a place for QALYs in public health. Even if QALYs do not capture the full range of relevant outcomes and require additional measures to capture such wider outcomes, they provide a powerful mechanism for illustrating the relative cost-effectiveness of PHIs designed to prevent ill health and disability, compared with medical interventions such as drugs used to treat and manage illness and disability (Owen et al., 2011).

In subsequent chapters of the book we explore the use of CBA and CCA as alternatives to CUA. Chapter 9 highlights that, with respect to public health, finding an appropriately broad and encompassing welfare measure is a key requirement to support evidence-based policy in addition to outlining the potential role of discrete choice experiment methods for valuing outcomes across sectors (Baba, 2016).

Chapter 11 addresses the potential for economic modelling in the evaluation of PHIs. Acknowledging the need for large numbers in RCTs of PHIs, often aimed at encouraging small changes across the population such as lowering salt or sugar consumption, we explain that there is a potentially vital role for modelling in public health economics. Many of the earlier examples came from modelling infectious diseases such as malaria and were developed for use in the developing world.

Chapter 12 returns to the principles of CBA and the method of SROI. We present case studies to illustrate how SROI is being used in the evaluation of PHIs to offer a triple bottom line: economic, social, and environmental. We present SROI with the caveats of the need for standardization and perhaps thresholds as are used in more traditional CEA (Fujiwara, 2015).

In Chapters 13 and 14 we turn to the issue of the need for priority setting mechanisms in spending decisions about public health resources, both within the NHS and across other sectors.

In Chapter 13 we discuss MCDA. In Chapter 14 we present a case study of the use of PBMA in public health. These techniques for priority setting allow for transparent, evidence-based, and consultative exploration of various options in public health spending within and across government sectors.

With respect to the publication and reporting of economic evaluations of public health interventions we argue in Chapter 3 that available guidance on reporting and presenting results (CHEERS) will only take us so far. We offer a checklist at the end of this, the final chapter, which is broader and may be more useful for economic evaluations of public health interventions, to be used alongside CHEERS (Huserau et al., 2013).

Checklist of additional factors to consider in the design, conduct, and reporting of economic evaluations in public health interventions

1 What is the appropriate theoretical framework for analysis (e.g. welfarist, extra-welfarist, capability theory)?

2 What is the setting of the public health intervention under evaluation (e.g. environmental change; infectious disease control; screening; supporting behaviour change; supporting government legislation or policy)?

3 Is this best described as a primary, secondary, or tertiary prevention intervention (i.e. upstream or downstream)?

4 What is the main agency (government; health service; local government; voluntary sector) responsible for implementation and who are the key stakeholders?

5 If this is an intervention aimed at behaviour change, what are the key levers of change (legislation; price; changing social norms; choice architecture; nudging)?

6 What is the appropriate time horizon of analysis and what is the most appropriate discount rate for costs and outcomes? Can we record costs and benefits in the first year as well as a longer time horizon to meet the needs of policy-makers within a political cycle of government?

7 If the public health intervention aims to 'shift the curve', are we most interested in the centre or tails of the distribution?

> **Checklist of additional factors to consider in the design, conduct, and reporting of economic evaluations in public health interventions (continued)**
>
> 8   How is this public health intervention likely to impact on inequalities in health?
>
> 9   Will subgroup analysis help identify the range of cost effectiveness estimates across different settings, delivery methods, and population groups?
>
> 10 What are the main final outcome measures of interest (e.g. QALYs/DALYs /capabilities) and what are any relevant intermediate or proxy outcomes (e.g. behaviour change, changes in social norms)?
>
> 11 How important is it to value costs, benefits, and returns in monetary terms? Is it reasonable to expect the intervention to be cost saving in the short, medium or long term?
>
> 12 How relevant will it be to compare an ICER with the NICE threshold of £20,000-30,000 or an international equivalent, or are there other sources of relevant societal payer thresholds?
>
> Source: Edwards et al., 2013.

Summary of Chapter 15

1. The rule of rescue (McCabe, 2018), means that sick people today will always take precedence over people who will get sick in the future, even when the latter is clearly preventable. Voters today will vote for health care today for sick people today—concepts of public health fit most closely with intergenerational concerns and policies for economic, environmental, and social sustainability in the longer run.

2. The debate over the appropriate cost per QALY threshold raised by Claxton and colleagues has essentially meant that we have devoted scarce NHS resources to high-cost drugs with an opportunity cost which has been the investment of resources into prevention (Claxton et al., 2013). A lower cost per QALY threshold of, for example, £13,000, if adopted, would shift focus more emphatically away from high-cost drugs towards investment in prevention.

3. Political time horizons mean that it is very important that health economists designing evaluations of PHIs capture immediate (e.g. in the first year), medium term (e.g. over a five-year period), and long term (e.g. ten to twenty years) benefits. The immediate outcomes, even if they are intermediate or proxy, and, for example, reflect positive behaviour change in relation to health-harming habits, are important to policy-makers focusing on short time horizons for spending decisions.

4. There is a real need for standardization of methods of ROI; that is, time period discount rates, sources of values, drop-off rates, and attribution methodology.

5. Multifaceted, cross-sectoral investment and working is arguably the only feasible way to change the factors that shape a population's lives and resulting health. Co-financing discussions are recommended as is happening with Scotland's recent health and social care integration. With a greater emphasis on joining up services and focusing on anticipatory and preventative care, integration within Scottish

health care aims to improve care and support for people who use services, their carers, and their families.

6. We need consensus on what outcomes are valued in PHI and how best we incorporate such outcomes within broad-ranging PHI economic evaluations.

7. Consideration need to be given to the role of broader frameworks such as CBA and how they can be integrated with systems modelling to provide the full evaluative picture.

References

Anopa, Y., McMahon, A., Conway, D., Ball, G., Mcintosh, E., and Macpherson, L., 2015. Improving child oral health: Cost analysis of a national nursery toothbrushing programme. *PLoS ONE*, 10.

Baba, C., 2016 Valuing the health and wellbeing aspects of community empowerment in an urban regeneration context using economic evaluation techniques PhD Thesis, University of Glasgow

Bate, A. and Bellis, A., 2017. The Troubled Families programme (England). Available at: <https://researchbriefings.parliament.uk/ResearchBriefing/Summary/CBP-7585#fullreport>

Bayer, R. and Galeo, S., 2015. Public health in the precision-medicine era. *New England Journal of Medicine*, 373: 499–501.

BBC Radio 4, Nov 2011. The Life Scientific: Sir Michael Marmot. Available at: <http://www.bbc.co.uk/programmes/b016ld4q> (Accessed 16 October 2018).

Brouwer, W.B., 2018. The Inclusion of Spillover Effects in Economic Evaluations: Not an Optional Extra. *Pharmacoeconomics*, 1–6.

Brouwer, W.B., Niessen, L.W., Postma, M.J., and Rutten, F.F., 2005. Need for differential discounting of costs and health effects in cost effectiveness analyses. *British Medical Journal*, 331(7514): 446–8.

Buck, D. and Maguire, D., 2015. *Inequalities in Life Expectancy*. Changes Over Time and Implications for Policy. London: King's Fund.

Butterfield, R., Henderson, J., and Scott, R., 2009. i Public Health and Prevention Expenditure in England. doi:10.1.1.372.1840&rep=rep1&type=pdf.

Caxton, K., Rice, N., Sculpher, M., Devlin, N., Soares, M., and Spackman, E., 2013. *Methods for Estimation of the Cost-Effectiveness Threshold of the NHS*. Available at: <https://www.york.ac.uk/media/che/documents/papers/researchpapers/CHERP81_methods_estimation_NICE_costeffectiveness_threshold_(Nov2013).pdf> (Accessed 11 November 2018).

Cookson, R. and Claxton, K., 2012. *The Humble Economist: Tony Culyer on Health. Health Care and Social Decision Making*. York: University of York.

Commission for Architecture and the Built Environment (CABE), 2009 Future health—sustainable places for health and well-being (full report). <https://www.thenbs.com/PublicationIndex/documents/details?Pub=CABE&DocID=293102> (Accessed 16 October 2018).

Colchero, M.A., Rivera, J.A., Popkin, B.M., and Ng, S.W., 2017. Sustained consumer response: evidence from two-years after implementing the sugar sweetened beverage tax in Mexico. *Health Affairs (Project Hope). 36*(3): 564–71.

Communities That Care Returns ¢9.74 per Dollar Invested by Preventing Youth Tobacco Use and Delinquency. <http://www.sdrg.org/ctcresource/Research%20Brief%20No%209%20-%20Jan%202012%20final.pdf> (Accessed 16 October 2018).

Cookson, R., Griffin, S., Norheim, and Culyer, A.J., (forthcoming). Distributional Cost-Effectiveness Analysis: A Handbook of Equity-Informative Health Economic Evaluation. Oxford: Oxford University Press.

Culyer, A.J. and Horisberger, B. eds., 2012. *Economic and Medical Evaluation of Health Care Technologies*. Springer Science & Business Media.

Culyer, A.J., 1989. The normative economics of health care finance and provision. *Oxford Review of Economic Policy, 5*(1): 34–58.

Dallat, M.A.T., Soerjomataram, I., Hunter, R.F., Tully, M.A., Cairns, K.J., and Kee, F., 2014. Urban greenways have the potential to increase physical activity levels cost-effectively. *European Journal of Public Health, 24*(2): 190–5.

Davies, A., Keeble E., Bhatia, T., and Fisher, E., 2016. Quality Watch: Focus on Public Health and Prevention, Nuffield Trust. Available at: <https://www.nuffieldtrust.org.uk/research/focus-on-public-health-and-prevention (Accessed 11 November 2018).

Day, L., Bryson, C., and White, C., Purdon, S., Bewley, H., Sala, L.K., and Portes, J., 2016. National Evaluation of the Troubled Families Programme: Final Synthesis Report. Department for Communities and Local Government Available at: <https://www.niesr.ac.uk/publications/national-evaluation-troubled-families-programme-final-synthesis-report>

Department of Health, 2010. Improving the Health and Well-being of People with Long-term Conditions. Available at: <https://www.gov.uk/government/publications/improving-care-for-people-with-long-term-conditions-at-a-glance-information-sheets-for-healthcare-professionals> (Accessed 11 November 2018).

Edwards, R.T., 2017. Valuing Nature in Public Health Economics and the role of Public Goods <http://cheme.bangor.ac.uk/blogs/Valuing%20nature%20in%20public%20health%20economics.RTE.16.3.17.pdf> (Accessed 16 October 2018).

<http://cheme.bangor.ac.uk/documents/transforming-young-lives/CHEME%20transforming%20Young%20Lives%20Full%20Report%20Eng%20WEB%202.pdfnature> (Accessed 16 October 2018).

Edwards, R.T. Bryning, L., and Lloyd-Williams, H., 2016. Transforming Young Lives across Wales: The Economic Argument for Investing in Early Years <http://cheme.bangor.ac.uk/documents/transforming-young-lives/CHEME%20transforming%20Young%20Lives%20Full%20Report%20Eng%20WEB%202.pdf> (Accessed 16 October 2018).

Edwards, R.T., Charles, J.M., and Lloyd-Williams, H., 2013. Public health economics: a systematic review of guidance for the economic evaluation of public health interventions and discussion of key methodological issues. *BMC Public Health, 13*(1): 1001.

Fields in Trust, 2018. Revaluing Parks and Green Spaces. <http://www.fieldsintrust.org/Upload/file/research/Revaluing-Parks-and-Green-Spaces-Report.pdf> (Accessed 16 October 2018).

Fujiwara, D., (2015). The Seven Principle Problems of SROI. Simetrica. Available from: <http://media.wix.com/ugd/9ccf1d_049e3b74664b436ca6e9e4fe219c1413.pdf> (Accessed 16 October 2018).

Gascon, M., Zijlema, W., Vert, C., White, M.P., and Nieuwenhuijsen, M.J., 2017. Outdoor blue spaces, human health and well-being: a systematic review of quantitative studies. *International Journal of Hygiene and Environmental Health, 220*(8):1207–21.

Healthcare Plastics Recycling Council, 2017. HPRC and the Circular Economy. <https://www.hprc.org/single-post/2016/06/22/HPRC-and-the-Circular-Economy> (Accessed 16 October 2018).

Heckman, J. and **Masterov, D.V., Masterov,** 2007. The productivity argument for investing in young children. *Review of Agricultural Economics, 29*(3):446–93.

Hoddinott, P., Morgan, H., MacLennan, G., Sewel, K., Thomson, G., Bauld, L., Yi, D., et al., 2014. Public acceptability of financial incentives for smoking cessation in pregnancy and breast feeding: a survey of the British public. *British Medical Journal Open, 4*(7): e005524.

Husereau, D., Drummond, M., Petrou, S., Carswell, C., Moher, D., Greenberg, D., Augustovski, F., et al., 2013. Consolidated Health Economic Evaluation Reporting Standards (CHEERS) statement. *BMC Medicine, 11*(346): f1049.

Juniper, T., 2013. *What has Nature Ever Done for Us? How Money Really Does Grow on Trees.* London: Profile Books.

Korytárová, J. and **Papežíková, P.,** 2015. Assessment of large-scale projects based on CBA. *Procedia Computer Science, 64:* 736–43.

Kuklinski, M.R., Briney, J.S., Hawkins, J.D., and **Catalano, R.F.,** 2012. Cost–benefit analysis of communities that care outcomes at eighth grade. *Prevention Science, 13:* 150–61.

Kuklinski, M.R., Fagan, A.A., Hawkins, J.D., Briney, J.S. and **Catalano, R.F.,** 2015. Benefit–cost analysis of a randomized evaluation of communities That Care: monetizing intervention effects on the initiation of delinquency and substance use through grade 12. *Journal of Experimental Criminology, 11*(2): 165–92.

Lacy, P. and **Rutqvist, J.,** 2016. *Waste to Wealth: The Circular Economy Advantage.* London: Palgrave Macmillan.

Levy-Lahad, E., Lahad, A., and **King, M.-C.,** 2015. Precision medicine meets public health: Population screening for BRCA1 and BRCA2. *Journal of the National Cancer Institute, 107:* dju420-dju420.

Malik, V.S., Popkin, B.M., Bray, G.A., Despres, J.P., Willett, W.C., and **Hu, F.B.,** 2010. Sugar-sweetened beverages and risk of metabolic syndrome and type 2 diabetes: a meta-analysis. *Diabetes Care, 33*(11): 2477–83.

Malik, V.S., Schulze, M.B., Hu, F.B., 2006. Intake of sugar-sweetened beverages and weight gain: a systematic review. *American Journal of Clinical Nutrition, 84*(2): 274–88.

Masters, R., Anwar, E., Collins, B., Cookson, R., and **Capewell, S.,** 2017. Return on investment of public health interventions: a systematic review. *Journal of Epidemiology and Community Health, 71:* 827–34.

Matrix, 2010. An economic evaluation of play provision. Play England, Final Report. Available at: <http://www.playengland.org.uk/media/227879/play%20england%20an%20economic%20evaluation%20of%20play%20provision.pdf> (Accessed 11 November 2018).

McCabe, C., 2018. Expanding the scope of costs and benefits for economic evaluations in health: Some words of caution. *Pharmacoeconomics,* 1–4.

Merkur, S., Sassi, F., and **McDaid, D.,** 2013. Promoting health, preventing disease: Is there an economic case? Policy summary, 6. Copenhagen: European Observatory on Health Systems and Policies.

National Evaluation of Sure Start Team, 2010. The Impact of Sure Start Local Programmes on Seven Year Olds and Their Families. London: Institute for the Study of Children, Families and Social Issues, Birkbeck, University of London.

National Institute of Health and Care Excellence, 2012. Methods for the development of NICE public health guidance (third edition). Available at: <https://www.nice.org.uk/

process/pmg9/resources/guide-to-the-methods-of-technology-appraisal-2013-pdf-2007975843781> and <https://www.nice.org.uk/process/pmg4/resources/methods-for-the-development-of-nice-public-health-guidance-third-edition-pdf-2007967445701> (Accessed 11 November 2018).

National Institute of Health and Care Excellence, 2013. Guide to the methods of technology appraisal 2013. Available at: nigreenways.com, 2017. <https://nigreenways.com/about/> (Accessed 16 October 2018).

Nissinen, A., Tuomilehto, J., Kottke, T.E., and Puska, P., 1986. Cost-effectiveness of the North Karelia Hypertension Program 1972–1977. *Medical Care*, 24(8): 767–80.

Owen, L., Morgan, A., Fischer, A., Ellis, S., Hoy, A., and Kelly, M.P., 2011. The cost-effectiveness of public health interventions. *Journal of Public Health*, 34(1):37–45.

parkrun.org, 2017. <http://www.parkrun.org.uk/> (Accessed 16 October 2018).

Public Health England, 2016. Available at: <https://www.gov.uk/government/publications/health-matters-midlife-approaches-to-reduce-dementia-risk/health-matters-midlife-approaches-to-reduce-dementia-risk> (Accessed 11 November 2018).

Puska, P., 2002. Successful prevention of non-communicable diseases: 25 year experiences with North Karelia Project in Finland. *Public Health Medicine*, 4(1):5–7.

Remme, M., Martinez-Alvarez, M., and Vassall, A. 2017. Cost-effectiveness thresholds in global health: Taking a multisectoral perspective. *Value in Health*, 20:699–704.

Rose, G. 1985. Sick individuals and sick populations. *International Journal of Epidemiology*, 14(1): 32–8

Rutter, M., 2006. Is Sure Start an effective preventive intervention? *Child and Adolescent Mental Health*, 11(3): 135–41.

Ryan, M., Yi, D., Avenell, A., Douglas, F., Aucott, L., Van Teijlingen, E., and Vale, L., 2015. Gaining pounds by losing pounds: preferences for lifestyle interventions to reduce obesity. *Health Economics, Policy and Law*, 10(02):161–82.

Sanders, G.D., Neumann, P.J., Basu, A., Brock, D.W., Feeny, D., Krahn, M., Kuntz, K.M., et al., (2016). Recommendations for conduct, methodological practices, and reporting of cost-effectiveness analyses: Second panel on cost-effectiveness in health and medicine. *Journal of the American Medical Association*, Sep 13;316(10): 1093–103.

Sælensminde, K., 2004. Cost–benefit analyses of walking and cycling track networks taking into account insecurity, health effects and external costs of motorized traffic. *Transportation Research Part A: Policy and Practice*, 38(8):5 93–606.

Sanghera, S., Frew, E., and Roberts, T., 2015. Adapting the CHEERS statement for reporting cost–benefit analysis. *Pharmacoeconomics*, 33(5): 533–4.

Sundararajan, A., 2016. *The Sharing Economy: The End of Employment and The Rise of Crowd-Based Capitalism*. Cambridge, MA: MIT Press.

Treasury, H.M., 2003. *The Green Book: Appraisal and Evaluation in Central Government*. London: HM Treasury.

Vaithinathan, A.G. and Asokan, V., 2017. Public health and precision medicine share a goal. *Journal of Evidence-Based Medicine*, 10:76–80.

Vos, T., Carter, R., Barendregt, J., Mihalopoulos, C., Veerman, L., Magnus, A., Cobiac, L., et al., 2010. Assessing cost-effectiveness in prevention: ACE–prevention September 2010 final report (Doctoral dissertation, University of Queensland).

Weatherly, H., Drummond, M., Claxton, K., Cookson, R., Ferguson, B., Godfrey, C., Rice, N., et al., 2009. Methods for assessing the cost-effectiveness of public health interventions: Key challenges and recommendations. *Health Policy*, 93(2): 85–92.

Index

Tables, figures and boxes are indicated by an italic *t*, *f*, and *b* following the paragraph number. Where more than two authors of reference sources are cited in the text, only the first named author is listed in the index.

dietary vitamin D supplementation 56–57
food production and labelling control 63, 72
in schools; *see also* children, PHIs for; PHIs in
    non-NHS settings
    health education 63
    school meals 9–10
sugar taxes
    in Australia 344–45
    in Mexico 346
    in the UK 346
    in the United States 346; *see also* United States
see also obesity management and prevention
Heberlein, Thomas A. 213
Heckman, James 19*f*, 19, 294
Hicks, John 208–9
HIV/AIDS, *see* sexually transmitted diseases
HM Treasury 146, 348, 354
Hospital Episode Statistics database 113–15; *see
    also* costing PHIs
Housing Associations' Charitable Trust 296–97
housing improvement PHIs:
    asthma control (CHARISMA trial),
        see CHARISMA trial of housing
        modification for asthma control
    Decent Homes scheme, Nottingham, *see*
        social return on investment (SROI),
        case study: Decent Homes housing
        improvement scheme (Nottingham)
Hulshof, Josée A. 308
human development index (HDI) (United
    Nations) 146, 147*f*; *see also* capability
    well-being theory applied to PHIs

immunization programmes 6, 64–65; *see also*
    communicable disease control
Incredible Years Parenting Programmes:
    in Birmingham, outcome measurement and
        evaluation case study 136–37; *see also*
        outcomes of PHIs, measurement and
        evaluation
    in Seattle 73
    in Wales, micro-costing case study 118, 119–
        21*b*, 121–24*t*; *see also* costing PHIs
    see also children, PHIs for;
incremental cost-effectiveness ratios, *see* cost-
    effectiveness analysis (CEA), incremental
    cost-effectiveness ratios (ICERs)
incremental cost-utility ratios (ICURs), *see*
    quality-adjusted life years (QALYs), CUA
    use (incremental cost-utility ratios)
inequalities in health, *see* health inequalities
infectious disease control, *see* communicable
    disease control

Jagosh, Justin 97–98
Jit, Mark 64–65
Jones, Alice, *see* social return on investment
    (SROI), case study: Decent Homes
    housing improvement scheme
    (Nottingham)
Jonsen, Albert R. 73–74

Kahneman, Daniel 145
Kaldor, Nicholas 208–9
Kaltenthaler, Eva 271–72
Keeney, Ralph L. 303, 305–6
Kelly, Michael P. 54, 65, 66*t*, 265
Kenkel, Donald S. 36

Levy-Lahad, Ephrat 352
local government:
    parks and playgrounds, need for economic
        evaluation 347; *see also* public health
        economics, future research priorities
    public health function in England 7
    public sector multi-agency perspective on
        public health 71–72, 110, 111–12, 148;
        see also perspectives of public health
        economics; PHIs in non-NHS settings
    ROI toolkit being developed for 14, 15, 296;
        see also return on investment (ROI)
Lorgelly, Paula 138, 142–43

McCabe, Christopher 53–54, 111,
    181–82, 349–50
MacCulloch, Robert 145–46
McDaid, David 78
McIntosh, Emma 136–37
McKie, John 73–74
macro-economic approach to public health
    economics, *see* systems approach to
    public health economics
Maguire, David 349
Margrain, Thomas H. 113, 114*f*
market failure of healthcare markets 63, 71, 355
    case study (Watts and Segal) 34–35
    market failure concept 33
    reasons for
        asymmetry of information between
            producers and consumers 33–34, 35
        free-rider problem 33–34
        irrational behaviour by consumers 33–34
        time preferences and discounting, *see* time
            factors
    see also micro-economic approach to public
        health economics
Marmot Review *(Fair society, healthy lives:
    Strategic review of health inequalities in
    England post-2010)* 8; *see also* health
    inequalities
Marmot, Sir Michael 8, 27, 354, 355
Marsh, Kevin 55
MCDA, *see* multi-criteria decision
    analysis (MCDA)
Medical Research Council guidance on studying
    complex interventions 59–61, 134,
    149–50, 259; *see also* guidance on public
    health economics; PHIs as complex
    interventions
meta-analysis, *see* evidence synthesis for PHI
    evaluation, meta-analysis
Mexico, taxation of unhealthy foods 346; *see
    also* healthy eating

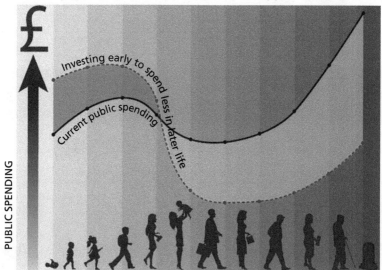

Applied Health Economics for Public Health Practice and Research

Shifting the curve towards prevention and early years investment

£

PUBLIC SPENDING

Investing early to spend less in later life

Current public spending

LIFE COURSE (birth to death)